C-EFM Exam Study Guide

600 Practice Questions + C-EFM Study Guide with Latest Review for the NCC Certification in Electronic Fetal Monitoring Exam

Brigham R. Riley
© 2023-2024
Printed in USA.

Disclaimer:

Contents

1. ELECTRONIC MONITORING EQUIPMENT:

    1.1 Fetal heart rate monitoring:

    1.2 Uterine monitoring:

    1.3 Equipment failure and troubleshooting:

2. PHYSIOLOGY:

    2.1 Uteroplacental:

    2.2 Factors affecting fetal oxygenation:

3. PATTERN RECOGNITION AND INTERVENTION:

    3.1 Fetal baseline heart rate:

    3.2 Fetal heart rate variability:

    3.3 Abnormal uterine activity:

    3.4 Fetal dysrhythmias:

    3.5 Maternal Complications:

    3.6 Uteroplacental complications:

    3.7 Fetal complications:

    3.8 Fetal heart rate accelerations:

    3.9 Normal uterine activity:

4. FETAL ASSESSMENT METHODS:

    4.1 Auscultation:

    4.2 Fetal movement and stimulation:

    4.3 Nonstress testing:

    4.4 Cord Blood Acid Base Testing:

    4.5 Biophysical profile:

    4.6 Fetal Acoustic Stimulation:

5. PROFESSIONAL ISSUES:

    5.1 Legal:

    5.2 Ethics:

    5.3 Patient safety:

    5.4 Quality Improvement:

C-EFM Exam Practice Questions

Answers with Detailed Explanation

Why do you need to be C-EFM Certified?

➤ Firstly, being C-EFM certified validates your expertise in the domain, enabling you to stand out among your peers and gain professional recognition. It showcases your commitment to continuous learning and staying updated with the latest advancements in the field.

➤ Additionally, the C-EFM certification signifies your ability to deliver safe and high-quality care to patients. This can enhance patient trust and satisfaction, and lead to improved patient outcomes.

➤ Furthermore, the C-EFM certification sets you apart in the job market, making you a sought-after candidate. Many employers prioritize hiring C-EFM certified candidates due to the added confidence in their skills and knowledge.

➤ Lastly, obtaining the C-EFM certification can open up opportunities for career advancement and higher salaries. Many healthcare organizations value the expertise and dedication of C-EFM certified candidates and may offer increased responsibilities and compensation packages accordingly.

Willing to Join Our Author Panel?

Dear,

We would like to invite you to join our 'Panel Of Authors'.

First of all, Thank you for your hard work and dedication to your patients. We know that the hours are long and the workload is demanding, but you do it with grace and dignity. Your compassion is evident in the way you treat your patients, and we are grateful for all that you do.

We believe that your expertise and experience will be a valuable contribution to our books. Our goal is to provide valuable content that helps our readers to step forward in their career development. This is a unique opportunity to share your expertise with others in need and help shape their future.

The requirements for joining our panel of authors are as follows:

- A minimum experience of 8 years

- Proper certification from a renowned organization

- Good writing and teaching skills

- Enthusiasm in sharing knowledge

If you meet these requirements and are interested in joining our panel, please send us your resume along with a writing sample for our review to propublisher@zohomail.com.

We would be happy to have you on board!

We are happy that our panel of authors can provide the best content because they are experienced and passionate in their own field. We would love for you to join our panel of authors and help us continue to provide quality content for our readers. You will also be able to connect with other experts in your domain from around the world and build a network of support. Undoubtedly, this will be a great opportunity for you to make a difference in your profession.

Thank You

Why is this book the right choice for you to clear the C-EFM Exam?

Latest Study Guide:

If you are looking for an up-to-date study guide for the C-EFM Exam, then look no further than this book. This book provides everything you need to know to ace the exam with tons of practice questions to help you prepare. This book is also constantly updated to ensure that it always covers the latest information on the exam as per the outline provided by the NCC ®.

C-EFM® TEST CONTENT OUTLINE

1. ELECTRONIC MONITORING EQUIPMENT
2. PHYSIOLOGY
3. PATTERN RECOGNITION AND INTERVENTION
4. FETAL ASSESSMENT METHODS
5. PROFESSIONAL ISSUES

Experienced Set of Authors:

There are many reasons to choose this book over others, but one of the most important is that it is written by experienced authors who are C-EFM Certified. The authors of this book have a wealth of experience in taking and passing exams, and we have used our knowledge to create a study guide that is comprehensive and easy to follow.
With our experienced authors and comprehensive coverage, our book is the best way to prepare for this important test.

Detailed rationale for the answer:

We provide an in-depth explanation for each question, so you can understand not only the correct answer but also why it is correct. This book also gives you an ample amount of practice to help you feel confident on exam day.

Similar Question Format as that in the actual exam:

One of the most important features of this book is that the questions and answers follow the same pattern as the actual exam. This is extremely important because you need to be familiar with the format of the exam to do well on it.

Fine Tunes your thinking:

Going through the questions, answers and explanations repeatedly will sharpen your thinking and understanding ability. This will help you to understand the root of the question in the C-EFM Exam and make the right selection of the answer.

Clear and Concise:

This C-EFM Prep is written in simple language and is not overly technical. This sets this book apart from other study materials because when you are studying for the C-EFM Exam, you need to be able to understand the material without getting bogged down in details. This book will help you do just that. This combination of easy-to-understand language and practical testing will help you be successful on the C-EFM exam.

Magical Steps to Pass the C-EFM Exam with Ease:

1. Belief: You must believe that you can pass the C-EFM exam with ease. This belief will help you stay focused and motivated throughout your studies. We help build your confidence by giving you the feel of attending virtual exams in our book, making you familiar with the type of questions that will be asked in the exam, and giving you a thorough idea about all the topics as specified by NCC®.

2. Visualization: Visualize yourself passing the C-EFM exam with flying colors. This will help you stay positive and focused on your goal. Taking multiple tests and solving various questions will help improve your positivity and confidence. We try our best to improve your positivity.

3. Study: Make sure to study all the material thoroughly. Quality Learning is more important than Quantity Learning. Time yourself when you take tests and try to complete them within the stipulated time.

4. Practice: The more you practice the more is the chance of passing the exam. By doing this, you will get a feel for the types of questions that will be asked and how to best answer them. We have an abundant number of questions for you to practice.

5. Relax: On the day of the exam, make sure to relax and stay calm. This will help you think more clearly and perform at your best.

Smart Learning with Trust in Yourself will make Success knock at your door! All the Best!

Magical Steps to Pass the C-EFM Exam With

ease.

Smart Learning with Trust in Yourself will make Success

Knock at your door." All the Best!

C-EFM

Guide

1   ELECTRONIC MONITORING EQUIPMENT:

Electronic monitoring equipment refers to the various devices and tools used to monitor and track electronic signals or activities. In the context of an Electronic Fetal Monitoring Specialist, electronic monitoring equipment is specifically used to monitor the fetal heart rate and uterine contractions during pregnancy and childbirth. This equipment plays a crucial role in assessing the well-being of the fetus and maternal progress during labor.

One of the main components of electronic monitoring equipment is the fetal heart rate monitor. This device is typically placed on the mother's abdomen and uses ultrasound technology to detect the fetal heart rate. The monitor provides real-time information about the baby's heartbeat, allowing the specialist to assess its regularity and detect any abnormal patterns or signs of distress. It helps in identifying oxygen deprivation or changes in fetal activity.

Another important aspect of electronic monitoring equipment is the uterine contraction monitor. This device measures the frequency, duration, and intensity of contractions during labor. It helps the specialist determine whether the contractions are strong enough to facilitate the progress of labor and whether they pose any risk to the baby's well-being. By closely monitoring and analyzing the data provided, the specialist can make informed decisions regarding the need for intervention or medical assistance.

Electronic monitoring equipment also includes additional features to enhance its functionality. These may include built-in alarms and alerts to notify the specialist of any significant changes or abnormalities detected during the monitoring process. These alerts ensure that prompt action can be taken to address any potential risks to the mother or baby.

Furthermore, advanced electronic monitoring equipment often incorporates wireless technology, allowing data to be transmitted and displayed on remote monitors or computer screens. This enables the specialist to closely monitor the fetal heart rate and uterine contractions from different locations, ensuring continuous and uninterrupted monitoring throughout labor.

To ensure accurate and reliable monitoring, electronic monitoring equipment must be properly maintained and calibrated. Regular calibration checks are necessary to verify the accuracy of the readings and ensure consistent performance. This maintenance is essential to guarantee the safety and well-being of both the mother and the baby.

In addition to the technical aspects, it is essential for an Electronic Fetal Monitoring Specialist to be trained in the proper use and interpretation of electronic monitoring equipment. This includes understanding the different parameters measured, interpreting the data provided, and making timely and informed decisions based on the information obtained. This specialized training is crucial to effectively monitor and assess the fetal well-being throughout pregnancy and childbirth. It enables the tracking and analysis of fetal heart rate and uterine contractions, providing critical information about the progress of labor and the well-being of both the mother and the baby. The accuracy, reliability, and proper use of this equipment are essential for ensuring optimal care and outcomes during pregnancy and childbirth.

1.1   Fetal heart rate monitoring:

Fetal heart rate monitoring is a crucial aspect of prenatal care and is performed using electronic monitoring equipment. This monitoring allows healthcare professionals to assess the well-being of the unborn baby by measuring the heart rate and detecting any abnormalities or distress.

One type of electronic monitoring equipment commonly used for fetal heart rate monitoring is a Doppler ultrasound device. This non-invasive tool uses sound waves to measure and display the baby's heart rate in real-time. It can be easily placed on the mother's abdomen and provides continuous monitoring throughout the pregnancy.

Another type of monitoring equipment is the electronic fetal monitor (EFM). This device consists of two separate components: a transducer to record the baby's heart rate and a tocometer to monitor the mother's uterine contractions. The information from both components is displayed on a computer screen or printed on a strip of paper, allowing healthcare professionals to assess the baby's heart rate in relation to the contractions.

Fetal heart rate monitoring is typically performed during routine prenatal visits, as well as during labor and delivery. During pregnancy, it helps to identify any potential issues such as fetal distress, inadequate oxygen supply, or irregular heart rhythms. In labor, it aids in the assessment of the baby's response to contractions and helps guide decisions regarding the need for interventions or cesarean delivery.

One important aspect of fetal heart rate monitoring is the interpretation of the heart rate patterns. Normal fetal heart rate patterns consist of baseline rate, variability, accelerations, and decelerations. The baseline rate refers to the average heart rate during periods of fetal well-being. Variability indicates the fluctuations in the heart rate, demonstrating the baby's ability to respond to stressors. Accelerations are temporary increases in the heart rate, which are usually a positive sign of a healthy baby. On the other hand, decelerations are temporary decreases in the heart rate, which can indicate poor oxygen supply or fetal distress.

There are different types of decelerations that healthcare professionals carefully evaluate. Early decelerations occur in response to the baby's head compression during contractions and are generally considered benign. Late decelerations, however, occur after the start of a contraction and can be a sign of oxygen deprivation. Variable decelerations happen unpredictably and can be a result of umbilical cord compression. These different patterns help guide clinical decision-making during labor.

It is important for electronic fetal monitoring specialists to be well-trained in interpreting these heart rate patterns to ensure optimal care for both the mother and the baby. Regular monitoring and prompt recognition of abnormal patterns can lead to timely interventions and improved outcomes. This monitoring allows healthcare professionals to assess the baby's well-being by measuring the heart rate and identifying any abnormalities or distress. Doppler ultrasound and electronic fetal monitors are commonly used tools for this purpose. Interpreting the heart rate patterns is crucial to identify deviations from normal and guide clinical decision-making. Fetal heart rate monitoring plays a vital role in ensuring the health and safety of both the mother and the baby throughout pregnancy and labor.

1.1.1   Internal:

Internal monitoring is a method used during fetal heart rate monitoring that involves the insertion of a small electrode into the scalp of the baby. This electrode is attached to a wire that is connected to an electronic monitoring device. It provides a more accurate and detailed assessment of the baby's heart rate than external monitoring methods.

One of the main advantages of internal monitoring is its ability to provide a continuous and direct measurement of the baby's heart rate. This allows healthcare providers to closely monitor any changes or abnormalities in the baby's heart rate, providing them with valuable information about the baby's well-being. It also allows for more accurate detection of fetal distress or signs of potential complications.

Internal monitoring also provides a more accurate assessment of the strength and duration of the baby's contractions. This information is important in determining the baby's response to labor and ensuring that adequate oxygen supply is provided to the baby during the birthing process.

The insertion of the electrode is usually performed by a healthcare provider, such as a nurse or doctor, during labor. They first clean the area and then insert the electrode into the baby's scalp. The process is relatively quick and usually does not cause significant discomfort to the mother or baby.

One potential drawback of internal monitoring is the increased risk of infection. Since it involves the insertion of an electrode into the baby's scalp, there is a small risk of introducing bacteria into the baby's bloodstream. However, this risk is usually minimal and can be mitigated by following strict sterile techniques during the insertion process.

Another consideration with internal monitoring is the need for ruptured membranes. In order to perform internal monitoring, the amniotic sac needs to rupture, either spontaneously or by artificial means. If the amniotic sac has not ruptured, healthcare providers may need to artificially rupture the membranes before proceeding with internal monitoring. It provides a more accurate and continuous assessment of the baby's heart rate and the strength and duration of contractions. While there may be some potential risks and considerations associated with internal monitoring, it is a valuable tool in ensuring the well-being of both the mother and the baby during labor and delivery.

1.1.2   External:

External fetal heart rate monitoring is a method used to assess the well-being of a fetus during labor and delivery. It involves placing sensors on the mother's abdomen to measure the fetal heart rate and track any changes or abnormalities. This type of monitoring is done using electronic monitoring equipment specifically designed for this purpose.

One of the main components of external fetal heart rate monitoring is the use of an ultrasound transducer. This transducer is a handheld device that emits ultrasonic waves and receives the echoes to capture the fetal heart rate. It is typically placed on the mother's abdomen, over the area where the baby's heart is located. The transducer picks up the sound waves reflecting off the fetal heart and converts them into an electronic signal that can be displayed on a monitor or recorded for further analysis.

Another important piece of equipment used in external fetal heart rate monitoring is the tocodynamometer. This device is placed on the mother's abdomen to measure and record uterine contractions. It works by sensing the pressure changes in the abdominal wall during contractions. The tocodynamometer helps assess the relationship between the fetal heart rate and the contractions, providing valuable information about the baby's response to labor.

The electronic monitoring equipment used in external fetal heart rate monitoring is connected to a central monitoring system. This system allows healthcare professionals to closely observe and analyze the fetal heart rate and uterine contractions. It provides a continuous tracing of the fetal heart rate pattern, which can be plotted on a graph for easier interpretation.

External fetal heart rate monitoring offers several advantages. It is non-invasive and does not require any surgical intervention. It allows for continuous monitoring, providing real-time information about the fetus's well-being. It is also a useful tool in detecting fetal distress, which can be indicative of oxygen deprivation or other complications.

However, there are some limitations to external fetal heart rate monitoring. The accuracy of the readings may be affected by maternal obesity, fetal position, or the presence of excessive amniotic fluid. It may also be challenging to obtain a clear signal if the baby is moving too much or if the mother has an anterior placenta. In such cases, internal fetal heart rate monitoring may be necessary. It involves using electronic monitoring equipment, such as ultrasound transducers and tocodynamometers, to measure the fetal heart rate and uterine contractions. This method provides valuable information about the baby's response to labor and helps detect fetal distress. While external fetal heart rate monitoring has some limitations, it remains a widely used and effective method for monitoring fetal well-being during childbirth.

1.2   Uterine monitoring:

Uterine monitoring is an essential aspect of electronic monitoring equipment for the field of electronic fetal monitoring. It involves the monitoring and recording of uterine contractions during pregnancy and labor. This monitoring is crucial in assessing the health and well-being of both the mother and the fetus.

One of the main goals of uterine monitoring is to evaluate the strength and frequency of contractions. This information provides valuable insights into the progress of labor and allows healthcare providers to make well-informed decisions regarding the management of childbirth. By monitoring uterine contractions, healthcare providers can determine if labor is progressing normally or if there are any irregularities that may require intervention.

There are several methods used for uterine monitoring, including external and internal techniques. The external method involves placing a tocodynamometer, a device that measures the pressure changes on the abdomen, to detect and record uterine contractions. This method is non-invasive and comfortable for the mother.

On the other hand, internal monitoring involves inserting a catheter or an intrauterine pressure catheter (IUPC) into the uterine cavity to measure the strength, frequency, and duration of contractions directly. This method provides more accurate and detailed information about uterine activity but is more invasive than the external method.

In addition to monitoring contractions, uterine monitoring can also assess the fetal heart rate (FHR). Changes in the FHR can indicate fetal distress or other complications. By combining uterine monitoring with FHR monitoring, healthcare providers can have a comprehensive understanding of the status of both the mother and the fetus during labor.

Continuous uterine monitoring is especially important for high-risk pregnancies or when complications are anticipated. It allows healthcare providers to detect any abnormalities promptly and take appropriate actions to ensure the safety of both the mother and the fetus. Timely interventions can help prevent potential complications and improve pregnancy outcomes.

Uterine monitoring equipment has advanced significantly over the years. Nowadays, electronic fetal monitoring machines are equipped with sophisticated technologies that can accurately measure uterine contractions. These machines provide real-time data and generate graphical representations of uterine activity, making it easier for healthcare providers to interpret and analyze the information. It involves the assessment of uterine contractions during pregnancy and labor to evaluate the progress of labor and the well-being of both the mother and the fetus. With the use of advanced electronic monitoring equipment, healthcare providers can obtain accurate and detailed information about uterine activity, aiding in the management of childbirth and ensuring optimal outcomes.

1.2.1   External:

External monitoring is a key aspect of electronic fetal monitoring equipment used by Electronic Fetal Monitoring Specialists. It involves the use of external devices to assess the well-being of the fetus during labor and delivery.

One important component of external monitoring is the use of ultrasound technology. This allows the specialist to obtain real-time images of the fetus and monitor its heart rate. The ultrasound transducer is placed on the mother's abdomen and emits sound waves that bounce off the fetus, creating a visual representation on a monitor. This enables the specialist to assess fetal movement, heart rate patterns, and any potential abnormalities.

Another aspect of external monitoring is the use of a tocodynamometer, which measures uterine contractions. This device is also placed on the mother's abdomen and uses pressure sensors to detect changes in the uterine muscle during contractions. By monitoring the frequency, duration, and intensity of these contractions, the specialist can assess the progress of labor and the well-being of the fetus.

External monitoring also involves the use of a fetal heart rate monitor, which is placed on the mother's abdomen to record the baby's heart rate. This device uses a transducer to detect the electrical signals produced by the fetal heart and converts them into audible or visual representations. By monitoring the heart rate patterns, the specialist can identify any signs of distress or abnormality.

One subtopic related to external monitoring is the use of external sensors to measure fetal scalp pH. This involves placing a small electrode on the baby's scalp during labor to obtain a sample of blood. The pH level of this blood sample provides valuable information about the fetus's well-being and helps the specialist determine the best course of action during delivery.

Another subtopic is the use of external monitoring in high-risk pregnancies. In cases where there are risk factors such as maternal diabetes, hypertension, or placental abnormalities, continuous external monitoring may be necessary to closely monitor the well-being of both the mother and the fetus.

It is important for Electronic Fetal Monitoring Specialists to have a thorough understanding of external monitoring and the different devices and techniques involved. They must be able to interpret the data obtained from these devices accurately and make informed decisions based on the information gathered. They must also ensure that the equipment is properly calibrated and applied to ensure accurate readings. It involves the use of external devices such as ultrasound transducers, tocodynamometers, and fetal heart rate monitors to assess fetal movement, heart rate patterns, uterine contractions, and **overall** fetal well-being. Understanding and effectively utilizing these external monitoring techniques and devices is essential for an Electronic Fetal Monitoring Specialist in providing safe and effective care during labor and delivery.

1.2.2   IUPC:

IUPC, or Intrauterine Pressure Catheter, is an essential tool used in electronic fetal monitoring to measure uterine contractions accurately. It is a thin catheter that is inserted into the uterine cavity and connected to a monitoring system. The IUPC provides valuable information about the strength, frequency, and duration of contractions, aiding in the assessment of uterine activity during labor.

One important aspect of IUPC is its placement. The catheter is carefully introduced into the amniotic cavity through the cervix during labor. Its position is verified by observing the characteristic waveform on the monitor. Accurate placement is crucial for reliable monitoring results.

A significant advantage of IUPC is its ability to measure uterine contractions directly. This method provides more precise information than other external monitoring techniques, such as tocodynamometry. By measuring the pressure changes within the uterus, IUPC allows for a more accurate assessment of the intensity and frequency of contractions.

The information obtained with the help of IUPC is crucial in various scenarios. For instance, it aids in determining the progress of labor and identifying abnormal uterine contractions that might require intervention. Monitoring uterine contractions can also provide insight into the effectiveness of medications used to induce or augment labor.

The IUPC waveform provides valuable data for interpretation. It shows the baseline resting tone of the uterus as well as the peaks representing contractions. The frequency and duration of contractions can be analyzed from the waveform, enabling healthcare providers to detect any irregularities or abnormalities.

Another important aspect to consider when using IUPC is the potential risks associated with its use. Although rare, complications such as uterine perforation or infection can occur. Therefore, trained professionals should perform the insertion procedure to minimize the chances of complications. It allows for accurate and direct measurement of uterine contractions, providing valuable information about labor progress and uterine activity. The placement of the catheter is crucial, and careful monitoring and interpretation of the obtained waveform are essential for effective utilization of IUPC. While the procedure has potential risks, when performed by trained professionals, the benefits outweigh the risks, making IUPC a valuable tool for the Electronic Fetal Monitoring Specialist.

1.3   Equipment failure and troubleshooting:

Equipment failure and troubleshooting in electronic monitoring equipment is a critical aspect of the role of an Electronic Fetal Monitoring Specialist. When working with electronic monitoring equipment, it is important to be prepared to handle any potential malfunctions or failures that may occur.

One common equipment failure is a loss of power. This can happen for various reasons, such as a blown fuse or a power outage. When faced with a loss of power, it is important to check the power source and ensure that all connections are secure. Additionally, having backup power supplies, such as battery-operated devices, can help in these situations.

Another equipment failure that may occur is a malfunction in the display screen. This can prevent the Electronic Fetal Monitoring Specialist from accurately monitoring the fetal heart rate and uterine contractions. To troubleshoot this issue, it is important to check all the connections between the display screen and the main unit. If the problem persists, contacting technical support or the manufacturer may be necessary.

Sensor failure is another common issue that Electronic Fetal Monitoring Specialists may encounter. This can occur if the sensors become disconnected or if they are not properly placed on the patient's abdomen. When troubleshooting sensor failure, it is important to check the connections and reposition the sensors if necessary. It is also important to ensure that the sensors are clean and free of any debris or fluids that may interfere with their functionality.

In some cases, alarms or alerts may not sound when they should, or they may go off unnecessarily. This can be caused by a malfunction in the alarm system or incorrect alarm settings. Troubleshooting this issue involves checking the alarm settings and ensuring that they are appropriately calibrated. If the problem persists, contacting technical support or the manufacturer is recommended.

Software glitches or malfunctions can also occur in electronic monitoring equipment. This can result in inaccurate data or the inability to access certain features. When faced with software issues, it is important to check for any available software updates and install them if necessary. If the problem persists, contacting technical support or the manufacturer may be required.

In addition to addressing specific equipment failures, Electronic Fetal Monitoring Specialists should also perform routine maintenance and testing to prevent or minimize equipment failures. This includes regularly inspecting the equipment for any visible damage, cleaning the equipment according to manufacturer guidelines, and conducting periodic calibration checks. By being prepared to handle various types of failures, such as loss of power, display screen malfunctions, sensor failures, alarm issues, and software glitches, professionals in this role can ensure the accurate and reliable monitoring of fetal heart rate and uterine contractions. Regular maintenance and testing also play a vital role in preventing equipment failures and maximizing the functionality and lifespan of the equipment.

1.3.1   Artifact Detection:

Artifact detection is a crucial aspect of electronic monitoring equipment, particularly in the field of electronic fetal monitoring. As an Electronic Fetal Monitoring Specialist, it is essential to understand the concept of artifact detection and its significance in ensuring accurate and reliable monitoring of fetal well-being.

Artifacts are undesired signals that interfere with the proper interpretation of electronic monitoring equipment. They can arise from various sources, including maternal or fetal movement, electrode displacement, electrical interference, or technical issues with the monitoring equipment itself. Detecting and addressing artifacts promptly is vital to avoid misinterpretation of fetal heart rate patterns and prevent unnecessary interventions.

One of the primary goals of artifact detection is to differentiate between true fetal heart rate patterns and artifacts. False alarms or misinterpretation of artifacts as abnormal patterns can lead to unnecessary interventions and potentially harm both the mother and the baby. Consequently, mastering artifact detection techniques is a critical skill for an Electronic Fetal Monitoring Specialist.

Several methods can help identify and differentiate artifacts from genuine fetal heart rate patterns. One such method involves carefully assessing the timing of the suspected artifact in relation to maternal or fetal movement. If the signal coincides with a known movement, it is likely an artifact rather than a true abnormality. Additionally, observing the waveform morphology can provide clues, as artifacts often appear different from actual fetal heart rate patterns.

Moreover, paying close attention to the appearance of baseline fluctuations can aid in artifact detection. Baseline shifts caused by artifacts tend to be sudden and unrelated to fetal well-being, whereas fluctuations associated with fetal compromise typically exhibit a gradual or persistent pattern.

In some cases, artifacts may result from electrode displacement or poor contact. Regularly checking and readjusting the placement of electrodes helps minimize such artifacts. Ensuring a secure attachment and proper hydration of the mother can also contribute to reliable monitoring.

Electrical interference from external sources, such as power lines or electronic devices, can introduce artifacts into the monitoring signal. Shielding the equipment and minimizing contact with potential sources of interference can help reduce these artifacts.

Regular maintenance and calibration of electronic monitoring equipment are essential to minimize technical issues that can lead to artifacts. Conducting routine checks on the cables, connectors, and sensors ensures their proper functioning and reduces the risk of false alarms due to technical malfunctions. As an Electronic Fetal Monitoring Specialist, understanding the various sources and characteristics of artifacts and mastering the techniques for artifact detection is paramount. By differentiating artifacts from genuine fetal heart rate patterns, **you** can ensure accurate interpretation and enhance the reliability of fetal monitoring. Additionally, proactive measures such as electrode placement, shielding, and equipment maintenance contribute to minimizing artifacts and optimizing the quality of monitoring.

1.3.2   Signal Ambiguity:

Signal ambiguity refers to situations in which the electronic monitoring equipment used in various fields, such as electronic fetal monitoring, encounters difficulties in clearly differentiating between different signals or readings. This can lead to a lack of clarity or confusion in interpreting the data provided by the equipment.

One of the main reasons why signal ambiguity occurs is equipment failure. This can happen due to technical malfunctions, such as faulty sensors or wiring issues. When the equipment fails, it may not accurately capture or transmit the signals it is designed to monitor, leading to ambiguous readings. In such cases, troubleshooting becomes essential to identify the source of the problem and resolve it promptly.

Troubleshooting is the process of identifying, isolating, and resolving issues that arise with electronic monitoring equipment. When it comes to signal ambiguity, troubleshooting involves examining the various components of the equipment to determine if there are any malfunctions or defects. This typically includes checking the connections, cables, sensors, and the main unit itself. By systematically evaluating each component, **expert**s can pinpoint the source of the ambiguity and take appropriate action.

In the context of electronic fetal monitoring, signal ambiguity can potentially have serious implications. This monitoring technique is used during pregnancy and labor to assess the well-being of the fetus. It relies on detecting and interpreting electrical signals generated by the fetal heart and uterine contractions. Therefore, any ambiguity in the signals can lead to incorrect assessments and potentially compromise the safety of both the mother and the baby.

To address signal ambiguity in electronic fetal monitoring, it is important to follow established protocols and guidelines. These protocols provide a systematic approach to troubleshooting and ensure that the equipment is functioning optimally. Regular maintenance and calibration of the equipment are also crucial to prevent and address signal ambiguity.

There are various factors that can contribute to signal ambiguity in electronic fetal monitoring. For example, movement artifacts caused by fetal or maternal movement can interfere with the accuracy of the readings. These artifacts can be minimized by ensuring that the sensors are properly positioned and secured. Additionally, environmental factors such as electromagnetic interference from other devices or power sources can also introduce signal ambiguity. Proper grounding and shielding techniques can help mitigate these issues.

Training and education play a vital role in the effective management of signal ambiguity. Electronic fetal monitoring specialists should be trained in troubleshooting techniques, equipment maintenance, and the interpretation of ambiguous signals. Ongoing education and staying up to date with advancements in technology are essential to ensure accurate and reliable monitoring. It can occur due to equipment failure, technical malfunctions, or external factors. Troubleshooting and adhering to established protocols are key in addressing signal ambiguity. Proper positioning, maintenance, and training are essential in minimizing the impact of ambiguity and ensuring the safety of patients. By being proactive in resolving these issues, electronic fetal monitoring specialists can provide accurate and reliable assessments during pregnancy and labor.

2   PHYSIOLOGY:

Physiology is the branch of biology that deals with the functions and processes of living organisms. It focuses on the study of how different parts of the body work together to maintain homeostasis, which is the stable internal environment of the body. In the context of being an Electronic Fetal Monitoring Specialist, understanding the physiology of pregnancy and fetal development is crucial.

The physiological changes that occur during pregnancy are quite remarkable. Hormonal fluctuations, such as an increase in estrogen and progesterone, play a vital role in preparing the body for pregnancy and maintaining fetal development. These hormones help to regulate the menstrual cycle, promote the growth of the uterus, and support the development of the placenta.

The cardiovascular system undergoes significant changes during pregnancy. The heart pumps more blood to meet the needs of the growing fetus, leading to an increase in cardiac output. Blood volume and plasma volume also increase to ensure an adequate supply of nutrients and oxygen to the developing baby. These changes can result in alterations in blood pressure and heart rate.

Respiratory changes are also observed during pregnancy. The growing uterus can put pressure on the diaphragm, making it harder for the mother to take deep breaths. Additionally, hormonal changes cause an increase in the levels of carbon dioxide in the blood, which stimulates the respiratory drive. As a result, pregnant women may experience shortness of breath and an increased respiratory rate.

The digestive system also goes through significant adaptations to support the developing fetus. Hormones, such as progesterone, relax the smooth muscles in the digestive tract, leading to a decrease in motility. This can result in symptoms like constipation and heartburn. The increased size of the uterus can also heighten the pressure on the stomach, leading to feelings of fullness and decreased appetite.

The urinary system is responsible for filtering waste products from the blood and maintaining fluid balance. During pregnancy, there is an increased blood flow to the kidneys, which leads to an increase in urine production. The growing uterus can also exert pressure on the bladder, causing more frequent urination.

Understanding the physiology of the fetal development is essential for an Electronic Fetal Monitoring Specialist. The development of the placenta, umbilical cord, and amniotic fluid is critical to ensuring the proper supply of oxygen and nutrients to the fetus. Monitoring fetal heart rate and uterine contractions are crucial in assessing the well-being and health of the baby during labor. It encompasses the numerous changes that occur in a woman's body during pregnancy and the development of the fetus. By understanding these physiological processes, an Electronic Fetal Monitoring Specialist can provide valuable insights and care to ensure the well-being of both the mother and the baby.

2.1   Uteroplacental:

The uteroplacental unit is a crucial component of pregnancy physiology. It involves the interaction between the uterus and the placenta, which allows the fetus to receive oxygen and nutrients for its growth and development. Understanding the dynamics of the uteroplacental unit is essential for electronic fetal monitoring specialists to assess fetal well-being during pregnancy.

The uterus plays a vital role in supporting the growth of the fetus. It undergoes various changes throughout pregnancy to accommodate the developing fetus. The uterine blood vessels, specifically the spiral arteries, undergo a process called trophoblastic invasion, which allows them to become larger and more efficient in delivering oxygen and nutrients to the placenta.

The placenta, a highly specialized organ, acts as a bridge between the mother and the fetus. It develops from the fertilized egg and attaches to the uterine wall. The placenta consists of maternal and fetal components. Maternal blood flows through the intervillous space, surrounding the fetal villi. The maternal blood supplies oxygen and nutrients to the fetus, while waste products are removed. The exchange of substances between the mother and the fetus occurs through the placental membrane. This membrane is selectively permeable, allowing for the passage of essential nutrients, gases like oxygen and carbon dioxide, and other necessary substances while preventing the transfer of harmful substances.

Blood flow through the uteroplacental unit is dynamic and regulated by various factors. Maternal blood flow to the placenta is mainly driven by changes in uterine artery resistance. Hormones such as progesterone and relaxin relax the smooth muscles of the uterine arteries, promoting blood flow. Additionally, maternal blood pressure and cardiac output play a role in regulating placental perfusion. Fetal blood flow within the placenta is regulated by the umbilical cord, which contains two arteries and one vein. The umbilical arteries carry deoxygenated blood and waste products from the fetus to the placenta, while the umbilical vein carries oxygen-rich blood and nutrients from the placenta to the fetus.

Several factors can impact the uteroplacental unit and potentially affect fetal well-being. These include maternal conditions such as hypertension, preeclampsia, and gestational diabetes, as well as placental abnormalities like placental insufficiency or placental abruption. Any disturbance in the uteroplacental unit can compromise the fetal oxygen and nutrient supply, leading to fetal distress.

Monitoring the uteroplacental unit's function is crucial for detecting any potential issues and ensuring optimal fetal well-being. Electronic fetal monitoring is a commonly used tool for assessing the fetal heart rate and uterine contractions. It provides valuable information about fetal oxygenation and helps identify fetal distress. Understanding its physiology and monitoring its function is essential for electronic fetal monitoring specialists to assess fetal well-being accurately. By comprehensively evaluating the uteroplacental unit, potential issues can be detected and managed promptly to ensure optimal outcomes for both the mother and the baby.

2.1.1   Uteroplacental circulation:

Uteroplacental circulation refers to the blood flow between the mother's uterus and the placenta during pregnancy. It is a vital process that ensures the exchange of oxygen and nutrients between the mother and developing fetus. This circulation occurs through a network of blood vessels known as the uteroplacental vascular bed.

The uteroplacental circulation begins when the embryo implants into the mother's uterus and the placenta develops. It is established primarily by the remodeling of the spiral arteries in the uterine wall. These arteries undergo significant changes to become wider and more efficient in delivering oxygen and nutrients to the placenta.

The placenta is a disc-shaped organ that acts as a bridge between the mother and the fetus. It is attached to the uterine wall and has a rich supply of blood vessels. These blood vessels are divided into two major components: maternal and fetal. Maternal blood is delivered to the placenta from the mother's arteries, while fetal blood is transported through the umbilical cord.

Maternal blood enters the uteroplacental vascular bed through the spiral arteries. These arteries carry oxygenated blood from the mother's heart into the placenta. Within the placenta, the maternal blood is channeled into numerous small vessels called intervillous spaces. These spaces are surrounded by finger-like projections called chorionic villi, which provide a large surface area for exchange of oxygen and nutrients.

The fetal blood, on the other hand, travels through the umbilical arteries from the fetus to the placenta. The umbilical arteries carry deoxygenated blood and waste products away from the fetus and into the placenta. In the placenta, the umbilical arteries branch into smaller vessels called chorionic arteries, which bring the fetal blood into close proximity with the maternal blood in the intervillous spaces.

Within the intervillous spaces, oxygen and nutrients diffuse from the maternal blood into the fetal blood, while waste products like carbon dioxide also pass from the fetal blood to the maternal blood. This exchange of substances allows the developing fetus to receive the necessary oxygen and nutrients for growth and development while eliminating waste products.

After the exchange of substances takes place, the blood is returned to the mother's circulation. The deoxygenated blood flows back through the chorionic veins, which merge to form larger vessels called the umbilical veins. The umbilical veins carry the oxygenated blood back to the fetus, supplying it with essential nutrients and oxygen.

The uteroplacental circulation is regulated by various factors, including hormonal changes during pregnancy. Hormones such as progesterone, estrogen, and human chorionic gonadotropin play crucial roles in maintaining the integrity and function of the uteroplacental vascular bed. It involves the remodeling of the spiral arteries, the transfer of substances in the intervillous spaces, and the return of blood to the maternal and fetal circulations. Understanding this circulation is crucial for an Electronic Fetal Monitoring Specialist, as it provides valuable insights into fetal well-being and can help detect any potential complications that may arise during pregnancy.

2.1.2   Fetal circulation:

Fetal circulation refers to the circulation of blood in a developing fetus, where the placenta plays a vital role in delivering nutrients and oxygen to the developing fetus. Understanding fetal circulation is crucial for Electronic Fetal Monitoring Specialists as it helps in assessing the well-being of the fetus during pregnancy and labor. In this article, we will delve into the important aspects of fetal circulation.

Fetal circulation begins in the placenta, where the mother's blood is enriched with oxygen and essential nutrients. Oxygenated blood from the placenta enters the fetus through the umbilical vein. The umbilical vein carries oxygen-rich blood and nutrient-rich substances to the liver of the fetus. At the liver, a portion of the blood flows through the hepatic circulation, while the rest bypasses the liver through a specialized blood vessel called the ductus venosus.

From the liver, the blood then enters the inferior vena cava, a large vein that carries deoxygenated blood from the lower part of the body. In the inferior vena cava, the oxygenated blood mixes with deoxygenated blood returning from the lower body.

The blood from the inferior vena cava enters the right atrium of the fetal heart. A portion of the blood flows directly into the left atrium through an opening called the foramen ovale. The foramen ovale helps bypass the non-functioning fetal lungs, as they receive oxygen directly from the placenta.

The remaining blood in the right atrium enters the right ventricle. From the right ventricle, it is pumped into the pulmonary trunk. However, the majority of blood in the pulmonary trunk bypasses the lungs through a vessel called the ductus arteriosus. This vessel connects the pulmonary trunk and the descending aorta, allowing the blood to bypass the non-functional lungs.

Next, the blood enters the fetal systemic circulation through the aorta. The blood is distributed to the various organs and tissues of the fetus, supplying oxygen and nutrients necessary for growth and development. Deoxygenated blood is then returned to the placenta through the two umbilical arteries, where it gets oxygenated again.

As the fetus develops and prepares for birth, certain changes occur in the fetal circulation. The foramen ovale, which allowed blood to bypass the fetal lungs, closes shortly after birth. The ductus arteriosus also constricts and eventually closes within a day or two after birth. These changes are triggered by the change in pressure and blood flow in the newborn's body. The placenta plays a vital role in facilitating this exchange. The fetal circulation bypasses the non-functioning lungs by utilizing specialized structures like the ductus venosus, foramen ovale, and ductus arteriosus. Understanding fetal circulation is essential for Electronic Fetal Monitoring Specialists to assess fetal well-being during pregnancy and childbirth.

2.1.3   Fetal heart regulation:

Fetal heart regulation is an essential aspect of uteroplacental physiology, and it involves the control and coordination of the fetal heart rate (FHR) during pregnancy. The fetal heart plays a crucial role in supplying oxygen and nutrients to the developing fetus, making its regulation vital for healthy fetal development. Various physiological mechanisms and factors contribute to the regulation of the fetal heart.

One of the primary regulators of the fetal heart is the autonomic nervous system. The autonomic nervous system consists of two branches: the sympathetic and parasympathetic nervous systems. These branches work in balance to control the FHR. The sympathetic system increases the heart rate, while the parasympathetic system slows it down. This balance ensures that the FHR remains within a normal range and responds appropriately to changes in the fetal environment.

The uteroplacental circulation also plays a significant role in fetal heart regulation. The placenta acts as the interface between the maternal and fetal circulations, allowing the exchange of oxygen and nutrients. Adequate blood flow through the uteroplacental circulation is essential for maintaining optimal fetal heart function. Any disruption in this blood flow, such as placental insufficiency or umbilical cord abnormalities, can adversely affect fetal heart regulation.

Another factor influencing fetal heart regulation is the fetal oxygen supply. Oxygen is critical for cells' energy production, including those in the fetal heart. When oxygen levels in the fetal blood decrease, it triggers a cascade of events that aim to increase oxygen delivery. As a result, the fetal heart rate increases to enhance blood flow and oxygenation. Conversely, when adequate oxygen levels are achieved, the fetal heart rate returns to baseline.

Fetal movements also have an impact on fetal heart regulation. Fetal movement serves as a stimulus to the fetal nervous system, activating the sympathetic branch of the autonomic nervous system and increasing the heart rate. This response ensures that the fetal heart is prepared for increased oxygen demand during periods of activity. After the movement ceases, the heart rate gradually returns to its baseline.

Maternal factors can also influence fetal heart regulation. Maternal emotions and stress can trigger the release of stress hormones, such as cortisol, which can then cross the placenta and affect the fetal heart rate. Maternal illnesses, medications, and substance use can also have an impact on fetal heart regulation. It is crucial for healthcare providers to monitor and address any maternal factors that may affect the fetal heart rate to ensure the well-being of the fetus.

Monitoring the fetal heart rate is an essential part of prenatal care. Electronic fetal monitoring (EFM) is a common technique used to assess fetal heart regulation. This monitoring involves the use of external devices or internal electrodes to continuously record the FHR during labor and delivery. It provides valuable information about the fetal heart rate patterns, helping healthcare providers identify any deviations from the normal range and intervene if necessary. The autonomic nervous system, uteroplacental circulation, fetal oxygen supply, fetal movements, and maternal factors all contribute to the regulation of the fetal heart rate. Understanding and monitoring fetal heart regulation are crucial for ensuring optimal fetal development and well-being. Electronic fetal monitoring is a valuable tool for assessing the fetal heart rate and detecting any abnormalities that may require medical intervention.

2.2   Factors affecting fetal oxygenation:

Factors affecting fetal oxygenation are crucial to understand for an Electronic Fetal Monitoring Specialist, as this knowledge helps in monitoring the well-being of the fetus during pregnancy and labor. Several factors can impact the oxygen supply to the fetus, ultimately affecting its health and development.

1. Placental function: The placenta plays a significant role in supplying oxygen to the fetus. Any abnormality in placental structure or function, such as placental insufficiency, can lead to inadequate oxygen transfer. Factors like placental abruption, placenta previa, or placental infections can compromise placental function and impact fetal oxygenation.

2. Maternal health conditions: Certain maternal health conditions can negatively affect fetal oxygenation. For example, maternal hypertension and preeclampsia can reduce blood flow to the placenta, diminishing oxygen supply. Diabetes, both pre-existing and gestational, can also contribute to impairment in fetal oxygenation.

3. Maternal smoking: Smoking during pregnancy can have detrimental effects on fetal oxygenation. The chemicals present in cigarettes, such as nicotine and carbon monoxide, reduce the amount of oxygen available in the maternal bloodstream. As a result, less oxygen reaches the fetus, potentially leading to oxygen deprivation and related complications.

4. Maternal anemia: Anemia, a condition characterized by low levels of red blood cells or hemoglobin in the blood, can impair the transportation of oxygen to the fetus. Maternal anemia can be caused by factors such as iron deficiency or excessive blood loss. Adequate treatment and management of anemia are vital for maintaining optimal fetal oxygenation.

5. Umbilical cord abnormalities: The umbilical cord serves as the lifeline between the mother and the fetus, carrying oxygen-rich blood to the fetus. However, certain abnormalities such as knots, twists, or compression can disrupt the oxygen supply. Prolonged cord compression can cause significant oxygen deprivation and may necessitate immediate medical intervention.

6. Maternal position: The position of the mother during labor can influence fetal oxygenation. When lying flat on the back, the weight of the uterus can exert pressure on major blood vessels, reducing blood flow to the placenta and affecting oxygenation. Encouraging the mother to change positions frequently or adopt a more upright position can help optimize fetal oxygenation.

7. Uterine contractions: Strong, frequent, or prolonged uterine contractions can hinder fetal oxygenation. These contractions can compress the blood vessels in the uterus, reducing blood flow to the placenta. Adequate rest periods between contractions and appropriate management of labor progress are essential to ensure sufficient oxygenation.

8. Fetal abnormalities: Certain fetal conditions can impact oxygenation directly. For instance, congenital heart defects or lung abnormalities can hinder the effective oxygen exchange. Diagnosis and timely intervention are crucial in managing these abnormalities to optimize fetal oxygenation. Monitoring and evaluating these factors during pregnancy and labor allow for early recognition and appropriate management of any potential complications, ensuring optimal oxygenation for the developing fetus.

2.2.1   Uterine activity:

Uterine activity refers to the contractions of the uterus during labor. This is an important aspect of fetal oxygenation as it directly affects the circulation of blood and oxygen to the developing fetus. Understanding uterine activity is crucial for electronic fetal monitoring specialists, as it helps them assess the well-being of the fetus and make informed decisions regarding the management of labor.

Uterine contractions can be categorized into two types: tonic contractions and phasic contractions. Tonic contractions are sustained contractions that are responsible for establishing a baseline tone in the uterus. These contractions usually occur during the early stages of labor and help to thin and dilate the cervix. Phasic contractions, on the other hand, are intermittent contractions that occur during active labor. These contractions play a vital role in pushing the fetus downward through the birth canal.

The frequency, duration, and intensity of uterine contractions are important parameters to monitor. Frequency refers to the time interval between the start of one contraction and the start of the next. Duration measures how long each contraction lasts. Intensity, also known as the strength of the contraction, is determined by palpation or by using an intrauterine pressure catheter (IUPC) during labor.

Uterine contractions can be influenced by various factors. One factor is hormonal changes, particularly the release of oxytocin, a hormone that stimulates uterine contractions. Oxytocin is produced by the pituitary gland and is responsible for initiating and maintaining labor. Another factor is the stretching and pressure on the uterine muscles caused by the growing fetus. As the fetus grows, it puts pressure on the cervix, which triggers uterine contractions.

The frequency and intensity of uterine contractions increase as labor progresses. In the early stages of labor, contractions may be mild and occur at longer intervals. However, as labor advances, contractions become more frequent, longer in duration, and more intense. This pattern helps facilitate cervical dilation and effacement, allowing the fetus to descend through the birth canal.

Monitoring uterine activity is crucial for assessing fetal well-being and oxygenation. By analyzing the patterns of uterine contractions, electronic fetal monitoring specialists can determine whether the fetus is receiving adequate oxygenation. If the contractions are too frequent or too intense, they may compromise blood flow to the placenta, leading to decreased oxygen supply to the fetus. Conversely, ineffective or insufficient contractions can impede the progress of labor and prolong fetal exposure to the stress of labor.

The assessment of uterine activity is typically done using an electronic fetal monitor (EFM), which records the frequency, duration, and intensity of uterine contractions. EFM is non-invasive and involves placing two sensors on the mother's abdomen: one to monitor fetal heart rate and another to detect uterine contractions. The information provided by the EFM helps guide the management of labor, ensuring the well-being of the fetus and facilitating a safe delivery. Understanding the patterns and characteristics of uterine contractions is vital for electronic fetal monitoring specialists. By assessing uterine activity, they can determine if the fetus is receiving adequate oxygenation and make informed decisions to ensure a safe delivery. Utilizing electronic fetal monitoring techniques, such as EFM, helps in accurately monitoring uterine contractions and fetal well-being throughout the labor process.

2.2.2   Maternal factors:

Maternal factors play a crucial role in affecting fetal oxygenation, which is vital for the well-being and development of the unborn baby. These factors include various aspects related to the mother's health and lifestyle choices throughout pregnancy.

One significant maternal factor is the mother's **overall** health. Chronic conditions such as diabetes, hypertension, and heart disease can negatively impact fetal oxygenation. These conditions may affect the mother's blood vessels, reducing the amount of oxygen-rich blood reaching the placenta. Similarly, maternal anemia, which is characterized by low levels of red blood cells or hemoglobin, can reduce the oxygen-carrying capacity of the blood.

Another essential aspect is the mother's respiratory function. Any condition that affects the lungs, such as asthma or respiratory infections, may compromise the exchange of oxygen and carbon dioxide between the mother and the fetus. Proper lung function is necessary to ensure an adequate oxygen supply to the developing baby.

The mother's lifestyle choices can also significantly influence fetal oxygenation. Smoking, for instance, exposes the fetus to harmful substances such as nicotine and carbon monoxide, which reduce the amount of oxygen that can reach the baby. Additionally, smoking can constrict the blood vessels, restricting blood flow and oxygen delivery.

Alcohol consumption during pregnancy is another significant maternal factor. When a pregnant woman drinks alcohol, it passes through the placenta, directly affecting the fetal blood supply. Alcohol can interfere with the baby's ability to extract oxygen from the mother's blood, leading to fetal hypoxia.

Drug abuse is yet another maternal factor that can impact fetal oxygenation. Illicit drugs like cocaine and methamphetamine can cause severe vasoconstriction, reducing blood flow and oxygen delivery to the fetus. These substances can also disrupt the normal functioning of the placenta, further compromising fetal oxygenation.

Maternal obesity is becoming increasingly common and is another important factor to consider. Obese mothers often have reduced circulation, which can limit oxygen supply to the fetus. The excess fat tissue can also lead to chronic inflammation, potentially affecting placental function and reducing fetal oxygenation.

Hypotension or low blood pressure in the mother can have adverse effects on the fetus as well. Insufficient blood pressure may result in reduced blood flow to the placenta, compromising oxygen delivery to the baby.

Infections in the mother, such as urinary tract infections or sexually transmitted diseases, can also impact fetal oxygenation. These infections can trigger an inflammatory response that can potentially compromise placental function and blood flow, reducing the supply of oxygen.

Additionally, maternal stress levels can influence fetal oxygenation. High levels of stress hormones, such as cortisol, can constrict blood vessels and decrease blood flow to the placenta, limiting oxygen delivery to the fetus. A mother's **overall** health, respiratory function, lifestyle choices, including smoking, alcohol consumption, and drug abuse, as well as obesity, hypotension, infections, and stress levels, can all impact the oxygen supply to the developing baby. Understanding and managing these factors are crucial for the well-being and healthy development of the fetus.

2.2.3   Anesthesia:

Anesthesia is a medical procedure used to induce temporary loss of sensation or consciousness. It is commonly used during surgical procedures to ensure the patient remains pain-free and still. In the context of fetal oxygenation and physiology, the administration of anesthesia can have significant effects on the well-being of the fetus.

There are various factors within anesthesia that can affect fetal oxygenation. One important aspect is the choice of anesthesia technique. General anesthesia, which involves the use of medications to induce complete unconsciousness, can decrease fetal oxygenation. This is because the medications used in general anesthesia can cross the placenta and directly affect the fetus. Regional anesthesia techniques, such as epidurals or spinal anesthesia, have been found to have less impact on fetal oxygenation compared to general anesthesia.

Another factor to consider is the timing of anesthesia administration. If anesthesia is given in the early stages of labor, it may cause a decrease in placental blood flow and subsequently reduce fetal oxygen supply. However, there is evidence to suggest that regional anesthesia techniques, when administered carefully and with close monitoring, can have minimal impact on fetal oxygenation even if given early in labor.

The specific medications used in anesthesia also play a role in fetal oxygenation. Certain anesthetic drugs can cause maternal hypotension, which can in turn lead to decreased placental perfusion and reduced oxygen supply to the fetus. It is crucial for the anesthesia provider to carefully monitor the mother's blood pressure and maintain adequate perfusion to prevent any adverse effects on fetal oxygenation.

Maternal factors such as maternal health conditions and medications can also influence fetal oxygenation during anesthesia. Some pre-existing medical conditions, such as hypertension or diabetes, can affect placental function and oxygen exchange. Medications taken by the mother can also have an impact on fetal oxygenation. The anesthesiologist must be aware of these factors and take them into consideration when planning and administering anesthesia.

In addition to the factors mentioned above, it is important to highlight the role of continuous electronic fetal monitoring during anesthesia. Fetal heart rate monitoring allows for real-time assessment of fetal well-being and helps identify any signs of fetal distress. Close monitoring of the fetal heart rate patterns during anesthesia can alert the healthcare team to any changes that may indicate compromised fetal oxygenation.

To mitigate the potential risks and optimize fetal oxygenation during anesthesia, a multidisciplinary approach involving obstetricians, anesthesiologists, and nurses is essential. Collaboration and effective communication among the healthcare team are crucial in ensuring the safety and well-being of both the mother and the fetus during anesthesia. When considering the factors affecting fetal oxygenation and physiology, it is important to carefully choose the anesthesia technique, consider the timing of administration, monitor maternal factors, and closely observe fetal well-being through continuous electronic fetal monitoring. By addressing these factors and implementing appropriate measures, healthcare providers can optimize fetal oxygenation and minimize any potential risks associated with anesthesia.

2.2.4   Drugs (Therapeutic & Recreational):

Drugs play a significant role in affecting fetal oxygenation, involving both therapeutic and recreational drugs. Understanding the impact of these drugs is essential for electronic fetal monitoring specialists.

Therapeutic drugs are medications prescribed to manage various conditions during pregnancy. They can be beneficial in treating illnesses and promoting the **overall** well-being of the mother. However, certain therapeutic drugs may indirectly affect fetal oxygenation.

One common therapeutic drug that can influence fetal oxygenation is opioid pain medication. These medications are often prescribed to manage severe pain, but they can cross the placental barrier and directly affect the fetus. Opioids can depress the central nervous system, leading to respiratory depression in both the mother and the unborn baby. This respiratory depression can reduce the amount of oxygen available to the fetus, potentially causing hypoxia.

Another therapeutic drug that can affect fetal oxygenation is certain antidepressants, such as selective serotonin reuptake inhibitors (SSRIs). While the **overall** effects of these drugs on fetal oxygenation are still being studied, some SSRIs have been associated with an increased risk of fetal hypoxia. It is important for electronic fetal monitoring specialists to monitor mothers taking these medications closely.

Moving on to recreational drugs, their impact on fetal oxygenation can be detrimental. Substances like cocaine, marijuana, and methamphetamine can have severe consequences for the unborn baby. These drugs can restrict blood vessels, leading to reduced blood flow to the placenta. This reduction in blood flow deprives the fetus of essential oxygen and nutrients, increasing the risk of fetal hypoxia.

Cocaine, in particular, is known to have neurotoxic effects on the fetal brain. It can cause vasoconstriction, leading to blood vessel narrowing and reduced oxygen supply. This constriction can trigger placental abruptions, which can further compromise fetal oxygenation. Electronic fetal monitoring specialists must be vigilant in monitoring pregnancies where recreational drug use is suspected.

When it comes to managing pregnancies involving drugs, communication between healthcare providers is crucial. Obstetricians, neonatologists, and electronic fetal monitoring specialists should collaborate to develop comprehensive care plans that consider the effects of therapeutic and recreational drugs on fetal oxygenation.

They need to assess the maternal drug usage, including dosage and frequency, to determine the potential risks to the fetus. Ongoing monitoring through electronic fetal monitoring can provide valuable insight into the well-being of the unborn baby, including signs of fetal distress or hypoxia. Opioid pain medications and certain antidepressants can indirectly affect oxygen levels, while recreational drugs like cocaine can directly cause vasoconstriction and compromise blood flow to the placenta. Electronic fetal monitoring specialists should stay up-to-date with current research and work closely with other healthcare providers to ensure the best outcome for both the mother and the unborn baby.

2.2.5   Placental factors:

Placental factors play a crucial role in the **overall** oxygenation of the fetus and can significantly impact its well-being. These factors refer to any condition or event that affects the function and health of the placenta, the organ responsible for providing oxygen and nutrients to the developing fetus. Understanding these factors is of utmost importance for an Electronic Fetal Monitoring Specialist in order to monitor and assess the fetal oxygenation accurately.

One of the primary placental factors that can affect fetal oxygenation is the placental insufficiency. This condition occurs when the placenta is unable to deliver an adequate supply of oxygen and nutrients to the fetus. Placental insufficiency can be caused by various factors, such as placental abnormalities, maternal conditions like high blood pressure or diabetes, or problems with the placental blood vessels. These factors can lead to a reduced blood flow to the fetus, compromising its oxygenation.

Another important placental factor is the presence of placental abruption. This occurs when the placenta detaches from the uterine wall before delivery, leading to bleeding and reduced oxygen supply to the fetus. Placental abruption can be caused by trauma, maternal hypertension, smoking, or drug use. Prompt detection and management of this condition are crucial to prevent fetal distress and potential complications.

Placenta previa is yet another placental factor that can affect fetal oxygenation. In this condition, the placenta partially or completely covers the cervix, obstructing the exit route for the baby. This can cause bleeding and compromise the blood flow to the fetus, leading to oxygen deprivation. Electronic fetal monitoring plays a crucial role in identifying signs of distress in these cases and guiding appropriate interventions.

Placental infection, known as chorioamnionitis, is also a significant placental factor affecting fetal oxygenation. This infection can lead to inflammation and damage to the placenta, impairing its ability to provide adequate oxygen to the fetus. Chorioamnionitis commonly occurs when bacteria from the vagina ascend into the uterus. Prompt identification and treatment of this condition are crucial to minimize the impact on the fetus.

Furthermore, placental factors related to umbilical cord abnormalities can also affect fetal oxygenation. Umbilical cord compression or prolapse can lead to restricted blood flow through the cord, compromising the oxygen supply to the fetus. Additionally, a nuchal cord, where the umbilical cord wraps around the baby's neck, can also lead to oxygen deprivation if it becomes too tight. Placental insufficiency, placental abruption, placenta previa, chorioamnionitis, and umbilical cord abnormalities are key factors that can compromise fetal well-being. As an Electronic Fetal Monitoring Specialist, it is essential to have a comprehensive knowledge of these factors, their manifestations, and the appropriate monitoring and management strategies to ensure the optimal oxygenation and well-being of the fetus.

2.2.6   Umbilical blood flow:

Umbilical blood flow is a crucial factor in fetal oxygenation, an essential process for the fetus's **overall** well-being. This flow refers to the movement of blood through the umbilical cord, which connects the fetus to the placenta. Understanding the various aspects of umbilical blood flow is vital for an Electronic Fetal Monitoring Specialist to assess the fetal condition accurately.

One key factor affecting umbilical blood flow is the diameter of the umbilical blood vessels. The umbilical artery carries deoxygenated blood from the fetus to the placenta, while the umbilical vein transports oxygenated blood back to the fetus. Any constriction or narrowing of these vessels can lead to decreased blood flow and compromised oxygenation. Similarly, any abnormalities in the umbilical cord's structure or position can also impact blood flow.

Another important aspect is the resistance in the placental vascular bed. The placenta acts as the interface between the maternal and fetal circulatory systems. Any changes in the resistance within the placental blood vessels can affect umbilical blood flow. Increased resistance can impair the delivery of oxygen-rich blood to the fetus, while decreased resistance can result in excessive blood flow that may strain the fetal cardiovascular system.

Maternal blood pressure also plays a role in umbilical blood flow. Elevated blood pressure can constrict the maternal blood vessels that supply the placenta, consequently reducing the oxygen and nutrients available for transfer to the fetus. On the other hand, low blood pressure can result in inadequate perfusion of the placenta, impacting umbilical blood flow.

The fetal heart rate is closely related to umbilical blood flow and serves as an indirect indicator of fetal well-being. Changes in the fetal heart rate pattern, as detected by electronic fetal monitoring, can indicate alterations in umbilical blood flow. For example, a decrease in the heart rate may suggest decreased oxygenation or compromised blood flow, while an increased heart rate could indicate fetal distress.

Hormonal factors, particularly those released during labor, can also influence umbilical blood flow. For instance, the release of oxytocin causes uterine contractions, which can temporarily reduce blood flow to the placenta during each contraction. This interruption in blood flow is necessary for the fetus to withstand the stress of labor but should be brief to minimize the risk of fetal compromise.

Other factors affecting umbilical blood flow include maternal smoking, which can constrict blood vessels and reduce oxygen supply to the fetus. Maternal positioning during labor also plays a role, as certain positions can restrict blood flow through the inferior vena cava and uterine vessels, affecting placental perfusion. Factors such as the diameter of umbilical vessels, resistance in the placental vascular bed, maternal blood pressure, fetal heart rate, hormonal influences, maternal smoking, and positioning during labor all contribute to the regulation of this flow. As an Electronic Fetal Monitoring Specialist, understanding these factors and their impact on umbilical blood flow is essential for accurate assessment and monitoring of the fetal condition.

2.2.7 Acid base and cord blood gases:

In the field of electronic fetal monitoring, understanding the factors that affect fetal oxygenation is crucial. One important aspect of this is the acid-base balance and cord blood gases.

The acid-base balance refers to the levels of acids and bases, specifically hydrogen ions (H+) and bicarbonate ions (HCO3-), in the body. It is a measurement of the body's ability to maintain a stable pH level. In the context of fetal oxygenation, the acid-base balance is important because it reflects the oxygenation status of the fetus.

Cord blood gases, on the other hand, are measurements taken from the blood in the umbilical cord immediately after birth. They provide valuable information about the fetus's oxygenation and acid-base balance during labor and delivery.

There are several factors that can affect the acid-base balance and cord blood gases in the fetus. One such factor is the duration and intensity of contractions. Prolonged or strong contractions can compress the blood vessels in the uterus, reducing blood flow to the fetus. This can lead to fetal hypoxia, a condition characterized by low oxygen levels in the fetal blood. In turn, fetal hypoxia can disrupt the acid-base balance and result in metabolic acidosis, where there is an accumulation of acid in the blood.

Another factor that can affect the acid-base balance is the fetal heart rate. Bradycardia, or a slow heart rate, can be a sign of fetal distress and inadequate oxygenation. This can lead to metabolic acidosis as well. Conversely, tachycardia, or a fast heart rate, can be a compensatory mechanism in response to fetal hypoxia. However, if tachycardia persists, it can indicate fetal acidosis.

The position of the fetus in the uterus can also impact the acid-base balance. For example, a prolapsed umbilical cord, where the cord slips ahead of the presenting part of the fetus, can lead to cord compression and compromised blood flow. This can cause fetal hypoxia and acidosis.

Maternal factors can also affect the acid-base balance and cord blood gases. Maternal hypotension, for instance, can impair blood flow to the placenta and reduce oxygen delivery to the fetus. This can result in fetal acidosis. Maternal hypoxemia, or low oxygen levels in the mother's blood, can also lead to fetal hypoxemia and acidosis.

Monitoring the acid-base balance and cord blood gases is essential during labor and delivery to assess the well-being of the fetus. By evaluating these measurements, healthcare professionals can identify signs of fetal distress and take appropriate interventions to optimize fetal oxygenation. These interventions may include repositioning the mother, administering oxygen, or performing a cesarean delivery. Factors such as contractions, fetal heart rate, fetal position, and maternal factors can all influence these measurements. By monitoring and interpreting these measurements, healthcare professionals can effectively assess fetal oxygenation and take the necessary steps to ensure the well-being of the fetus during labor and delivery.

3 PATTERN RECOGNITION AND INTERVENTION:

Pattern recognition and intervention are important aspects of being an Electronic Fetal Monitoring Specialist. By understanding and being able to recognize patterns in fetal heart rate tracings, specialists can identify potential complications and take appropriate actions to intervene and ensure the well-being of both the mother and the baby.

One of the main patterns that Electronic Fetal Monitoring Specialists look for is variability in the fetal heart rate. Variability refers to the fluctuations in the heart rate, and it is a sign of a healthy baby. A lack of variability can indicate fetal distress or compromise, and immediate intervention may be needed to prevent further complications.

Another pattern that specialists pay close attention to is decelerations in the fetal heart rate. Decelerations are temporary drops in the heart rate, and they can occur for various reasons. Early decelerations are typically benign and are a normal response to contractions. Late decelerations, on the other hand, can be a sign of fetal distress, usually caused by uteroplacental insufficiency. Immediate intervention, such as repositioning the mother or administering oxygen, may be necessary in these cases.

Variable decelerations, which are sharp and sudden drops in the heart rate, are also important patterns to recognize. They can be caused by cord compression or umbilical cord prolapse, which can restrict the baby's oxygen supply. In such situations, the specialist may need to take immediate action to relieve cord compression or prepare for an emergency cesarean section.

Additionally, specialists consider the baseline heart rate when analyzing patterns. The baseline is the average heart rate of the baby during periods of relative stability. It provides crucial information about the **overall** well-being of the fetus. A high or low baseline heart rate can indicate an underlying issue that requires intervention.

Interventions taken by Electronic Fetal Monitoring Specialists may include notifying the attending healthcare provider, adjusting the mother's position, administering intravenous fluids, providing oxygen, or preparing for an emergency delivery. Timely recognition of abnormal patterns and appropriate interventions can significantly improve outcomes for both the mother and the baby.

Apart from pattern recognition and intervention, Electronic Fetal Monitoring Specialists also play a vital role in documentation. Accurate documentation of fetal heart rate tracings and the interventions performed is essential for continuity of care and legal purposes. Specialists must clearly communicate their findings and actions to the healthcare team to ensure the best possible care for the mother and the baby. By understanding the different patterns in fetal heart rate tracings and taking appropriate actions, specialists can identify potential complications and intervene in a timely manner. This allows for the best possible outcomes for both the mother and the baby. Accurate documentation and effective communication are also crucial aspects of the specialist's role in ensuring quality care.

3.1 Fetal baseline heart rate:

Fetal baseline heart rate is a crucial aspect of electronic fetal monitoring, which plays a significant role in recognizing and intervening in fetal distress during labor. The baseline heart rate refers to the average number of fetal heartbeats per minute, measured continuously. This information helps healthcare professionals assess the well-being of the unborn baby and make informed decisions regarding interventions, if necessary.

One important aspect of fetal baseline heart rate is determining its normal range. The average baseline heart rate usually falls between **110** and **160** beats per minute (bpm), with minor fluctuations considered normal variations. However, it is important to understand that each fetus is unique, and factors such as gestational age and maternal characteristics can influence the baseline heart rate.

To accurately recognize deviations from the normal baseline, medical professionals also consider short-term and long-term variability. Short-term variability refers to the fluctuations in the fetal heart rate from beat to beat, while long-term variability represents the changes over longer periods of time. Both types of variability provide insight into the fetal autonomic nervous system's ability to respond to various stimuli, indicating normal neurological development.

In addition to variability, healthcare professionals also analyze accelerations and decelerations in the fetal baseline heart rate. Accelerations are temporary increases, often associated with fetal movement, indicating a responsive and healthy nervous system. Conversely, decelerations reflect temporary decreases in the heart rate, which can be classified into different categories.

Early decelerations occur in response to head compression during contractions and are generally considered benign. On the other hand, late decelerations, which occur after the contraction begins, may indicate insufficient oxygen supply to the fetus and require intervention. Variable decelerations are another type, resulting from umbilical cord compression, and their severity can range from mild to severe, necessitating close monitoring and possibly interventions.

Monitoring the fetal baseline heart rate and its accompanying patterns allows medical professionals to identify signs of fetal distress and intervene promptly. Appropriate interventions may include changing the mother's position, providing oxygen therapy, adjusting intravenous fluids, or preparing for an urgent delivery, such as through cesarean section.

It is crucial for electronic fetal monitoring specialists to thoroughly understand the concept of fetal baseline heart rate and its patterns. They must be able to recognize variations, interpret their significance accurately, and communicate effectively with the healthcare team, including obstetricians, nurses, and other specialists.

Continuous assessment of the fetal baseline heart rate during labor provides valuable information for tracking the well-being of the baby. It ensures that any signs of fetal distress are promptly identified, which can significantly contribute to positive birth outcomes. By maintaining a clear understanding of the subject, electronic fetal monitoring specialists play a vital role in assisting healthcare providers in detecting potential complications and providing appropriate interventions when required.

3.1.1   Bradycardia:

Bradycardia is a condition characterized by a slow fetal baseline heart rate, which falls below the normal range of **110** to **160** beats per minute. It is one of the important aspects in the field of fetal baseline heart rate, pattern recognition, and intervention for Electronic Fetal Monitoring Specialists.

Bradycardia can be classified into two types: early, or baseline bradycardia, and late, or decelerative bradycardia. Early bradycardia is identified by a heart rate below **110** beats per minute that persists over a period of time. On the other hand, late bradycardia is characterized by a gradual decrease in the fetal heart rate following a uterine contraction.

Several factors can contribute to the occurrence of bradycardia in a fetus. These include fetal hypoxia, which is a lack of oxygen supply to the fetus, placental abruption, where the placenta detaches from the uterine wall, umbilical cord prolapse, where the umbilical cord slips through the cervix before the baby, and maternal hypotension, which is low blood pressure in the mother.

Electronic fetal monitoring plays a crucial role in identifying and monitoring bradycardia. This monitoring technique involves placing sensors on the mother's abdomen to measure the fetal heart rate and uterine contractions. By keeping a close watch on the fetal heart rate pattern, changes in baseline, and the presence of decelerations, bradycardia can be detected.

When bradycardia is detected, it is important for the Electronic Fetal Monitoring Specialist to intervene promptly. The first step is to assess the mother's vital signs and make any necessary adjustments to improve oxygen and blood flow to the fetus. This may involve repositioning the mother to maximize blood flow or administering fluids or medications to increase blood pressure.

If interventions to improve oxygenation and blood flow prove ineffective, the next step may be to prepare for an emergency delivery. This could involve preparing for a cesarean section or having the necessary personnel and equipment ready for a vaginal delivery with adequate fetal monitoring.

It is essential for the Electronic Fetal Monitoring Specialist to communicate effectively with other members of the healthcare team, including obstetricians, nurses, and neonatologists, to ensure a coordinated and timely response to bradycardia. It is characterized by a slow fetal heart rate and can be caused by various factors. Electronic fetal monitoring plays a vital role in identifying and monitoring bradycardia. Prompt intervention and effective communication with the healthcare team are essential for optimal management of bradycardia in order to ensure the best possible outcome for the fetus and the mother.

3.1.2   Tachycardia:

Tachycardia refers to a condition where the fetal heart rate is abnormally high. It is an important aspect of fetal baseline heart rate pattern recognition and intervention in electronic fetal monitoring.

Tachycardia in a fetus is defined as a baseline heart rate greater than **160** beats per minute (bpm) for a duration of at least **10** minutes. This elevated heart rate can be a sign of fetal distress or an underlying medical issue. It is crucial for an electronic fetal monitoring specialist to accurately identify tachycardia and take appropriate actions to ensure the well-being of the baby.

There are two types of tachycardia that can occur in a fetus: sinus tachycardia and supraventricular tachycardia.

Sinus tachycardia is when the fetal heart rate increases above the normal range. It can occur due to various factors such as maternal fever, maternal dehydration, maternal anxiety, or fetal hypoxia. The specialist should evaluate the **overall** clinical picture and potential causes to determine the appropriate intervention.

Supraventricular tachycardia, on the other hand, is a more severe form of tachycardia. It is characterized by a rapid and regular fetal heart rate, often exceeding **200** bpm. This condition is usually caused by abnormal electrical pathways in the heart. Prompt intervention is necessary to prevent further complications.

When tachycardia is detected during electronic fetal monitoring, the specialist must take certain steps. Firstly, they should assess the mother's vital signs and clinical history to identify any potential causes or risk factors. This may involve checking for signs of maternal fever or dehydration, as well as evaluating the **overall** condition of the fetus.

The next step is to assess the fetal well-being through additional tests. This may include performing a non-stress test, which measures the baby's heart rate in response to its movements. A biophysical profile may also be conducted to assess other parameters such as fetal breathing, movement, muscle tone, and amniotic fluid volume.

If the tachycardia persists or worsens, the specialist may consider interventions to address the underlying cause and improve fetal well-being. This can involve administering maternal oxygen, IV fluids, or medications to control maternal fever or anxiety. In severe cases of supraventricular tachycardia, the specialist may consider more aggressive interventions such as fetal cardioversion or maternal anesthesia.

Throughout the monitoring process, continuous assessment and documentation of the fetal heart rate and response to interventions are essential. This allows for the evaluation of any changes or improvements in the fetal condition. The specialist should also communicate effectively with the healthcare team, providing updates and seeking input as needed. The specialist plays a crucial role in identifying and managing tachycardia, assessing the underlying causes, and intervening appropriately to ensure the well-being of the fetus. By following established protocols and guidelines, the specialist can make informed decisions and provide optimal care for both the mother and the baby.

3.1.3   Variability:

Variability in fetal baseline heart rate is an important aspect of electronic fetal monitoring. It refers to the irregular fluctuations in the fetal heart rate over time. Variability is categorized into three types: absent variability, minimal variability, and moderate to marked variability.

Absent variability occurs when there is a flat baseline with little to no fluctuations in the fetal heart rate. This can indicate fetal distress or a compromised central nervous system. Minimal variability is characterized by small fluctuations of less than 5 beats per minute. It can be caused by fetal sleep, medications, or certain medical conditions. Moderate to marked variability is considered normal and signifies a healthy, responsive fetus.

Variability is evaluated by assessing the beat-to-beat changes in the fetal heart rate pattern. It is an essential part of pattern recognition during electronic fetal monitoring. Pattern recognition involves identifying different patterns in the fetal heart rate to determine if they are reassuring or non-reassuring.

Interventions are necessary when non-reassuring patterns are identified. These patterns may include prolonged decelerations, late decelerations, or bradycardia. Variability plays a crucial role in determining the urgency of the intervention. For example, absent or minimal variability accompanied by other non-reassuring patterns may require immediate action.

Several factors can influence fetal heart rate variability, including gestational age, fetal sleep cycles, medications, maternal position, and contractions. Gestational age affects the maturation of the fetal autonomic nervous system, leading to changes in heart rate variability. Fetal sleep cycles can also impact variability, as the heart rate tends to be more stable during periods of fetal sleep. Medications administered to the mother can affect fetal heart rate variability. Some medications, such as narcotics, can decrease variability, while others, like terbutaline, can increase it. Maternal position, particularly lying on the back, may reduce blood flow to the fetus and impact heart rate variability. Contractions can also influence variability, especially if they are frequent or prolonged.

Monitoring and understanding variability can help the electronic fetal monitoring specialist make informed decisions regarding the well-being of the fetus. Continuous assessment of variability combined with pattern recognition allows for early detection of potential fetal distress. This, in turn, enables prompt intervention to ensure the best possible outcome for both the mother and the baby. It provides valuable information about the fetal autonomic nervous system's function and **overall** well-being. Understanding and interpreting variability patterns is crucial for an electronic fetal monitoring specialist to recognize reassuring and non-reassuring patterns accurately. Prompt intervention is essential when non-reassuring patterns are identified. By incorporating variability assessment into electronic fetal monitoring, healthcare professionals can optimize care and improve outcomes for pregnant patients and their babies.

3.1.4   Sinusoidal:

Sinusoidal is a term used in the context of fetal baseline heart rate, pattern recognition, and intervention. It refers to a specific pattern seen on electronic fetal monitoring (EFM) tracings. Sinusoidal pattern is characterized by a smooth, undulating waveform that resembles the curves of a sine wave. This pattern is different from the normal irregular variability observed in fetal heart rate.

The sinusoidal pattern appears as a regular, symmetric waveform with a consistent amplitude and frequency. It often has a baseline heart rate of around 120-160 beats per minute. This pattern typically persists for at least 20 minutes and can last for hours.

Recognition of the sinusoidal pattern is crucial as it may indicate an underlying fetal condition that requires immediate medical intervention. It is considered an abnormal finding on EFM tracing and is associated with significant fetal distress. Therefore, it is essential for electronic fetal monitoring specialists to be able to identify this pattern accurately.

There are several distinct characteristics of the sinusoidal pattern that differentiate it from other EFM patterns. These include a smooth waveform with defined peaks and troughs, a regular frequency of oscillation, and a lack of variability. It is important to note that sinusoidal pattern is not affected by fetal movements, contractions, or external stimuli.

The possible causes of sinusoidal pattern include fetal anemia, severe fetal hypoxia, fetal hemorrhage, maternal drug administration (such as narcotic analgesics), and certain congenital abnormalities. It is crucial for specialists to investigate the underlying cause and determine appropriate interventions promptly.

When the sinusoidal pattern is identified, interventions should be implemented promptly to ensure the well-being of the fetus. The first step is to reposition the mother to optimize blood flow to the placenta and relieve any potential compression on the umbilical cord. This can be achieved by changing the maternal position or providing oxygen therapy to the mother.

Close monitoring of maternal vital signs and fetal heart rate is necessary to assess the response to interventions. In some cases, a biophysical profile or Doppler ultrasound may be performed to further evaluate fetal well-being.

If interventions fail to improve the sinusoidal pattern or if there are signs of fetal distress, more aggressive measures need to be taken. This may include immediate delivery, either by vaginal delivery or cesarean section, depending on the circumstances and gestational age of the fetus. It is associated with significant fetal distress and requires prompt recognition and intervention by electronic fetal monitoring specialists. Understanding the characteristics of this pattern and its potential underlying causes is crucial for ensuring the best possible outcomes for both the fetus and the mother.

3.2 Fetal heart rate variability:

Fetal heart rate variability refers to the natural fluctuations in the rate at which the baby's heart beats. It is an important aspect of fetal monitoring as it provides valuable information about the wellbeing of the fetus. The patterns observed in fetal heart rate variability can indicate the presence of certain conditions or complications during pregnancy.

There are two main types of fetal heart rate variability: short-term and long-term variability. Short-term variability refers to the beat-to-beat changes in the fetal heart rate over a short period of time. This can be measured using a fetal monitor, which records the baby's heart rate over a specific timeframe. Long-term variability, on the other hand, refers to larger changes in the fetal heart rate over a longer period of time, usually measured in minutes.

Fetal heart rate variability is influenced by various factors, including the baby's age, gestational age, and **overall** health. It can also be affected by the mother's activity level, position, and heart rate. Additionally, medications, maternal stress, and certain medical conditions can affect fetal heart rate variability.

The presence of normal fetal heart rate variability is a favorable sign and indicates that the baby is able to adapt and respond to its environment. It suggests that the baby's nervous system is functioning properly and that there is an adequate supply of oxygen and nutrients. On the other hand, decreased fetal heart rate variability may suggest fetal distress or compromise. This could be due to factors such as fetal hypoxia, a non-reassuring fetal heart rate pattern, or certain medications.

Monitoring fetal heart rate variability is an essential part of electronic fetal monitoring, which is commonly used during labor and delivery. It allows healthcare providers to assess the baby's wellbeing and make informed decisions regarding the need for intervention or further evaluation. The American College of Obstetricians and Gynecologists recommends that continuous electronic fetal monitoring be used for high-risk pregnancies and during labor for the early detection of fetal distress.

When assessing fetal heart rate variability, healthcare providers look for specific patterns. A normal baseline fetal heart rate is typically between **110** and **160** beats per minute. Variability within this range is considered reassuring. Absent or minimal variability, on the other hand, may be indicative of fetal distress or compromise.

In addition to the baseline fetal heart rate and variability, healthcare providers also consider other factors, such as the presence of accelerations or decelerations. Accelerations are temporary increases in the fetal heart rate, often associated with fetal movement, and are considered a sign of fetal well-being. Decelerations, on the other hand, are temporary decreases in the fetal heart rate and are categorized into different types, depending on their shape and timing.

Overall, fetal heart rate variability provides valuable information about the baby's health and well-being during pregnancy and labor. It is an important tool for healthcare providers in monitoring the fetus and making timely interventions when necessary. By understanding the patterns and interpreting the significance of fetal heart rate variability, electronic fetal monitoring specialists play a crucial role in ensuring the safe delivery of healthy babies.

3.2.1 Identification:

Identification is a crucial aspect within the broader **topic** of fetal heart rate variability in the context of pattern recognition and intervention. It involves the process of accurately determining the unique characteristics and patterns related to the fetal heart rate. The first step in identification is establishing a baseline for the fetal heart rate. This baseline serves as a reference point and helps healthcare professionals identify any deviations or abnormalities. By monitoring the heart rate over a specific period, patterns can be recognized and deviations from the baseline can be identified.

One important aspect of identification is recognizing accelerations in the fetal heart rate. Accelerations are temporary increases in the heart rate and are considered a positive sign of fetal well-being. They often occur in response to fetal movement and are an encouraging indication of fetal health. By identifying these accelerations, healthcare professionals can ensure the well-being of the fetus.

Decelerations, on the other hand, are temporary decreases in the heart rate. They can be categorized as early, variable, or late decelerations, each having different implications. Early decelerations are usually harmless and occur as a result of the head compression during contractions. Variable decelerations are more concerning as they can be caused by umbilical cord compression. Late decelerations, occurring after the peak of a contraction, may indicate impaired placental function and can be a sign of fetal distress. Identifying the type of deceleration and understanding its implications is crucial for appropriate intervention. Another important aspect of identification is recognizing patterns such as periodic changes in the heart rate. Periodic patterns can be recurrent and predictable, indicating normal variation, or they may be non-recurring and irregular, signaling potential problems. Identifying these patterns can help healthcare professionals intervene appropriately and provide necessary interventions to ensure the well-being of the fetus.

Identification also involves observing the duration and frequency of contractions. Contractions play a vital role in the fetal heart rate variability, and abnormalities in contraction patterns can affect the fetal well-being. By accurately identifying the duration and frequency of contractions, healthcare professionals can assess the impact on the fetus and determine if intervention is necessary. It involves establishing a baseline, recognizing accelerations and decelerations, identifying patterns, and observing the duration and frequency of contractions. By accurately identifying these aspects, healthcare professionals can intervene appropriately to ensure the well-being of the fetus.

3.2.2 Causes:

Causes of fetal heart rate variability can be categorized into various factors that affect the pattern recognition and intervention in electronic fetal monitoring.

One major cause of fetal heart rate variability is fetal distress. This can occur due to conditions such as inadequate oxygen supply to the fetus or a decrease in fetal blood flow. These conditions can be caused by problems with the placenta, umbilical cord, or maternal health issues like high blood pressure or diabetes.

Another cause of variability in fetal heart rate is fetal movement. Fetal movement can cause momentary changes in the heart rate, leading to fluctuations in variability. This is a normal physiological response and is generally not a cause for concern.

Maternal factors can also contribute to changes in fetal heart rate variability. Maternal health conditions like fever, infection, or drug use can affect the fetal heart rate pattern. Certain medications, such as those used for pain relief during labor, can also impact fetal heart rate variability.

Medical interventions during labor and childbirth can influence fetal heart rate variability as well. For example, the administration of certain medications like Pitocin, which is used to induce or augment labor, can affect the fetal heart rate pattern. Anesthesia or surgical procedures during labor and delivery can also have an impact.

In some cases, abnormal fetal heart rate patterns may be caused by fetal congenital anomalies. These anomalies can affect the normal development and function of the fetal heart, leading to variations in the heart rate pattern.

Other factors that can contribute to changes in fetal heart rate variability include maternal position, uterine contractions, and external factors like noise or stress. The position of the mother, such as lying on her back or side, can influence blood flow to the fetus, potentially affecting the heart rate pattern.

Uterine contractions during labor can also impact fetal heart rate variability. Strong or frequent contractions can temporarily decrease blood flow to the fetus, leading to changes in the heart rate.

External factors, such as noise or stress, can also affect the fetal heart rate pattern. Loud noises or stressful situations can cause temporary changes in the heart rate, but these changes are generally short-lived and do not indicate a significant problem. These include fetal distress, fetal movement, maternal factors, medical interventions, congenital anomalies, maternal position, uterine contractions, and external factors. Understanding these causes is essential for accurate pattern recognition and appropriate intervention in electronic fetal monitoring.

Remember, it is crucial to analyze the **overall** context and additional clinical information to accurately interpret fetal heart rate patterns and determine the appropriate course of action.

3.3   Abnormal uterine activity:

Fetal heart rate variability is an important concept in electronic fetal monitoring that falls under the broad **topic** of pattern recognition and intervention. It refers to fluctuations in the fetal heart rate over time, which can provide valuable information about the well-being of the fetus. Understanding and interpreting these variations play a crucial role in assessing fetal health during labor and delivery.

Fetal heart rate variability is measured by analyzing the changes in intervals between successive heartbeats. It is influenced by various factors such as fetal age, gestational age, levels of fetal oxygenation, fetal activity, and autonomic nervous system control. These factors contribute to the natural fluctuations in the fetal heart rate, reflecting the adaptability and integrity of the fetal central nervous system.

There are two main types of fetal heart rate variability: short-term and long-term variability. Short-term variability refers to rapid fluctuations in the fetal heart rate that occur over one-minute intervals. It is primarily influenced by the autonomic nervous system, particularly the sympathetic and parasympathetic branches. This type of variability is considered a sign of fetal well-being and indicates a healthy and responsive nervous system.

Long-term variability, on the other hand, refers to slower oscillations in the fetal heart rate that occur over a span of several minutes. It is influenced by factors such as fetal sleep cycles, fetal movements, and uterine contractions. Long-term variability provides insights into the fetal sleep-wake cycles and **overall** fetal activity level. A decrease in long-term variability may indicate fetal compromise or distress.

Based on the patterns and features observed in fetal heart rate variability, healthcare professionals can recognize abnormal patterns and identify potential issues with fetal well-being. These patterns are classified as non-reassuring or abnormal, which may require further intervention or monitoring.

For example, decreased or absent fetal heart rate variability, along with other abnormal patterns like decelerations or tachycardia, can indicate fetal distress. In such cases, prompt intervention is necessary to mitigate any potential risks to the fetus. This intervention may include repositioning the mother, increasing maternal hydration, administering oxygen, or considering more invasive measures like fetal scalp stimulation or umbilical cord blood sampling.

Conversely, a reassuring fetal heart rate variability pattern, characterized by regular fluctuations and quick response to fetal movement, suggests a well-oxygenated and healthy fetus. This pattern indicates that the fetus can effectively adapt to intrauterine stressors and is less likely to experience complications during labor and delivery.

Monitoring and interpreting fetal heart rate variability during labor and delivery require **expert**ise and knowledge in electronic fetal monitoring. The electronic fetal monitoring specialist plays a crucial role in assessing and documenting these patterns, assisting healthcare providers in making informed decisions regarding the management of labor. It provides valuable insights into the well-being of the fetus and helps healthcare professionals identify abnormal patterns that may require intervention. Understanding the different types of variability, their significance, and their interpretation is essential for electronic fetal monitoring specialists in providing optimal care and ensuring the safety of both the mother and the fetus.

3.3.1   Decreased blood flow:

Decreased blood flow in the context of fetal heart rate variability, pattern recognition, and intervention refers to a reduction in the amount of blood reaching the fetus, which can have significant implications for the well-being of the baby. This **topic** covers various important aspects related to decreased blood flow during pregnancy and the potential interventions that can be undertaken.

One of the primary causes of decreased blood flow is placental insufficiency, which means that the placenta is not functioning optimally. The placenta is responsible for exchanging nutrients and oxygen between the mother and the fetus. When it fails to perform this task efficiently, the fetus may not receive an adequate supply of oxygen and nutrients, leading to slowed blood flow. Another factor that can contribute to decreased blood flow is maternal conditions such as hypertension or preeclampsia. These conditions can narrow the blood vessels, impairing the flow of blood to the fetus. Additionally, certain fetal conditions like growth restriction or cardiac abnormalities may also impact blood flow.

Detecting decreased blood flow is crucial for early intervention. This is often done through electronic fetal monitoring, which involves measuring the fetal heart rate. A reduction in the fetal heart rate variability, particularly a decreased short-term variability, can indicate compromised blood flow.

Intervention strategies for decreased blood flow aim to improve the blood circulation to the fetus and ensure its well-being. One common intervention is maternal repositioning, where the expecting mother changes her position to alleviate any pressure on the blood vessels and promote better blood flow. For example, shifting from the supine to the lateral position can relieve compression on the vena cava, a major blood vessel.

In more severe cases, medical interventions may be necessary. These can include administering medications to improve blood flow or even performing an emergency cesarean section if the fetus is at risk of further compromise. An important aspect of intervention is the timely recognition of decreased blood flow and prompt decision-making to ensure the best outcome for both the mother and baby.

Monitoring fetal blood flow is a multidimensional process that involves the evaluation of various parameters, including umbilical artery Doppler studies, middle cerebral artery Doppler studies, and fetal biophysical profile testing. These assessments assist in determining the severity of the decreased blood flow and guiding the appropriate course of action.

It is worth noting that decreased blood flow can have long-term consequences for the baby's health. It can increase the risk of developmental delays, low birth weight, and even intrauterine fetal demise. Therefore, it is imperative for electronic fetal monitoring specialists to be vigilant and proactive in detecting signs of decreased blood flow to provide timely interventions and prevent potential complications. Electronic fetal monitoring plays a critical role in identifying this condition, allowing for timely intervention to optimize blood flow and ensure a healthy pregnancy. The involvement of healthcare professionals, particularly electronic fetal monitoring specialists, is crucial in recognizing the signs, implementing appropriate interventions, and ultimately improving outcomes for both the mother and the baby.

3.3.2   Response to hypertonus:

Response to hypertonus refers to the physiological and clinical reactions observed in the fetal heart rate (FHR) when the uterus experiences increased tone or contractions. Hypertonus occurs when the frequency, duration, or intensity of uterine contractions exceeds normal ranges. It is an important aspect of fetal heart rate variability and requires a prompt response and appropriate intervention to ensure the well-being of the fetus.

One of the first responses to hypertonus is an increase in fetal heart rate. This is known as tachycardia and can be an early sign of fetal distress. Tachycardia is characterized by a FHR above **160** beats per minute and can be a result of inadequate placental perfusion due to excessive uterine contractions. Monitoring the FHR in response to hypertonus is crucial in detecting tachycardia. Another response to hypertonus is a decrease in fetal heart rate, known as bradycardia. This is usually temporary and resolves once the hypertonus is relieved. Bradycardia can occur due to reduced blood flow to the fetus when the uterine contractions are too intense or prolonged. It is essential to recognize and address bradycardia promptly to prevent fetal compromise.

Besides changes in heart rate, hypertonus can also cause alterations in the FHR pattern. These patterns can be recognized using pattern recognition technology. The patterns associated with hypertonus include decelerations, accelerations, and variability changes. Decelerations can be either early, late, or variable, and their presence and characteristics provide important clues about the fetal response to hypertonus.

Early decelerations are usually benign and occur in response to head compression during contractions. Late decelerations, on the other hand, indicate compromised placental perfusion and fetal oxygenation. Variable decelerations are rapid decreases in heart rate caused by cord compression. These decelerations are significant indicators of fetal hypoxia and distress.

Accelerations, which are increases in the FHR, can also be observed in response to hypertonus. These accelerations are generally reassuring and reflect good fetal health. They indicate the absence of acute fetal compromise and are an encouraging sign during hypertonus. Monitoring the presence and characteristics of accelerations is essential for determining the fetal response to hypertonus.

Additionally, hypertonus can affect fetal heart rate variability, which is an important indicator of fetal well-being. Variability refers to the beat-to-beat fluctuations in the FHR and can be reduced or absent during hypertonus. The absence of variability indicates fetal distress and requires immediate intervention. Monitoring the variability of the FHR allows for the early identification of fetal compromise during hypertonus.

Interventions for hypertonus aim to relieve the excessive uterine contractions and restore normal fetal well-being. These interventions include repositioning the mother to relieve any pressure on the uterus, hydrating the mother to promote uterine relaxation, and administering medications to decrease contractions. Continuous electronic fetal monitoring plays a critical role in assessing the effectiveness of these interventions and ensuring the safety of the fetus. It involves changes in the FHR, including tachycardia, bradycardia, decelerations, accelerations, and variability alterations. Prompt recognition and appropriate interventions are necessary to address hypertonus and prevent fetal distress. Electronic fetal monitoring specialists play a vital role in monitoring these responses and ensuring the well-being of both the mother and the fetus.

3.3.3   Tachysystole:

Tachysystole is a term used in fetal monitoring to describe an abnormally high frequency of contractions during labor. It refers to the occurrence of more than five contractions in a **10**-minute period, averaged over a **30**-minute window. Tachysystole can have significant implications for both the mother and the baby, making it an important aspect to understand for an Electronic Fetal Monitoring Specialist.

One important aspect to consider when dealing with tachysystole is fetal heart rate variability. Normally, during labor, the fetal heart rate fluctuates, with accelerations and decelerations reflecting the well-being of the fetus. When tachysystole occurs, the frequency of contractions may lead to decreased variability in the fetal heart rate. This can be a possible sign of fetal distress, as the baby may not be receiving enough oxygen and nutrients during contractions.

Pattern recognition is another crucial aspect in evaluating tachysystole. By analyzing the pattern of contractions, monitoring specialists can identify whether the high frequency is sustained or intermittent. Sustained tachysystole refers to a continuous presence of high-frequency contractions, whereas intermittent tachysystole involves periods of normal contractions interspersed with episodes of excessive frequency. This differentiation is important as sustained tachysystole is more likely to impact fetal well-being and may require prompt intervention.

Intervention is an essential component when managing tachysystole. It involves a series of steps taken to ensure the safety and well-being of both the mother and the baby. Initially, if tachysystole is detected, the monitoring specialist may begin by repositioning the mother, as sometimes the positioning of the mother can affect the frequency of contractions. Additionally, hydration and providing pain relief may be considered to alleviate stress and reduce contractions.

If these measures do not resolve the tachysystole, further interventions may be necessary. This can include administering tocolytic medications, which work to suppress uterine contractions and restore a more normal pattern. Intravenous fluids may also be given to maintain hydration and prevent dehydration-induced contractions.

Continued assessment is crucial when managing tachysystole. Close monitoring of the fetal heart rate and contraction pattern is essential to determine the effectiveness of interventions. If the interventions do not result in improvement or if the fetal heart rate continues to show signs of distress, more invasive interventions such as amnioinfusion or cesarean delivery might be necessary to ensure the well-being of the baby. It involves the evaluation of fetal heart rate variability, pattern recognition, and intervention. Recognizing tachysystole requires analyzing the frequency and pattern of contractions, while intervention strategies aim to alleviate stress on the fetus and restore a more normal contraction pattern. Continued assessment is crucial to ensure the effectiveness of interventions and the **overall** well-being of both the mother and the baby.

3.4   Fetal dysrhythmias:

Fetal dysrhythmias refer to abnormal heart rhythms in the developing fetus. As an Electronic Fetal Monitoring Specialist, it is important to recognize and intervene promptly in cases of fetal dysrhythmias. These abnormalities can have various causes and may indicate an underlying medical condition or complication.

There are different types of fetal dysrhythmias, with the most common being sinus arrhythmia, which refers to irregular heartbeats. Another type is bradycardia, where the fetal heart rate drops below the normal range. Tachycardia, on the other hand, is an abnormally fast heart rate. Other dysrhythmias include premature atrial contractions, premature ventricular contractions, and atrial fibrillation.

Understanding the patterns associated with fetal dysrhythmias is crucial in order to provide appropriate interventions. Close monitoring of the fetal heart rate is essential using electronic fetal monitoring (EFM) techniques. This involves placing a device on the mother's abdomen to record the electrical activity of the fetal heart.

One important aspect of pattern recognition in fetal dysrhythmias is assessing the baseline heart rate. The baseline is the average heart rate over a **10**-minute period, excluding accelerations and decelerations. It is typically between **110** and **160** beats per minute. Significant deviations from this range may indicate the presence of a dysrhythmia.

In addition to the baseline, the presence of variability is also assessed. Variability refers to fluctuations in the fetal heart rate pattern and is considered a sign of a healthy functioning nervous system. Absent or minimal variability may suggest fetal distress.

Accelerations and decelerations are another important aspect of fetal heart rate patterns. Accelerations are temporary increases in the heart rate and are generally a reassuring sign. Decelerations, on the other hand, are transient decreases in the heart rate and can be early, late, or variable.

Early decelerations are typically benign and occur in response to the fetal head compression during contractions. Late decelerations, however, may be indicative of uteroplacental insufficiency and require immediate intervention. Variable decelerations have an abrupt onset and are typically associated with cord compression.

When a fetal dysrhythmia is identified, it is important to initiate appropriate interventions to optimize the fetal well-being. The interventions may involve changing the mother's position, administering oxygen to the mother, or providing intravenous fluids. In some cases, emergency interventions such as an emergency cesarean section may be required.

Continuous monitoring and regular reassessment of the fetal heart rate pattern are crucial in managing fetal dysrhythmias. An ongoing assessment allows for the identification of any changes or worsening of the condition, enabling prompt intervention. As an Electronic Fetal Monitoring Specialist, understanding the various types of dysrhythmias and recognizing their patterns is essential. This involves assessing the baseline heart rate, variability, and the presence of accelerations and decelerations. Timely interventions are necessary to ensure the well-being of the fetus. Continuous monitoring and reassessment are vital in managing fetal dysrhythmias effectively.

3.4.1   Supraventricular tachycardia:

Supraventricular Tachycardia (SVT) is a type of fetal dysrhythmia, which refers to irregular heart rhythms in the fetus. It can be categorized under the broader **topic** of pattern recognition and intervention in electronic fetal monitoring. SVT is characterized by a rapid heart rate greater than **220** beats per minute.

One important aspect to understand about SVT is its etiology or cause. SVT in fetuses can be the result of abnormalities in the electrical conduction system of the heart, such as the presence of accessory pathways. These pathways cause abnormal electrical impulses that can lead to tachycardia.

The diagnosis of SVT typically involves the use of electronic fetal monitoring, specifically a cardiotocography (CTG) monitor. This device records the fetal heart rate patterns and allows healthcare providers, like an electronic fetal monitoring specialist, to identify irregularities in the heart rhythm. A sustained heart rate greater than **220** beats per minute may indicate SVT.

Once SVT is diagnosed, intervention is necessary to prevent potential complications. There are several options for managing SVT in the fetus, including pharmacological treatment or in some cases, fetal cardiac interventions. Medications such as adenosine or digoxin can be administered to the mother to slow down the fetal heart rate. In more severe cases, fetal cardiac interventions, such as radiofrequency ablation, may be necessary to correct the abnormal electrical pathways.

Monitoring and follow-up are crucial in managing SVT in the fetus. After intervention, continuous electronic fetal monitoring is essential to monitor the response to treatment and ensure the heart rate remains within a normal range. The specialist should assess for any signs of fetal distress or recurrence of SVT during monitoring.

Recognizing the signs and symptoms of SVT is vital for an electronic fetal monitoring specialist. Common signs include an accelerated heart rate, decreased heart rate variability, and the absence of beat-to-beat variability. Additionally, the specialist should investigate any irregularities noticed during ultrasound examinations, such as atrial flutter or hydrops fetalis, which may be associated with SVT. Understanding the causes, diagnosis, interventions, and monitoring protocols for SVT is crucial for an electronic fetal monitoring specialist. Early detection and appropriate management of SVT can prevent potential complications and improve outcomes for the fetus.

3.4.2   Congenital heart block:

Congenital heart block is a type of fetal dysrhythmia that occurs when the electrical signals in the baby's heart are interrupted or blocked. This condition is typically present at birth and can have serious implications for the baby's health.

There are several causes of congenital heart block, but the most common cause is the presence of maternal antibodies that can cross the placenta and attack the baby's electrical system. These antibodies are often associated with autoimmune disorders such as systemic lupus erythematosus (SLE), which can be present in the mother. Other potential causes include certain medications taken by the mother during pregnancy, genetic factors, and structural abnormalities of the fetal heart.

The diagnosis of congenital heart block is usually made through fetal echocardiography, a specialized ultrasound that can visualize the baby's heart. This test can identify abnormalities in the rhythm and structure of the heart, confirming the presence of a heart block. Other diagnostic tests, such as a fetal electrocardiogram (ECG) or Doppler ultrasound, may also be performed to further evaluate the baby's condition.

The severity of congenital heart block can vary, ranging from a mild condition with minimal symptoms to a complete blockage of the electrical signals, leading to a slow and irregular heartbeat. In some cases, the heart block may progress over time, worsening the baby's symptoms.

Treatment options for congenital heart block depend on the severity of the condition and the baby's **overall** health. In mild cases, close monitoring may be sufficient, with regular follow-up appointments to assess the baby's heart rhythm and growth. In more severe cases, medication may be prescribed to regulate the heartbeat.

In certain situations, intervention may be necessary to improve the baby's heart function. This may involve the placement of a permanent pacemaker, a small device that helps regulate the heart's electrical signals. The pacemaker is typically implanted after birth or during the baby's early infancy, and regular monitoring is required to ensure its proper functioning.

The long-term outlook for babies with congenital heart block can vary depending on the severity of the condition and the presence of any underlying causes or associated conditions. Some babies may require ongoing medical management and monitoring of their heart health, while others may go on to lead relatively normal lives with minimal intervention. It is often caused by maternal antibodies that attack the baby's electrical system. Diagnosis is typically made through fetal echocardiography, and treatment options range from close monitoring to the placement of a pacemaker. The long-term outlook varies and depends on the severity of the condition.

3.4.3   Ectopic beats:

Ec**topic** beats, also known as premature beats, are an abnormal rhythm of the heart that can occur in the fetus. These beats originate from a location other than the normal pacemaker of the heart, which is the sinoatrial (SA) node. Instead, they arise from other regions of the heart, such as the atria or the ventricles.

Ec**topic** beats can be identified through electronic fetal monitoring (EFM), which is a technique used to monitor the fetal heart rate (FHR) and rhythm during pregnancy and childbirth. This monitoring is essential for recognizing any abnormalities and ensuring the well-being of the fetus.

There are two types of ec**topic** beats: premature atrial contractions (PACs) and premature ventricular contractions (PVCs). PACs occur when the atria contract earlier than normal, causing an irregularity in the heart rhythm. PVCs, on the other hand, occur when the ventricles contract prematurely. Both types of ec**topic** beats can disrupt the normal rhythm of the fetal heart.

Ec**topic** beats can have various causes. In some cases, they are benign and pose no significant threat to the fetus. However, other causes can indicate underlying health issues that require further investigation. Factors contributing to ec**topic** beats include maternal stress, medications, maternal health conditions like diabetes or hypertension, or structural abnormalities of the fetal heart.

When ec**topic** beats are detected during electronic fetal monitoring, it is crucial for an Electronic Fetal Monitoring Specialist to assess their frequency, duration, and potential impact on the fetus. PACs and PVCs may occur sporadically and resolve on their own, or they can persist and require intervention.

In mild cases, lifestyle modifications, such as reducing maternal stress, may be sufficient to resolve the issue. However, if the ec**topic** beats are more frequent or prolonged, medical intervention may be necessary. The Electronic Fetal Monitoring Specialist might recommend additional tests, such as an ultrasound or a fetal echocardiogram, to evaluate the structural integrity of the fetal heart.

Since some ec**topic** beats can be a sign of an underlying health condition, it is crucial to assess the **overall** well-being of the fetus. The Electronic Fetal Monitoring Specialist will evaluate the fetal heart rate patterns, as well as the presence of any other fetal dysrhythmias, to determine the appropriate course of action.

Monitoring the fetus continues during labor and delivery, as ec**topic** beats can sometimes persist or increase in frequency during this critical period. The Electronic Fetal Monitoring Specialist will closely monitor the fetal heart rate for any changes and adjust the monitoring accordingly. These premature beats can arise from different areas of the heart and can be caused by various factors. While some ec**topic** beats may resolve on their own, others may require further investigation and potential medical intervention. The **expert**ise of an Electronic Fetal Monitoring Specialist is essential in recognizing and managing ec**topic** beats to ensure the well-being of the fetus.

3.5   Maternal Complications:

Maternal complications refer to health issues that can occur during pregnancy, labor, and the postpartum period. These complications can arise due to various factors such as pre-existing medical conditions, pregnancy-related conditions, or unexpected events. It is crucial for an Electronic Fetal Monitoring Specialist to be aware of these complications as they directly impact the health and well-being of both the mother and the fetus.

One common maternal complication is gestational diabetes, which is characterized by high blood sugar levels during pregnancy. This condition requires proper monitoring and management to prevent adverse effects on both the mother and the baby. Another complication is preeclampsia, a condition that results in high blood pressure and can damage organs such as the liver and kidneys. It poses a risk to the mother and can also affect fetal growth and development.

In some cases, maternal complications can arise from pre-existing medical conditions like hypertension or diabetes. These conditions require careful monitoring and management throughout pregnancy to ensure the well-being of both the mother and the baby. Maternal infections, such as urinary tract infections or sexually transmitted infections, can also lead to complications if not diagnosed and treated in a timely manner.

During labor, complications can include abnormal bleeding, which may occur due to issues with the placenta or uterus. In some cases, a condition called placenta previa can occur, where the placenta covers the cervix partially or completely. This condition can cause heavy bleeding and may require immediate medical intervention.

Postpartum complications can also arise after childbirth. These may include postpartum hemorrhage, which is excessive bleeding after delivery, or postpartum infections, such as endometritis or mastitis. These complications need to be promptly recognized and treated to prevent further health issues for the mother.

It is vital for an Electronic Fetal Monitoring Specialist to be knowledgeable about the signs and symptoms of maternal complications. This **expert**ise allows them to recognize potential problems and provide appropriate interventions. Monitoring vital signs, including blood pressure, heart rate, and temperature, can aid in identifying any abnormalities or warning signs.

Furthermore, the Electronic Fetal Monitoring Specialist should be familiar with appropriate interventions and procedures to address maternal complications. This may involve collaborating with other healthcare professionals, such as obstetricians or nurses, to ensure optimal care for the mother. These interventions may include administering medication, managing pain, or performing emergency procedures, like a cesarean section, when necessary.

Overall, understanding and recognizing maternal complications is essential for an Electronic Fetal Monitoring Specialist. By staying informed about these potential issues, they can play a crucial role in promoting the health and well-being of both the mother and the fetus. By closely monitoring and promptly intervening in case of any complications, they can help ensure a safe and healthy childbirth experience for all involved.

3.5.1   Preterm Labor:

Preterm labor is a condition in which a woman begins to experience regular contractions and cervical changes before **37** weeks of gestation. This is an important **topic** to understand for electronic fetal monitoring specialists because it can have significant implications for both the mother and the baby.

One important aspect of preterm labor is the etiology or causes behind it. There isn't always a clear cause, but some common factors include a history of preterm birth, multiple pregnancies (such as twins or triplets), infections in the genital tract, cervical insufficiency, certain medical conditions like diabetes or high blood pressure, and certain lifestyle factors like smoking or drug use. Understanding these causes can help specialists identify women who may be at higher risk and provide appropriate interventions.

Another important aspect of preterm labor is the signs and symptoms that women may experience. These can vary, but may include regular contractions that occur every ten minutes or more frequently, cramping or abdominal pain, lower backache, pelvic pressure, changes in vaginal discharge, and a feeling of the baby's head pushing down. Recognizing these signs and symptoms is crucial for specialists so that they can promptly initiate interventions.

The diagnosis of preterm labor involves several assessments and tests. These may include assessing the frequency and duration of contractions, checking the cervix for changes such as dilation or effacement, and determining if there is an infection present. Electronic fetal monitoring is also an important tool in the diagnosis process. It involves placing sensors on the mother's abdomen to monitor the baby's heart rate and the frequency and duration of contractions. This helps specialists assess the well-being of the baby and determine the appropriate course of action.

Interventions for preterm labor aim to either stop or delay the labor process to allow for further fetal development. One common intervention is administering medications called tocolytics, which can help relax the uterus and slow down or temporarily stop contractions. Another intervention may involve administering corticosteroids to help mature the baby's lungs in case preterm birth is inevitable. Bed rest and hydration may also be recommended to help alleviate symptoms and prevent further cervical changes.

In some cases, despite interventions, preterm labor may progress and result in preterm birth. This can lead to a range of complications for the baby, such as respiratory distress syndrome, feeding difficulties, jaundice, and increased risk of infections. Therefore, it is crucial for electronic fetal monitoring specialists to closely monitor the baby's well-being during labor and provide appropriate care and support. Recognizing the signs and symptoms, diagnosing the condition accurately, and implementing appropriate interventions can greatly improve outcomes for both the mother and the baby. By staying informed about the latest research and guidelines, specialists can provide comprehensive care and support to women experiencing preterm labor.

3.5.2   Hypertension:

Hypertension, also known as high blood pressure, is a common maternal complication during pregnancy that requires pattern recognition and intervention by an Electronic Fetal Monitoring Specialist. It is characterized by persistently elevated blood pressure, typically defined as a systolic blood pressure of **140** mmHg or higher and a diastolic blood pressure of **90** mmHg or higher.

Pregnancy-induced hypertension, also known as gestational hypertension, is a form of high blood pressure that arises during pregnancy. It usually develops after the **20**th week of gestation and is accompanied by the absence of protein in the urine. Pre-existing hypertension, on the other hand, refers to high blood pressure that existed before pregnancy or was diagnosed before the **20**th week of gestation.

Hypertension during pregnancy can have serious implications for both the mother and the fetus. It increases the risk of developing complications such as preeclampsia, eclampsia, placental abruption, and preterm birth. These complications can lead to maternal organ damage, fetal growth restriction, stillbirth, and neonatal complications.

Monitoring blood pressure is crucial in the management of hypertension during pregnancy. An Electronic Fetal Monitoring Specialist plays a vital role in recognizing patterns of blood pressure readings and identifying any trends or abnormalities. Regular blood pressure measurements are essential to monitor the progression and severity of hypertension.

Intervention strategies for hypertension during pregnancy may vary depending on the severity of the condition and the gestational age of the fetus. Lifestyle modifications, such as maintaining a healthy diet, engaging in regular physical activity, and avoiding tobacco and alcohol, are often recommended as initial interventions. These interventions aim to control blood pressure and reduce the risk of further complications.

In some cases, medication may be necessary to manage hypertension. Antihypertensive drugs, such as methyldopa, labetalol, and nifedipine, are commonly prescribed to control blood pressure. Close monitoring of both the mother and the fetus is essential when medication is used, as certain drugs may have potential adverse effects.

Frequent prenatal visits are crucial for women with hypertension during pregnancy. Regular assessment of fetal well-being, including monitoring fetal heart rate and growth, is necessary to ensure the optimal management of the condition. An Electronic Fetal Monitoring Specialist plays a crucial role in interpreting fetal heart rate patterns and identifying any signs of distress or compromise.

If preeclampsia or severe hypertension develops, the management approach may involve hospitalization, close monitoring, and delivery of the baby. In such cases, an Electronic Fetal Monitoring Specialist may be involved in continuous electronic fetal monitoring during labor to assess fetal well-being and response to uterine contractions. Close monitoring of blood pressure, lifestyle modifications, and medication when necessary are important strategies in managing hypertension. Regular prenatal visits and continuous fetal monitoring are essential to identify any complications and ensure the well-being of both the mother and the fetus.

3.5.2.1   Gestational hypertension:

Gestational hypertension is a common complication in pregnancy, characterized by high blood pressure that typically develops after the **20**th week of gestation. It is important for Electronic Fetal Monitoring Specialists to be knowledgeable about this condition as it can have significant implications for both the mother and the fetus.

One of the primary concerns with gestational hypertension is the potential progression to preeclampsia, a more severe form of hypertension during pregnancy that is accompanied by organ damage and other complications. Therefore, early identification and proper management of gestational hypertension are crucial.

The exact cause of gestational hypertension is often unknown, but it is believed to be related to problems with the placenta, the organ that provides oxygen and nutrients to the fetus. In women with gestational hypertension, the blood vessels in the placenta may not develop properly, leading to reduced blood flow and oxygen supply to the fetus.

The symptoms of gestational hypertension can vary, but commonly include high blood pressure (**140/90** mmHg or higher), swelling in the hands, face, or legs, and proteinuria (the presence of excess protein in the urine). If left untreated, gestational hypertension can lead to complications such as preterm birth, low birth weight, and placental abruption.

To diagnose gestational hypertension, medical professionals monitor blood pressure levels and conduct urine tests to detect the presence of protein. Regular prenatal check-ups are essential for detecting any signs of hypertension and ensuring appropriate intervention.

The management of gestational hypertension focuses on monitoring blood pressure levels, assessing fetal well-being, and preventing the progression to preeclampsia. Lifestyle modifications, such as maintaining a healthy diet, engaging in regular physical activity, and minimizing stress, are typically recommended.

In some cases, medication may be prescribed to control blood pressure. However, it is essential to choose medications that are safe for both the mother and the fetus. Electronic Fetal Monitoring Specialists should collaborate with other healthcare providers to ensure the selected medications do not have adverse effects on fetal well-being.

Regular fetal monitoring is crucial for assessing the well-being of the fetus. This can be done through various methods such as non-stress tests, biophysical profiles, and Doppler ultrasound. These tests help evaluate fetal heart rate patterns, amniotic fluid levels, and blood flow through the umbilical cord.

Regular follow-up visits are essential to monitor blood pressure, assess organ function, and identify any signs of worsening hypertension or preeclampsia. In severe cases, where the health of the mother or the fetus is compromised, early delivery may be necessary to prevent further complications. It can have significant implications for both the mother and the fetus if left untreated or if it progresses to preeclampsia. Early identification, proper management, and regular monitoring are essential for ensuring optimal maternal and fetal outcomes. Electronic Fetal Monitoring Specialists play a critical role in the comprehensive care of women with gestational hypertension, collaborating with other healthcare providers to ensure the well-being of both the mother and the fetus.

3.5.2.2   Preeclampsia-eclampsia:

Preeclampsia-eclampsia is a condition that affects pregnant women and is characterized by high blood pressure and organ dysfunction. It is a significant cause of maternal and perinatal morbidity and mortality worldwide. This condition typically occurs after **20** weeks of gestation and is a leading cause of maternal complications during pregnancy.

Preeclampsia-eclampsia is a complex disorder that involves multiple systems in the body. It is believed to be caused by problems with the development of the placenta, which leads to a systemic inflammatory response and blood vessel dysfunction. The exact cause of this condition is still unknown, but there are several risk factors that increase a woman's chances of developing it, including a history of preeclampsia in previous pregnancies, hypertension prior to pregnancy, obesity, and certain medical conditions such as diabetes and kidney disease.

The symptoms of preeclampsia can vary from mild to severe and may include high blood pressure, protein in the urine, swelling of the hands and face, headaches, blurred vision, and abdominal pain. If left untreated, preeclampsia can progress to eclampsia, which is characterized by seizures or convulsions. Eclampsia is a life-threatening condition for both the mother and the unborn baby. Early detection and timely intervention are crucial in managing preeclampsia-eclampsia. Regular prenatal care and monitoring of blood pressure and urine protein levels are essential. Other diagnostic tests such as blood tests, ultrasound, and fetal monitoring may also be performed to assess the mother and baby's health.

Once preeclampsia-eclampsia is diagnosed, the primary goal of management is to prevent complications and ensure the well-being of both the mother and the baby. This typically involves closely monitoring blood pressure, urine protein levels, and fetal well-being. Medications may be prescribed to lower blood pressure and prevent seizures. Hospitalization may be necessary in severe cases to closely monitor the mother and provide specialized care.

In some cases, delivery may be the most appropriate course of action to resolve preeclampsia-eclampsia. This decision is made based on the severity of the condition, the gestational age of the baby, and the health of the mother. The timing and mode of delivery will be determined by the healthcare team, taking into consideration the risks and benefits for both the mother and the baby. After delivery, most women will see a resolution of their symptoms. However, it is important for women who have had preeclampsia-eclampsia to be aware of their increased risk for future cardiovascular diseases and to closely monitor their blood pressure and **overall** health. Early detection, regular prenatal care, and appropriate management are crucial in ensuring the best outcomes for both the mother and the baby. Close monitoring, medication, and potential delivery may be required to prevent complications and resolve the condition. Women who have had preeclampsia-eclampsia should continue to monitor their health after delivery due to increased risks for future cardiovascular diseases.

3.5.2.3   HELLP syndrome:

HELLP syndrome is a rare but serious complication that can occur during pregnancy. It is a variant of preeclampsia, a condition characterized by high blood pressure and damage to organs such as the liver and kidneys. The acronym HELLP stands for Hemolysis, Elevated Liver Enzymes, and Low Platelet count, which are the key features of this syndrome.

HELLP syndrome often occurs in the third trimester of pregnancy, but it can also develop earlier. Its exact cause is still unknown, but it is believed to be related to problems with the placenta. It is more common in women who have a history of preeclampsia, are older, have multiple pregnancies, or have a family history of the condition.

One of the first signs of HELLP syndrome is often right upper quadrant pain that is caused by liver swelling. Other symptoms can include headache, nausea, vomiting, and visual disturbances. In severe cases, symptoms can progress rapidly to include seizures, pulmonary edema, and kidney failure.

Diagnosing HELLP syndrome can be challenging because its symptoms are similar to other conditions. However, a combination of high blood pressure, abnormalities in liver function tests, low platelet count, and presence of hemolysis can indicate the presence of this syndrome. Further tests may also be done, such as a liver biopsy or ultrasound, to confirm the diagnosis and assess the severity of the condition.

Treatment for HELLP syndrome typically involves immediate delivery of the baby, regardless of gestational age. This is because the syndrome can worsen rapidly and pose serious risks to the mother and baby. In some cases, if the baby is not yet mature enough for delivery, medications may be given to help prolong the pregnancy while closely monitoring the mother's condition.

In severe cases, where the mother's health is at immediate risk, an emergency cesarean section may be performed. After delivery, the symptoms of HELLP syndrome usually resolve within a few days to weeks. However, close monitoring of the mother's blood pressure, organ function, and platelet count may be necessary.

While the exact cause of HELLP syndrome is unknown, there are some factors that may increase the risk of developing this condition. These include a history of preeclampsia or HELLP syndrome in a previous pregnancy, being overweight or obese, having a family history of the condition, being pregnant with multiples, and having certain underlying medical conditions such as chronic hypertension or autoimmune diseases.

Complications of HELLP syndrome can be serious and potentially life-threatening if not promptly treated. These can include liver rupture, liver hematoma, kidney failure, placental abruption, and disseminated intravascular coagulation. Therefore, it is crucial for pregnant women and healthcare providers to be aware of the signs and symptoms of HELLP syndrome and seek medical attention if necessary. Its symptoms can mimic other conditions, so a high index of suspicion is necessary for diagnosis. Immediate delivery of the baby is often the mainstay of treatment, with close monitoring of the mother's condition postpartum. Early recognition and intervention are crucial in improving outcomes for both the mother and baby.

3.5.2.4   Chronic (essential):

Chronic (essential) hypertension is a medical condition characterized by high blood pressure that persists over a long period of time. It is considered essential when there is no identifiable cause for the elevated blood pressure. This condition is often diagnosed in pregnant women and can lead to various maternal complications.

One important aspect of chronic (essential) hypertension is its prevalence in pregnant women. It is estimated that about 1 to 5% of pregnancies are affected by this condition. The exact cause of chronic (essential) hypertension is not fully understood, but various factors such as genetics, obesity, and certain lifestyle choices may contribute to its development.

When a pregnant woman has chronic (essential) hypertension, it can increase the risk of maternal complications. One of the common complications is preeclampsia, which is characterized by high blood pressure and damage to organs such as the liver and kidneys. Preeclampsia can be dangerous for both the mother and the baby, and it requires close monitoring and management.

Another important aspect of chronic (essential) hypertension is the management of the condition during pregnancy. Pregnant women with this condition often require regular check-ups to monitor their blood pressure and assess the well-being of the baby.

Medications may be prescribed to help control blood pressure, and lifestyle modifications such as a healthy diet and regular exercise may also be recommended.

It is crucial for an Electronic Fetal Monitoring Specialist to be aware of the potential complications associated with chronic (essential) hypertension in order to provide appropriate care and monitoring for pregnant women. They should have a thorough understanding of the signs and symptoms of preeclampsia, as well as the methods for managing and controlling blood pressure.

In addition, an Electronic Fetal Monitoring Specialist should be knowledgeable about the different patterns that may be observed on electronic fetal monitoring when a pregnant woman has chronic (essential) hypertension. They should be able to recognize abnormal patterns that may indicate fetal distress or compromise, and take appropriate interventions to ensure the well-being of the baby.

Furthermore, it is important for an Electronic Fetal Monitoring Specialist to work closely with other healthcare professionals, such as obstetricians and nurses, to ensure a comprehensive approach to the management of chronic (essential) hypertension. They should be able to communicate effectively and provide timely updates on the fetal heart rate and any changes in the monitoring patterns. It is essential for an Electronic Fetal Monitoring Specialist to have a thorough understanding of this **topic**, including the potential complications, management strategies, and patterns observed on electronic fetal monitoring. By being knowledgeable and vigilant, they can contribute to the effective care and monitoring of pregnant women with chronic (essential) hypertension, ultimately ensuring the health and well-being of both the mother and the baby.

3.5.3   Postdates Pregnancy:

Postdates pregnancy refers to a condition where a pregnancy extends beyond the expected due date, which is typically around **40** weeks gestation. It is also known as post-term or prolonged pregnancy. This condition may pose certain risks to both the mother and the baby, making it important to closely monitor and manage postdates pregnancies.

One of the major concerns with postdates pregnancy is the risk of fetal distress. As the pregnancy progresses beyond the due date, the placenta may begin to age and deteriorate, affecting its ability to adequately supply the baby with nutrients and oxygen. This can lead to a decrease in the baby's well-being, causing fetal distress. Therefore, regular fetal monitoring is crucial in identifying any signs of distress.

Electronic fetal monitoring (EFM) is an essential tool for monitoring postdates pregnancies. It involves the use of special sensors placed on the mother's abdomen to record the baby's heart rate and uterine contractions. By analyzing the patterns and variability of the fetal heart rate, healthcare professionals can assess the baby's well-being and detect any potential problems.

In addition to monitoring the fetal heart rate, other interventions may be employed to manage postdates pregnancies. One common intervention is induction of labor. This involves using medications or other methods to stimulate uterine contractions and initiate labor. Induction may be recommended when the risks of continuing the pregnancy outweigh the risks of inducing labor. It is important to carefully assess each individual case and make a decision based on the **overall** well-being of both the mother and the baby.

Another aspect to consider in postdates pregnancies is the potential for complications during labor and delivery. As the pregnancy progresses beyond the due date, the baby may grow larger in size, making vaginal delivery more challenging. This can increase the risk of shoulder dystocia, a condition where the baby's shoulder gets stuck behind the mother's pelvic bone during delivery. In such cases, a healthcare provider may consider interventions like cesarean section to ensure a safe delivery.

Closely monitoring fluid levels is another important aspect of managing postdates pregnancies. As the pregnancy advances, the amniotic fluid levels may gradually decrease. This can lead to complications such as cord compression, fetal distress, or meconium aspiration syndrome if the baby passes meconium (a dark green substance) due to stress. Regular ultrasounds and assessments of the amniotic fluid index can help healthcare providers identify any abnormalities and take appropriate actions.

Postdates pregnancy can be associated with an increased risk of stillbirth. However, the exact timing of when the risk significantly increases is still a **topic** of debate among healthcare professionals. Some guidelines recommend offering induction of labor at or beyond **41** weeks, while others suggest waiting until **42** weeks. Individual factors such as the mother's age, medical history, and **overall** well-being should be taken into consideration when making a decision regarding the timing for induction. It carries certain risks for both the mother and the baby, including fetal distress, complications during labor, and an increased risk of stillbirth. Close monitoring through electronic fetal monitoring, assessment of amniotic fluid levels, and consideration of interventions like induction of labor or cesarean section can help manage postdates pregnancies effectively and ensure the well-being of both mother and baby.

3.5.4   Diabetes:

Diabetes is a medical condition characterized by elevated levels of blood glucose, also known as blood sugar. It occurs when the body is unable to properly utilize or produce insulin, a hormone that helps regulate blood sugar levels.

Diabetes can be classified into two main types: type **1** and type **2**. Type **1** diabetes is an autoimmune disease where the immune system mistakenly attacks and destroys the insulin-producing cells in the pancreas. This results in little to no insulin production and requires daily insulin injections. Type **2** diabetes, on the other hand, is more common and generally develops later in life. It is characterized by insulin resistance, where the body's cells do not respond properly to insulin, combined with a relative insulin deficiency.

During pregnancy, women with diabetes are at an increased risk of developing complications, which can affect both the mother and the baby. These complications fall under the broader **topic** of maternal complications and necessitate pattern recognition and intervention by an electronic fetal monitoring specialist.

One of the main concerns for pregnant women with diabetes is the risk of gestational diabetes, which develops during pregnancy and usually resolves after delivery. Gestational diabetes can lead to high birth weight, premature birth, or the need for a cesarean section. Monitoring blood sugar levels is crucial in managing gestational diabetes and minimizing these risks.

Pre-existing diabetes, whether type **1** or type **2**, can also pose risks during pregnancy. Poorly controlled blood sugar levels can increase the chances of birth defects, miscarriage, preeclampsia, and complications during childbirth. It is essential for women with pre-existing diabetes to closely monitor their blood glucose levels and work closely with their healthcare team to maintain optimal control.

Gestational diabetes and pre-existing diabetes can also affect the baby's health. Babies born to mothers with diabetes may have a higher risk of jaundice, respiratory distress syndrome, low blood sugar levels, and an increased likelihood of developing type 2 diabetes later in life.

To ensure the well-being of both the mother and the baby, electronic fetal monitoring plays a critical role. This monitoring involves the use of specialized devices to track the baby's heart rate and the mother's contractions. It allows healthcare providers to assess the baby's condition and make informed decisions about any necessary interventions.

During labor, electronic fetal monitoring helps detect any signs of distress or abnormal patterns in the baby's heart rate. This information helps guide interventions, such as changing the mother's position, administering oxygen, or even performing an emergency cesarean section if needed. Maternal complications associated with diabetes call for the **expert**ise of an electronic fetal monitoring specialist to recognize patterns, monitor the baby's well-being, and intervene when necessary. By closely monitoring blood sugar levels and employing electronic fetal monitoring techniques, healthcare providers can provide optimal care and improve outcomes for pregnant women with diabetes.

3.5.4.1   (Gestational, Type 1, Type 2):

Gestational diabetes, Type 1 diabetes, and Type 2 diabetes are three different types of diabetes that can occur during pregnancy. Each type has its own unique characteristics and management strategies. Understanding these types is important for an Electronic Fetal Monitoring Specialist to provide appropriate care and support to pregnant women with diabetes.

Gestational diabetes is a type of diabetes that develops during pregnancy and usually resolves after childbirth. It occurs when the body cannot produce enough insulin to meet the increased demands of pregnancy. This leads to high blood sugar levels, which can pose risks to both the mother and the baby. Gestational diabetes is typically diagnosed through glucose tolerance tests and is managed through lifestyle changes such as healthy eating, regular physical activity, and monitoring blood sugar levels. In some cases, insulin therapy may be necessary to control blood sugar levels.

Type 1 diabetes is an autoimmune disease in which the immune system attacks the pancreas, leading to little or no production of insulin. This type of diabetes is usually diagnosed in childhood or early adulthood but can occur during pregnancy as well. Women with Type 1 diabetes have a higher risk of complications during pregnancy, including preeclampsia, preterm birth, and birth defects. Managing Type 1 diabetes during pregnancy involves close monitoring of blood sugar levels, insulin therapy, and regular check-ups with healthcare providers specializing in diabetes management.

Type 2 diabetes is a metabolic disorder characterized by insulin resistance, meaning the body does not respond effectively to insulin. It is often associated with lifestyle factors such as obesity and lack of physical activity. Type 2 diabetes can be present before pregnancy or can develop during pregnancy, similar to gestational diabetes. Women with Type 2 diabetes have an increased risk of complications during pregnancy, including high blood pressure, cesarean delivery, and gestational hypertension. Management of Type 2 diabetes during pregnancy involves lifestyle modifications, such as healthy eating and regular exercise, as well as medications like metformin or insulin therapy if necessary.

Distinguishing between these three types of diabetes is crucial as each type requires different management approaches. For an Electronic Fetal Monitoring Specialist, being aware of these distinctions allows for tailored care and monitoring, ensuring the well-being of both the mother and the baby. Close monitoring of the mother's blood sugar levels through regular testing and assessment is essential to identify any risks or complications. Additionally, healthcare providers may collaborate to provide comprehensive care, including obstetricians, endocrinologists, and diabetes educators, to optimize outcomes for women with diabetes during pregnancy.

Identifying the type of diabetes a pregnant woman has is important for providing appropriate care and support throughout her pregnancy journey. Through close monitoring and a multidisciplinary approach, an Electronic Fetal Monitoring Specialist can contribute to the **overall** health and well-being of both the mother and the baby.

3.5.5   Multiple gestations:

Multiple gestations refer to pregnancies in which there are two or more fetuses. It is a unique situation that presents certain challenges and considerations for both the mother and the healthcare team involved. This **topic** falls under the broad **topic** of maternal complications and specifically pertains to pattern recognition and intervention in the context of electronic fetal monitoring.

One important aspect to consider in multiple gestations is the increased risk of complications compared to singleton pregnancies. The mother may experience a higher likelihood of developing gestational diabetes, hypertension, and preeclampsia. Additionally, there is an increased risk of preterm labor, placenta previa, and cesarean delivery. These potential complications necessitate vigilant monitoring and timely interventions.

Electronic fetal monitoring plays a vital role in the management of multiple gestations. It allows healthcare providers to assess the fetal heart rate patterns and uterine contractions to ensure the well-being of each fetus. The main objective is to identify any signs of fetal distress or oxygen deprivation. This information helps guide clinical decisions and interventions to optimize outcomes.

One important consideration in electronic fetal monitoring is the ability to differentiate between the heart rates of the multiple fetuses. This can be achieved by placing separate sensors or transducers on each fetus to accurately monitor their individual heart patterns. This allows for early detection of any deviations or abnormalities, enabling prompt intervention.

Another aspect to consider is the uterine activity monitoring. Multiple gestations often have a higher likelihood of experiencing excessive uterine contractions, which can put both the mother and the fetuses at risk. Electronic monitoring helps assess the frequency, duration, and intensity of contractions, enabling the healthcare team to intervene if necessary.

In cases where one fetus shows signs of distress or compromise, interventions may be required to optimize the conditions for all fetuses. This may involve repositioning the mother, increasing intravenous fluids, or administering medications to suppress uterine activity. These interventions aim to safeguard the well-being of all fetuses and prevent potential adverse outcomes.

Close monitoring of the cervical length is also crucial in multiple gestations. The cervix plays a vital role in maintaining a healthy pregnancy and preventing preterm birth. Serial ultrasounds can assess the cervical length over time and detect any shortening or changes that may increase the risk of preterm labor. Early recognition of cervical changes allows for interventions such as cerclage placement or progesterone supplementation to prevent or delay preterm birth.

Regular antenatal visits and consultations with a multidisciplinary team are essential in managing multiple gestations. This team may include obstetricians, perinatologists, fetal medicine specialists, neonatologists, and nurses experienced in caring for multiple pregnancies. Collaborative decision-making and a proactive approach to monitoring and intervention contribute to the best possible outcomes for both the mother and the fetuses. Electronic fetal monitoring plays a central role in pattern recognition and intervention, allowing healthcare providers to identify fetal distress, monitor uterine activity, and make timely decisions to optimize outcomes. Regular assessments, close surveillance, and a multidisciplinary approach form the foundation of successful management in multiple gestations.

3.5.6   Infections:

Infections can pose significant complications during pregnancy and childbirth, which fall under the broader **topic** of "Maternal Complications, Pattern Recognition, and Intervention" in the field of electronic fetal monitoring. Understanding and effectively managing infections is crucial for an Electronic Fetal Monitoring Specialist.

Infections during pregnancy can be of various types, including urinary tract infections (UTIs), sexually transmitted infections (STIs), bacterial vaginosis, and intra-amniotic infections. These infections can lead to adverse effects on both the mother and the developing fetus if not promptly diagnosed and treated.

Urinary tract infections, for instance, are common during pregnancy due to hormonal changes and increased pressure on the bladder. These infections can cause significant discomfort for the mother and may lead to complications such as kidney infections if left untreated. Therefore, it is essential for Electronic Fetal Monitoring Specialists to recognize the symptoms of UTIs, including frequent urination, pain or burning during urination, and lower abdominal pain, and intervene by referring the mother for appropriate medical treatment.

Sexually transmitted infections, such as chlamydia, gonorrhea, herpes, and syphilis, can be transmitted from mother to baby during childbirth. These infections can have serious consequences, including premature rupture of membranes, preterm birth, low birth weight, and even congenital infections in the newborn. Recognizing the risk factors and ensuring proper screening and treatment are crucial in minimizing the impact on both the mother and the baby.

Bacterial vaginosis is another common infection during pregnancy, characterized by an imbalance in the vaginal bacteria. While it may not always cause noticeable symptoms, it has been associated with an increased risk of preterm birth and other complications. Electronic Fetal Monitoring Specialists should be aware of the potential impact of bacterial vaginosis and collaborate with healthcare providers to ensure appropriate testing, diagnosis, and treatment.

Intra-amniotic infections, also known as chorioamnionitis, occur when bacteria enter the uterus and infect the amniotic fluid and fetal membranes. These infections can arise before or during labor and may lead to serious maternal and neonatal complications if not promptly addressed. Signs of intra-amniotic infections may include fever, increased heart rate in the mother or the baby, uterine tenderness, and foul-smelling amniotic fluid. Timely recognition and immediate medical intervention, including antibiotics, may be necessary to minimize the risks associated with these infections.

Electronic Fetal Monitoring Specialists should also be familiar with preventive measures to reduce the risk of infections during pregnancy. Promoting good hygiene practices, encouraging regular prenatal care visits, and advocating safe sexual practices can significantly reduce the likelihood of infections and their potential complications. Electronic Fetal Monitoring Specialists play a vital role in recognizing the signs and symptoms of infections, collaborating with healthcare providers for timely diagnosis and treatment, and advocating preventive measures. By ensuring effective pattern recognition and intervention, these specialists contribute to improving maternal and neonatal outcomes.

3.5.7   Maternal obesity:

Maternal obesity is a significant concern in the field of maternal complications and pattern recognition. It refers to the condition where a pregnant woman has a body mass index (BMI) of **30** or higher. This issue has gained attention due to its potential impact on both the mother and the unborn child.

One of the key aspects to consider in understanding maternal obesity is its prevalence. The rates of obesity worldwide have been rising steadily over the past few decades, and this trend is reflected in pregnant women as well. The National Institute for Health and Care Excellence (NICE) in the UK reports that around **20**% of pregnant women in the country are obese.

Maternal obesity is associated with various complications during pregnancy and childbirth. Firstly, obese pregnant women are at a higher risk of developing gestational diabetes, a condition where blood sugar levels become elevated during pregnancy. This not only poses risks to the mother's health but also increases the chances of the baby experiencing certain birth defects.

Additionally, maternal obesity increases the probability of high blood pressure and preeclampsia, a condition characterized by high blood pressure and damage to organs such as the liver and kidneys. Preeclampsia can have serious consequences for both the mother and the baby, potentially leading to preterm birth or even stillbirth.

Obese pregnant women may also face difficulties during labor and delivery. Due to their excess weight, they are more likely to require interventions such as induced labor, assisted delivery, or cesarean section. These interventions carry their own set of risks and may contribute to longer recovery times for the mother.

Furthermore, maternal obesity has long-term consequences for the child's health. Offspring of obese mothers are at a higher risk of developing obesity, type **2** diabetes, and cardiovascular diseases later in life. This highlights the importance of addressing maternal obesity not only during pregnancy but also in promoting future health outcomes for the child.

Intervention strategies play a crucial role in managing maternal obesity. Healthcare professionals should prioritize early identification of obese pregnant women and provide tailored support and education. This may involve dietary counseling, exercise recommendations, and monitoring of weight gain throughout pregnancy. Collaborative care involving obstetricians, nutritionists, and midwives can help optimize the management of maternal obesity.

It is crucial to raise awareness among pregnant women about the potential risks associated with obesity and provide them with resources to adopt a healthier lifestyle. Encouraging regular prenatal healthcare visits and offering support groups for pregnant women struggling with obesity can enhance their **overall** experience and improve outcomes. Its prevalence and associated complications necessitate attention and intervention strategies. By addressing maternal obesity through effective prenatal care, healthcare professionals can mitigate risks and promote healthier outcomes for both mothers and babies.

3.6   Uteroplacental complications:

Uteroplacental complications refer to a wide range of conditions that affect the placenta and its functioning during pregnancy. The placenta plays a vital role in providing oxygen and nutrients to the developing fetus, and any abnormalities or disruptions in its function can have significant implications for both the mother and the baby.

One of the most common uteroplacental complications is placenta previa, where the placenta partially or completely covers the cervix. This condition can cause bleeding during pregnancy, especially in the third trimester, and may necessitate medical interventions such as bed rest or cesarean delivery.

Another condition is placental abruption, where the placenta separates from the uterine wall before delivery. This can lead to severe bleeding, blood clot formation, and compromise the baby's oxygen and nutrient supply. Placental abruption requires immediate medical attention and may necessitate emergency delivery.

Uterine rupture is a rare but serious complication where the uterine wall tears, often along a previous cesarean scar. This can result in heavy bleeding, fetal distress, and requires immediate surgical intervention to prevent maternal and fetal complications.

Gestational hypertension and preeclampsia are also uteroplacental complications that can develop after **20** weeks of pregnancy. These conditions are characterized by high blood pressure, protein in the urine, and other organ dysfunction. They can affect the placental blood flow and lead to inadequate oxygen and nutrient supply to the fetus. Close monitoring, medication, and early delivery may be necessary to manage these conditions.

Intrauterine growth restriction (IUGR) is another uteroplacental complication where the baby fails to reach its expected growth potential. This can occur due to various factors, such as reduced blood flow through the placenta, genetic abnormalities, or maternal health conditions. Regular ultrasound scans and monitoring of the baby's growth are essential to detect IUGR and manage it appropriately.

Placenta accreta, increta, and percreta are conditions where the placenta adheres too deeply to the uterine wall, potentially invading nearby organs. These complications pose risks of severe bleeding, infection, and organ damage. They often require specialized care and a planned delivery approach to minimize complications.

In some cases, the placenta may develop cysts or tumors, such as placental chorioangioma or hydatidiform mole, respectively. These conditions can lead to abnormal placental functioning and can have adverse effects on the developing fetus. Appropriate monitoring, ultrasound evaluations, and, in some cases, medical or surgical interventions may be required.

To diagnose and manage uteroplacental complications, obstetricians rely on various tools and tests. Electronic fetal monitoring is one such tool, which involves continuously tracking the baby's heart rate and the mother's contractions during labor. This helps identify any signs of distress or compromise in the baby's oxygen and nutrient supply. These complications can have significant implications for both the mother and the baby and may require close monitoring, interventions, and, in some cases, early delivery to ensure optimal outcomes. It is essential for electronic fetal monitoring specialists to be knowledgeable about these complications to provide appropriate care and interventions during pregnancy and labor.

3.6.1   (previa, abruption):

Uteroplacental complications, specifically placenta previa and placental abruption, are important **topic**s that Electronic Fetal Monitoring Specialists need to understand. Placenta previa occurs when the placenta partially or completely covers the cervix, while placental abruption is the premature separation of the placenta from the uterus.

Placenta previa can be categorized into three types: complete, partial, and marginal. In complete previa, the cervix is entirely covered by the placenta, while in partial previa, only a portion of the cervix is covered. Marginal previa, on the other hand, occurs when the placenta is located near the cervix but does not cover it completely. This condition can cause painless vaginal bleeding during the second or third trimester. It is important for Electronic Fetal Monitoring Specialists to be aware of this as bleeding can affect fetal well-being and require intervention.

Placental abruption, on the other hand, occurs when the placenta detaches from the uterine wall before delivery. This can cause heavy bleeding and severe abdominal pain. There are two types of abruption: overt and concealed. Overt abruption is characterized by external bleeding, while concealed abruption occurs when the blood is trapped between the placenta and the uterine wall, leading to internal bleeding. Electronic Fetal Monitoring Specialists should be aware that this condition can result in fetal distress and potentially lead to fetal death if not recognized and managed promptly.

To recognize and intervene in cases of uteroplacental complications like previa and abruption, Electronic Fetal Monitoring Specialists should be familiar with the signs and symptoms. In placenta previa, bleeding is the primary symptom, but some patients may also experience painless contractions or an unusual fetal heart rate pattern. Placental abruption, on the other hand, is characterized by vaginal bleeding, abdominal pain, and changes in the fetal heart rate pattern.

Electronic Fetal Monitoring Specialists should closely monitor the fetal heart rate patterns to detect any abnormalities that may indicate uteroplacental complications. An abnormal heart rate pattern may include persistent late or variable decelerations, decreased variability, or sinusoidal pattern. Recognition of these patterns is crucial for the well-being of the fetus, and intervention may include immediate delivery via cesarean section or other medical interventions depending on the severity of the situation. Placenta previa can result in painless vaginal bleeding, while placental abruption can lead to heavy bleeding and severe abdominal pain. Monitoring fetal heart rate patterns, recognizing signs and symptoms, and intervening promptly are crucial in ensuring the well-being of both the mother and fetus.

3.6.2   Uterine rupture/scar dehiscence:

Uterine rupture and scar dehiscence are uteroplacental complications that can occur during pregnancy and childbirth. These conditions involve the separation or tearing of the uterus, which can be life-threatening for both the mother and the baby. Recognizing the signs and symptoms of uterine rupture and scar dehiscence is crucial for timely intervention and optimal outcomes.

Uterine rupture refers to a complete tear or separation of the uterine wall, often in a previous C-section scar. Scar dehiscence, on the other hand, is a partial separation of the uterine wall, typically in a previous uterine surgery scar. Both conditions pose significant risks, but uterine rupture is considered more severe and can lead to extensive bleeding, injury to nearby organs, and fetal distress. The most common cause of uterine rupture is a prior C-section, particularly in cases where a vertical incision was made on the uterus. Other risk factors include previous uterine surgery, such as a myomectomy or removal of fibroids, multiple previous C-sections, prior uterine rupture, or use of high-dose oxytocin during labor. Scar dehiscence, on the other hand, is more commonly associated with prior lower-segment uterine surgeries.

The symptoms of uterine rupture and scar dehiscence can vary, but some common signs include severe abdominal pain, abnormal fetal heart rate patterns, cessation of contractions, vaginal bleeding, and a palpable bulge or mass in the abdomen. In cases of complete uterine rupture, the baby may be pushed into the abdominal cavity, causing a distinctive "ballottement" sensation on palpation.

Early recognition and prompt intervention are crucial in managing these complications. Electronic fetal monitoring (EFM) plays a vital role in detecting abnormal fetal heart rate patterns, which can be an early sign of uterine rupture or scar dehiscence. Close monitoring of the mother's vital signs, such as blood pressure and heart rate, is also essential.

If uterine rupture or scar dehiscence is suspected, an emergency cesarean section is usually the recommended course of action. This intervention allows for immediate access to the uterus, control of bleeding, and delivery of the baby. In some cases, a hysterectomy may be necessary to prevent further complications and ensure the mother's well-being.

Prevention of uterine rupture and scar dehiscence involves careful consideration of the risks associated with previous uterine surgeries. Healthcare providers should thoroughly evaluate the uterine scar and assess the potential for complications during subsequent pregnancies. In some cases, a vaginal birth after cesarean (VBAC) may be considered, but it carries its own set of risks and should be carefully discussed with the patient. EFM is a valuable tool in monitoring fetal well-being and detecting early signs of these conditions. Timely surgical intervention, such as an emergency cesarean section, is crucial for ensuring the safety of both the mother and the baby. Healthcare providers play a vital role in preventing these complications by carefully assessing previous uterine surgeries and discussing the risks and benefits of different delivery options with their patients.

3.7   Fetal complications:

Fetal complications are a significant concern in obstetrics, and early recognition and intervention play a crucial role in ensuring the well-being of the fetus. These complications can arise due to various factors and can have significant implications for both the mother and the baby.

One of the most common fetal complications is fetal distress, which refers to any abnormality in the baby's heart rate during labor. This can be caused by factors such as insufficient oxygen supply, placental abnormalities, or umbilical cord compression. Electronic fetal monitoring (EFM) is often used to detect fetal distress by continuously monitoring the baby's heart rate and uterine contractions.

In cases of fetal distress, prompt intervention is necessary to prevent further complications. This may involve changing the mother's position, administering oxygen to the mother, stopping certain medications that may be affecting the baby's heart rate, or even performing an emergency cesarean section if the condition worsens.

Another fetal complication that can arise is intrauterine growth restriction (IUGR). This condition occurs when the baby does not grow at the expected rate inside the womb. It can be caused by maternal factors such as high blood pressure, chronic illnesses, or poor nutrition, as well as fetal factors such as chromosomal abnormalities or placental problems. EFM can help identify signs of IUGR by monitoring the baby's growth trajectory and detecting abnormal changes in the baby's heart rate patterns.

When IUGR is diagnosed, close monitoring and intervention are necessary to prevent further complications. Depending on the severity of IUGR, interventions may include more frequent ultrasounds to assess the baby's growth, Doppler studies to evaluate blood flow to the placenta, or early delivery if the fetus is at risk of further growth restriction.

Placental abruption is another fetal complication that can have serious consequences. This occurs when the placenta detaches from the uterine wall before delivery, leading to decreased blood supply to the baby. Placental abruption can be caused by trauma, high blood pressure, or certain medical conditions, and it is characterized by symptoms such as vaginal bleeding, abdominal pain, and changes in the baby's heart rate. EFM can help detect these changes and alert healthcare providers to the possibility of placental abruption.

When placental abruption is suspected, immediate intervention is necessary to prevent fetal harm. This may involve close monitoring of the mother and baby, administration of intravenous fluids, blood transfusions if necessary, and, in severe cases, emergency delivery to save the baby's life.

Other fetal complications that may require recognition and intervention include umbilical cord prolapse, meconium-stained amniotic fluid, and fetal anomalies. Each of these conditions requires careful monitoring and timely intervention to ensure the best possible outcome for the baby. EFM serves as a valuable tool in identifying fetal distress, intrauterine growth restriction, placental abruption, and other complications, allowing healthcare providers to intervene promptly and appropriately. By understanding the importance of early recognition and intervention, electronic fetal monitoring specialists play a vital role in ensuring the optimal care of pregnant women and their babies.

3.7.1   Injury:

Injury is a significant concern when it comes to fetal complications and pattern recognition during electronic fetal monitoring. It is crucial for an Electronic Fetal Monitoring Specialist to be aware of the various types of fetal injuries that can occur during pregnancy and childbirth. Understanding these injuries can help the specialist interpret the monitoring data accurately and make quick interventions when needed.

One type of fetal injury that can occur is head molding, which happens when pressure is applied to the fetal skull during labor and delivery. This can result in an elongated or distorted head shape. Another common injury is caput succedaneum, which is the swelling of the scalp due to pressure from the birth canal. Both of these injuries usually resolve on their own within a few days or weeks.

More severe types of fetal injuries include skull fractures and intracranial hemorrhages. These injuries can be caused by prolonged or difficult labor, the improper use of delivery instruments, or trauma during birth. Skull fractures can lead to long-term complications such as brain damage or neurological disorders. Intracranial hemorrhages, on the other hand, occur when blood vessels in the baby's brain rupture, leading to potentially serious consequences.

Another type of injury that an Electronic Fetal Monitoring Specialist should be aware of is brachial plexus injury. This occurs when the nerves that control the movement of the baby's arms and hands are stretched or damaged during delivery. It is most commonly associated with shoulder dystocia, a condition where the baby's shoulder becomes stuck behind the mother's pubic bone. Brachial plexus injuries can result in weakness or paralysis of the affected arm.

In addition to these specific injuries, there are general complications that can arise from fetal distress. These may include oxygen deprivation, which can lead to brain damage or even death if not promptly addressed. Hypoxia is a term used to describe low oxygen levels in the baby's blood, which can occur during labor or delivery. An Electronic Fetal Monitoring Specialist must closely monitor the fetal heart rate patterns to detect signs of distress and intervene accordingly.

When it comes to pattern recognition and intervention, an Electronic Fetal Monitoring Specialist should be proficient in interpreting the fetal heart rate tracings. They should be able to identify patterns that indicate fetal distress, such as decelerations or abnormal baseline rates. Timely intervention could involve repositioning the mother, administering oxygen, or deciding on an emergency delivery, such as a cesarean section.

Furthermore, the specialist should be knowledgeable about the appropriate use and limitations of interventions such as fetal scalp sampling or umbilical artery blood sampling. These procedures can provide valuable information about the baby's well-being but should be performed with caution.

Overall, injury is a significant aspect of fetal complications, pattern recognition, and intervention. An Electronic Fetal Monitoring Specialist plays a crucial role in monitoring the fetus during labor and delivery, being vigilant for signs of injury or distress. With a deep understanding of the different types of injuries and complications that can occur, along with the ability to interpret monitoring data accurately, the specialist can make informed decisions to optimize the health and safety of both mother and baby.

3.7.2   Cord compression:

Cord compression is a term used to describe a condition in which the umbilical cord of a fetus is compressed, leading to potential complications and risks during pregnancy and childbirth. It is an important aspect to consider in the field of fetal monitoring and intervention.

Cord compression can occur due to various reasons. One common cause is when the fetus moves or changes position, resulting in the cord getting entangled or compressed between the baby's body and the walls of the uterus. Another cause can be the presence of excessive amniotic fluid, which can create loops or knots in the cord, leading to compression.

There are certain signs and symptoms that can indicate cord compression. These include changes in the fetal heart rate pattern, such as decelerations or a decrease in variability. Other signs may include reduced fetal movement, meconium-stained amniotic fluid (indicating fetal distress), and changes in the mother's blood pressure or heart rate.

Electronic fetal monitoring is a crucial tool in identifying cord compression. It involves the use of sensors placed on the mother's abdomen to monitor the fetal heart rate and uterine contractions. The monitoring can be done externally or internally, depending on the situation. By observing the patterns on the monitor, healthcare professionals, especially Electronic Fetal Monitoring Specialists, can detect any abnormalities, including cord compression.

When cord compression is suspected, prompt intervention is necessary to mitigate potential risks. The first step is often repositioning the mother to relieve the pressure on the cord. Changing the mother's position can alleviate the compression and improve blood flow to the fetus. In some cases, if the compression persists, an amnioinfusion may be performed. This involves the introduction of sterile fluid into the uterus to relieve the pressure on the cord.

In more severe cases, where the baby's well-being is compromised, an emergency cesarean section may be required. This is particularly necessary if fetal distress is evident, and there is a significant risk to the health and safety of both the mother and the baby.

Prevention of cord compression is not always possible, as it can occur spontaneously. However, measures can be taken to minimize the risk. Regular monitoring during pregnancy can help detect any potential problems early on. Additionally, maintaining optimal amniotic fluid levels and encouraging fetal movement through activities like regular exercise may help reduce the chances of cord compression. Electronic fetal monitoring plays a crucial role in recognizing patterns indicative of cord compression. Early intervention and appropriate management are essential to ensure the well-being of both the mother and the fetus. By understanding the causes, symptoms, and interventions related to cord compression, Electronic Fetal Monitoring Specialists can provide the necessary care and support to ensure safe outcomes for both mother and baby.

3.7.3   Hypoxemia:

Hypoxemia is a condition characterized by low levels of oxygen in the blood. It is one of the fetal complications that can occur during pregnancy, labor, or delivery. Understanding hypoxemia is crucial for electronic fetal monitoring specialists as they play a significant role in recognizing and intervening to ensure the well-being of the fetus.

During fetal development, the placenta provides oxygen and nutrients to the fetus through the umbilical cord. However, various factors can lead to a decreased oxygen supply to the fetus, resulting in hypoxemia. These factors may include a compromised placenta, reduced blood flow to the placenta, or issues with the umbilical cord.

Electronic fetal monitoring (EFM) is a tool used by specialists to assess the fetal heart rate (FHR) and uterine contractions during labor. It helps in the early detection of fetal distress, including hypoxemia. EFM can be done externally, using a device placed on the mother's abdomen, or internally, with a probe inserted into the uterus.

When monitoring the FHR, specialists look for specific patterns that may indicate the presence of hypoxemia. Variations in the baseline heart rate, decelerations, or prolonged bradycardia can be signs of fetal distress. Prompt recognition of these patterns is essential to intervene and prevent further complications.

Interventions to address hypoxemia include providing supplemental oxygen to the mother, changing the mother's position, or increasing intravenous fluid administration. These interventions aim to improve oxygen delivery to the fetus and alleviate the hypoxemic state. In some cases, delivery may be expedited through cesarean section if the fetus's well-being is severely compromised.

During labor, intermittent auscultation is also crucial. This involves listening to the fetal heart rate at regular intervals using a handheld Doppler or stethoscope. Intermittent auscultation can help detect changes in the FHR and guide interventions if necessary.

In addition to EFM and intermittent auscultation, electronic fetal monitors can also provide valuable information through other parameters. For example, the analysis of fetal pulse oximetry can provide insight into the fetal oxygen saturation levels directly. This can be an important tool in the assessment and management of hypoxemia.

While being aware of the signs and interventions for hypoxemia is essential, it is equally important for electronic fetal monitoring specialists to consider the limitations of these monitoring techniques. False positive or false-negative results can occur, highlighting the need for clinical judgment and experience in interpreting the collected data. Electronic fetal monitoring specialists play a vital role in recognizing and intervening in cases of hypoxemia for the well-being of the fetus. Through EFM, intermittent auscultation, and other parameters, they can detect patterns indicating fetal distress and promptly initiate interventions to improve oxygen delivery to the fetus. Understanding the various aspects of hypoxemia and its management is crucial for the effective practice of an electronic fetal monitoring specialist.

3.7.4   Demise:

Demise refers to the unfortunate event of the death of a fetus in the womb. It is a devastating outcome that can occur during pregnancy and has various causes and implications. Understanding the reasons behind fetal demise is crucial for Electronic Fetal Monitoring Specialists in order to identify patterns, recognize warning signs, and intervene appropriately.

One of the primary causes of fetal demise is placental insufficiency, where there is an inadequate supply of oxygen and nutrients to the fetus. This can happen due to conditions such as preeclampsia, gestational diabetes, or problems with the placenta itself. It is essential for specialists to monitor the fetal heart rate continuously to detect any signs of distress or abnormalities.

Another significant cause of fetal demise is congenital anomalies or birth defects. These may be structural abnormalities or genetic disorders that affect the development of the fetus. Detecting such anomalies early on through ultrasound or genetic testing can help specialists in making informed decisions regarding management and intervention.

Infections during pregnancy can also lead to fetal demise. Intrauterine infections, such as toxoplasmosis, rubella, or cytomegalovirus, can severely affect the health of the fetus. Electronic Fetal Monitoring Specialists should be vigilant in monitoring for any signs of infection and take appropriate measures to prevent adverse outcomes.

Poor maternal health, such as chronic hypertension or substance abuse, can contribute to fetal demise. These conditions can compromise the well-being of the fetus and increase the risk of complications. Close monitoring of maternal vital signs and laboratory investigations can provide valuable information for intervention strategies.

In some cases, fetal demise may occur without any apparent cause. This is known as unexplained fetal demise or sudden fetal death syndrome. It is a challenging and distressing situation both for the parents and healthcare providers. Investigation and analysis of medical records, along with counseling and emotional support, are essential aspects of managing such cases.

To prevent or reduce the risk of fetal demise, Electronic Fetal Monitoring Specialists play a vital role in recognizing abnormal patterns in fetal heart rate tracings. Decelerations, bradycardia, tachycardia, or prolonged decelerations may indicate fetal distress and require immediate intervention. Communication with the healthcare team and prompt decision-making are crucial in such situations.

When a fetal demise occurs, it is important for the Electronic Fetal Monitoring Specialist to provide compassionate care to the parents and offer support throughout the grieving process. This includes explaining the possible causes, answering questions, and discussing future reproductive options. By recognizing patterns, intervening promptly, and providing emotional support, these specialists can significantly contribute to improving outcomes and minimizing the occurrence of such tragic events.

3.8   Fetal heart rate accelerations:

Fetal heart rate accelerations are a crucial aspect of electronic fetal monitoring. This **topic** falls under the broad scope of pattern recognition and intervention. Fetal heart rate accelerations refer to temporary increases in the fetal heart rate, which are considered to be a positive sign of fetal well-being. Understanding the various aspects of fetal heart rate accelerations is vital for an electronic fetal monitoring specialist.

One important aspect of fetal heart rate accelerations is their significance in determining fetal well-being. When a fetus experiences an acceleration, this indicates that the oxygen supply to the fetus is adequate, and the fetal central nervous system is functioning properly. These accelerations are often associated with fetal movements, indicating a healthy and responsive fetus.

Fetal heart rate accelerations can be further categorized based on their duration and magnitude. Short-term accelerations last for less than **30** seconds, while long-term accelerations persist for more than **30** seconds. The magnitude of accelerations is defined by an increase in the fetal heart rate above the baseline rate. Accelerations of at least **15** beats per minute and lasting for at least **15** seconds are considered significant.

Furthermore, the timing of fetal heart rate accelerations provides valuable information. Early accelerations occur in response to fetal movements and are generally a positive sign. Late accelerations, on the other hand, occur after a contraction and may indicate fetal distress. Variability in the timing and characteristics of accelerations can help the electronic fetal monitoring specialist identify the **overall** fetal well-being or any potential complications.

In addition to analyzing accelerations in isolation, it is essential to consider their presence in conjunction with other fetal heart rate patterns. For example, accelerations along with a reassuring baseline heart rate and normal variability are considered a reassuring pattern. Conversely, accelerations in the presence of decelerations or reduced variability may warrant further evaluation and possibly intervention.

As an electronic fetal monitoring specialist, it is crucial to accurately recognize and interpret fetal heart rate accelerations. The specialist must possess a thorough understanding of the different patterns, their significance, and their implications for fetal well-being. This knowledge enables the specialist to make informed clinical decisions and intervene appropriately if necessary. Interventions may vary depending on the clinical context and the specific patterns observed. If accelerations are absent or minimal, interventions may include repositioning the mother, administering IV fluids, or providing supplemental oxygen to enhance fetal oxygenation. If accelerations are present but accompanied by concerning features, further assessment, such as fetal scalp sampling or fetal blood sampling, may be required to evaluate the fetal condition more comprehensively. They provide valuable information about fetal well-being and can indicate the proper functioning of the fetal central nervous system. A comprehensive understanding of the duration, magnitude, timing, and associated patterns of accelerations is crucial for an electronic fetal monitoring specialist. By accurately recognizing and interpreting accelerations, the specialist can make informed decisions and intervene promptly if necessary to ensure the best possible outcomes for both the mother and the fetus.

3.8.1 Early:

Early decelerations refer to a pattern of fetal heart rate changes that occur during labor. These decelerations are typically symmetrical and mirror the contractions of the uterus. They are considered a normal response to the physiological stress of labor and are usually not associated with any adverse fetal outcomes.

Early decelerations occur as a result of vagal stimulation caused by the pressure applied to the fetal head during contractions. This pressure activates the vagus nerve, leading to a decrease in fetal heart rate. However, since the decelerations mirror the contractions, they are usually benign and do not pose a significant risk to the fetus.

In terms of appearance, early decelerations have a gradual onset, reaching their nadir around the same time as the peak of the contracting uterus. The heart rate then returns to baseline as the contraction resolves. The shape of the deceleration is often described as a mirror image of the contraction, with a similar duration and amplitude.

One important aspect to note about early decelerations is that they are a sign of fetal well-being, indicating a healthy response to labor. They are commonly associated with term gestation and are rarely seen in preterm pregnancies.

The main concern when reviewing early decelerations is to differentiate them from other types of decelerations that may indicate fetal distress. One way to make this distinction is by examining the timing of the decelerations in relation to the contractions. Early decelerations occur simultaneously with contractions, while late or variable decelerations are typically offset in their timing.

It's essential for an electronic fetal monitoring specialist to recognize early decelerations accurately as this will guide the appropriate management and intervention. Since early decelerations are benign and indicate fetal well-being, they do not require any specific intervention. However, continuous monitoring and ongoing assessment of the fetal heart rate pattern are necessary to ensure the well-being of the fetus throughout labor. They are typically symmetrical and mirror the contractions of the uterus. Early decelerations have a gradual onset, reaching their nadir around the same time as the peak of the contraction. They do not pose a significant risk to the fetus, and no specific intervention is required. However, continuous monitoring and assessment are necessary to ensure the ongoing well-being of the fetus. It's crucial for an electronic fetal monitoring specialist to differentiate early decelerations from other types of decelerations to guide appropriate clinical management.

3.8.2 Variable:

Variable decelerations are an essential aspect of fetal heart rate monitoring. These decelerations represent a decrease in the fetal heart rate that is not related to contractions. They are known as "variable" decelerations because they can occur at any time during the labor process.

Variable decelerations can be caused by a variety of factors, including compression of the umbilical cord or a decrease in blood flow to the fetus. When the umbilical cord is compressed, it reduces the flow of oxygen and nutrients to the baby, leading to a decrease in the heart rate. This can be a concerning sign and may require intervention to ensure the well-being of both the fetus and the mother.

There are several patterns that can be recognized when monitoring variable decelerations. These include early decelerations, late decelerations, and variable decelerations. Early decelerations are typically symmetrical and mirror the contractions, while late decelerations occur after the peak of the contraction and can be a sign of fetal distress. Variable decelerations, on the other hand, have an abrupt onset and can occur at any time during the labor process.

When recognizing variable decelerations, it is important for an Electronic Fetal Monitoring Specialist to take prompt action. This may include repositioning the mother to relieve pressure on the umbilical cord, administering oxygen to increase the oxygen supply to the baby, or performing an emergency cesarean delivery if the baby's well-being is severely compromised.

To effectively intervene in cases of variable decelerations, Electronic Fetal Monitoring Specialists must have a thorough understanding of the causes and potential complications associated with this condition. They must be able to recognize the signs of distress and respond quickly and appropriately.

In addition to recognizing and intervening in cases of variable decelerations, Electronic Fetal Monitoring Specialists play a crucial role in preventing these events from occurring in the first place. This can be done through proper positioning of the mother during labor, ensuring adequate hydration and nutrition, and closely monitoring the progress of the labor.

Overall, variable decelerations are an important aspect of fetal heart rate monitoring. Electronic Fetal Monitoring Specialists must be able to recognize the different patterns of decelerations and intervene as necessary to ensure the well-being of both the fetus and the mother. By closely monitoring and promptly addressing these decelerations, the chances of a positive birth outcome can significantly increase.

3.8.3 Late:

Late decelerations refer to a specific pattern observed in electronic fetal monitoring, which is used to assess the well-being of the fetus during labor. These decelerations are characterized by a slow decrease in the fetal heart rate that corresponds to uterine contractions.

Late decelerations typically occur due to inadequate oxygen supply to the fetus. They are associated with uteroplacental insufficiency, which can be caused by various factors such as maternal hypotension, placental abruption, or uterine hyperstimulation. It is crucial for an Electronic Fetal Monitoring Specialist to recognize and intervene promptly when late decelerations occur.

When analyzing the fetal heart rate pattern, the specialist should pay attention to the timing, shape, and duration of the decelerations. Late decelerations usually start after the peak of the contraction and return to the baseline after the contraction has ended. Their shape is usually uniform with a smooth descent and ascent. The duration of the decelerations can vary but should not exceed **3** minutes.

Late decelerations indicate fetal compromise and can be a sign of fetal hypoxia or acidosis. The decreased oxygen supply to the fetus during contractions leads to the activation of the fetal autonomic nervous system, resulting in vagal stimulation and subsequent deceleration of the heart rate. This response aims to redistribute oxygen to vital organs but can also be a sign of fetal distress.

When late decelerations are observed, it is essential to intervene promptly to prevent further compromise to the fetus. The first step is to address any underlying causes such as maternal hypotension by repositioning the mother, administering fluids, or providing oxygen. Maternal position changes, particularly from a supine to a lateral position, can help improve uteroplacental blood flow and relieve pressure on the vena cava.

If the decelerations persist despite these interventions, it may be necessary to consider more aggressive measures. This can include discontinuing oxytocin administration if hyperstimulation is present, as well as assessing the need for expedited delivery through methods such as vacuum extraction or cesarean section.

Continuous monitoring and close observation are essential when managing late decelerations. The specialist should closely monitor the fetal heart rate pattern, uterine contractions, and the **overall** well-being of both the mother and the fetus. Repeated assessments will help determine the effectiveness of the interventions and guide further management decisions. Prompt recognition and intervention are crucial to ensure the well-being of the fetus. Identifying and addressing the underlying causes, as well as considering more invasive interventions if necessary, can help prevent further fetal distress. Continuous monitoring and close observation are vital components of managing late decelerations.

3.8.4   Prolonged:

Prolonged decelerations in fetal heart rate are an important aspect of pattern recognition and intervention in electronic fetal monitoring. These decelerations are characterized by a decrease in the fetal heart rate that lasts longer than **2** minutes but less than **10** minutes.

When monitoring the fetal heart rate, it is essential to understand the different types of decelerations and their significance. Prolonged decelerations are considered to be non-reassuring patterns that may indicate fetal distress. They can occur in response to various factors such as cord compression, uterine hyperstimulation, maternal hypotension, or placental insufficiency.

One sub**topic** to consider when discussing prolonged decelerations is the potential causes. Cord compression is a common cause of prolonged decelerations, where the umbilical cord becomes compressed, limiting the blood flow to the fetus. This can be caused by factors such as cord prolapse, nuchal cord (cord wrapped around the fetus's neck), or cord entanglement.

Another sub**topic** to explore is the management and interventions for prolonged decelerations. When a prolonged deceleration is identified, it is crucial to assess the underlying cause and intervene promptly to ensure the well-being of the fetus. This may involve repositioning the mother, administering intravenous fluids to treat maternal hypotension, or providing supplemental oxygen to the mother.

Additionally, if cord compression is suspected as the cause of the prolonged deceleration, measures can be taken to relieve the compression. This may include manually elevating the fetal presenting part or performing a cesarean section if necessary.

It is essential for an Electronic Fetal Monitoring Specialist to be able to identify and differentiate prolonged decelerations from other deceleration patterns. This can be done by carefully analyzing the fetal heart rate tracing and noting the duration of the deceleration. By recognizing prolonged decelerations, appropriate interventions can be implemented to optimize fetal well-being and prevent potential complications. They are non-reassuring patterns that may indicate fetal distress and can have various causes such as cord compression or placental insufficiency. Prompt intervention and appropriate management are crucial to ensure the well-being of the fetus. As an Electronic Fetal Monitoring Specialist, it is important to be able to identify and differentiate prolonged decelerations from other deceleration patterns to provide effective care.

3.9   Normal uterine activity:

Normal uterine activity refers to the pattern of contractions that occur in the uterus during pregnancy. These contractions play a vital role in the progress of labor and delivery. Monitoring and recognizing the normal uterine activity is essential for an electronic fetal monitoring specialist to ensure the well-being of both the mother and the baby.

One important aspect of normal uterine activity is the frequency of contractions. Typically, during the early stages of labor, contractions may occur around every **10** to **20** minutes. As labor progresses, the frequency increases to approximately every **2** to **3** minutes. Monitoring this frequency helps determine the stage of labor and the progress being made.

Another aspect to consider is the duration of the contractions. Normal contractions usually last between **45** and **90** seconds. Constant monitoring of the duration helps identify any abnormalities that may require intervention.

The intensity of uterine contractions is another significant factor. The strength of these contractions can be assessed by measuring the intrauterine pressure (IUP) using an intrauterine catheter or an external tocodynamometer. The intensity of contractions is important for the progress of labor as stronger contractions facilitate effacement and dilation of the cervix.

It is also crucial to monitor the resting tone of the uterus between contractions. The resting tone refers to the state of relaxation of the uterine muscles when there are no contractions. A normal resting tone indicates an adequate uteroplacental blood flow, which ensures the oxygen supply to the baby. Continuous monitoring of the resting tone helps detect any uterine hypertonicity or hyperstimulation that could compromise fetal well-being.

In addition to these factors, monitoring the pattern of uterine contractions is important. Normal uterine activity exhibits a regular, coordinated pattern characterized by increasing intensity and frequency as labor progresses. Deviations from this pattern may indicate potential complications, such as uterine hyperstimulation or inadequate uteroplacental perfusion. Monitoring and recognizing these patterns allow for prompt intervention if necessary.

To ensure accurate monitoring of uterine activity, an electronic fetal monitoring specialist uses various tools and techniques. The most common method is external monitoring, which involves placing a tocodynamometer on the mother's abdomen to measure uterine contractions. Internal monitoring may also be used, where an intrauterine catheter is inserted to directly measure the uterine activity.

Understanding and interpreting the patterns of normal uterine activity plays a crucial role in the management of labor and delivery. By closely monitoring the frequency, duration, intensity, resting tone, and pattern of contractions, an electronic fetal monitoring specialist can identify any deviations from the norm and initiate appropriate interventions. This ensures the well-being of both the mother and the baby throughout the labor process.

3.9.1   <u>Resting tone:</u>

Resting tone refers to the baseline tone or tension of the uterine muscles in a pregnant woman when she is not experiencing any contractions. The measurement of resting tone is an important component of electronic fetal monitoring, which is used to assess the well-being of the fetus during labor. Understanding the significance of resting tone and interpreting its variations can help an Electronic Fetal Monitoring Specialist identify potential issues and intervene if necessary.

Resting tone is typically measured in millimeters of mercury (mmHg) and is recorded continuously throughout labor. It reflects the uterine muscle's ability to relax between contractions and plays a crucial role in maintaining a healthy blood flow to the placenta, providing oxygen and nutrients to the fetus.

The average resting tone during labor ranges from **5** to **20** mmHg, depending on various factors such as gestational age, maternal position, and individual variations. A normal resting tone within this range indicates a well-functioning uterus, ready to contract and deliver the baby.

A high resting tone, also known as uterine hypertonia, is characterized by a sustained elevation in the baseline tone beyond the normal range. This can indicate uterine overactivity, which can potentially compromise blood flow to the placenta and cause fetal distress. Uterine hypertonia can be caused by factors such as excessive use of uterotonic drugs (e.g., oxytocin), dehydration, or maternal anxiety. Prompt intervention may be required to address the underlying cause and prevent potential harm to the fetus.

Conversely, a low resting tone, also referred to as uterine hypotonia, is characterized by a baseline tone that falls below the normal range. This may suggest inadequate contractions and poor blood flow to the placenta. Causes of uterine hypotonia include maternal exhaustion, uterine fatigue after a prolonged labor, or the use of medications that relax the uterine muscles. Interventions such as encouraging maternal rest, rehydration, or administering medications to enhance uterine activity may be employed to address uterine hypotonia.

Monitoring resting tone in conjunction with other parameters such as fetal heart rate patterns and contractions helps the Electronic Fetal Monitoring Specialist assess the **overall** well-being of the fetus and make informed decisions regarding further management. Any sudden or persistent changes in resting tone should be carefully evaluated to identify potential complications and ensure appropriate intervention. Monitoring and interpreting variations in resting tone help Electronic Fetal Monitoring Specialists identify potential issues such as uterine hypertonia or hypotonia and intervene accordingly. By staying vigilant and proactive, these specialists can contribute to ensuring a safe and healthy delivery for both the mother and the baby.

3.9.2   <u>Contractions:</u>

Contractions are a crucial aspect of normal uterine activity and play a significant role in the pattern recognition and intervention during the monitoring process in electronic fetal monitoring.

Contractions refer to the periodic tightening and relaxation of the uterine muscles. These contractions help facilitate the progress of labor and the eventual delivery of the baby. They can be categorized into two types - uterine contractions and fetal movements.

Uterine contractions are the contractions of the uterine muscle. They can be further classified as either spontaneous or stimulated. Spontaneous contractions are a natural occurrence during the course of labor, while stimulated contractions can be induced through medical interventions like oxytocin.

Monitoring uterine contractions is vital during labor, as it helps assess the progress of labor and the well-being of both the mother and the baby. The frequency, intensity, and duration of the contractions are important parameters to consider. Frequency refers to the time between the beginning of one contraction to the beginning of the next. Intensity measures the strength of the contractions, while duration refers to the length of each contraction.

Electronic fetal monitoring plays a crucial role in assessing the pattern of contractions. It involves the use of sensors placed on the mother's abdomen to detect and record the contractions graphically. The resulting pattern can be analyzed to identify any deviations from the normal pattern and intervene if necessary.

Understanding the normal pattern of contractions is essential for an electronic fetal monitoring specialist. Typically, contractions during labor follow a characteristic pattern. They start with mild intensity, gradually increase in intensity, reach a peak, and then decrease in intensity. This pattern is known as the "mountain-shaped" contraction pattern.

However, there can be variations in the contraction patterns, such as hypertonic or hypotonic contractions. Hypertonic contractions occur when the uterine muscles contract excessively and fail to relax properly between contractions. This can lead to ineffective labor and potential fetal distress. Hypotonic contractions, on the other hand, are weak and fail to produce adequate progress in labor.

Recognizing abnormal contraction patterns is crucial for timely intervention. If contractions are too frequent, too intense, or too long, it can be a sign of uterine hyperactivity or other complications. Conversely, insufficient contractions may indicate uterine hypotonia, which can prolong labor or result in a higher risk of interventions.

Early intervention in response to abnormal contractions can help optimize labor progress and ensure the safety of both the mother and the baby. Interventions may include changes in the mother's position, administering medications to augment or decrease contractions, or even considering a cesarean delivery if necessary. By monitoring the frequency, intensity, and duration of contractions, specialists can identify deviations from the normal pattern and intervene appropriately to ensure a safe and successful delivery. Accurate pattern recognition and timely interventions are essential for optimizing labor progress and promoting the well-being of both the mother and the baby.

3.9.2.1   Frequency:

Frequency is a key aspect when it comes to electronic fetal monitoring, especially in the context of contractions, normal uterine activity, pattern recognition, and intervention.

In the field of electronic fetal monitoring, frequency refers to the rate at which contractions occur and the rate at which the baby's heart rate changes. It is an important parameter to evaluate the well-being and health of the fetus. By monitoring the frequency, healthcare professionals can assess the **overall** progress of labor and the baby's response to it.

When talking about contractions, frequency represents how often they occur within a certain time frame. It is typically measured in minutes and indicates the time elapsed between the start of one contraction and the start of the next. A frequency of three contractions in a span of **10** minutes, for example, indicates a more regular pattern compared to two contractions in the same timeframe.

Monitoring the frequency of contractions is essential to assess whether a woman is in active labor and progressing as expected. It helps identify any abnormalities or irregularities in the pattern of contractions, as well as potential risks for the baby's well-being. If the frequency of contractions is too high or too low, intervention may be necessary to ensure a safe childbirth.

Similarly, when assessing the normal uterine activity, the frequency of contractions plays a crucial role. It provides valuable insights into the strength and regularity of contractions, indicating whether they are optimal for an efficient labor process. Consistent and appropriate frequency of contractions is essential to ensure adequate blood flow to the placenta and oxygen supply to the fetus.

In the context of pattern recognition and intervention, frequency helps determine if contractions are occurring regularly or irregularly. By analyzing the patterns formed by the frequency of contractions, healthcare professionals can identify potential issues such as hypertonic or weak contractions, which may require intervention to avoid complications during labor.

It is essential for an electronic fetal monitoring specialist to be able to accurately assess and interpret the frequency of contractions and other uterine activities. This includes identifying variations in frequency and patterns that may indicate distress or abnormality. Monitoring the frequency allows specialists to intervene in a timely manner, whether it involves providing medication to stimulate contractions or taking measures to reduce their intensity. It helps healthcare professionals determine the progress of labor, assess the well-being of the fetus, and make informed decisions regarding necessary interventions. A thorough understanding of frequency is vital for an electronic fetal monitoring specialist to ensure the safety and well-being of both the mother and the baby during childbirth.

3.9.2.2   Duration:

Duration is an important aspect of electronic fetal monitoring that is used to assess the length of contractions and uterine activity during pregnancy and labor. It refers to the length of time that a contraction or a period of uterine activity lasts. Understanding the duration of contractions is crucial in identifying any abnormalities or potential complications during labor.

During electronic fetal monitoring, the duration of each contraction is measured and recorded. This information helps healthcare professionals assess the strength and frequency of contractions and monitor the well-being of the baby. The duration of a contraction is typically measured from the beginning of one contraction to the end of the same contraction. This allows healthcare providers to observe the contraction pattern and determine if they are within the normal range.

Normal uterine activity consists of contractions that have a regular pattern and are of appropriate duration. In a normal labor, contractions typically last around **30-60** seconds, with a frequency of **2-5** contractions every **10** minutes. This pattern allows for proper oxygenation of the baby during the contraction and relaxation periods. It is important to note that the duration of contractions can vary between individuals, but deviations from the normal range may indicate potential issues.

Monitoring the duration of contractions allows healthcare professionals to recognize any deviations from the normal pattern. Prolonged contractions, which are contractions lasting longer than **90** seconds, may indicate a condition called uterine tachysystole. This condition can lead to decreased blood flow to the baby and may require intervention to prevent complications. On the other hand, very short contractions, lasting less than **20** seconds, may suggest ineffective contractions that could hinder progress in labor.

In addition to monitoring the duration of contractions, healthcare providers also consider other factors, such as the strength and frequency of contractions, in order to assess the **overall** uterine activity. This comprehensive evaluation helps determine if the labor is progressing normally or if intervention is needed.

Overall, duration is a critical parameter in electronic fetal monitoring that helps healthcare professionals assess the normality of contractions and uterine activity. By monitoring the duration of contractions, healthcare providers can identify potential issues and intervene when necessary to ensure the well-being of both the mother and the baby. Regular monitoring and evaluation of the duration, in conjunction with other factors, enable proper pattern recognition and intervention if required.

3.9.2.3   Intensity:

Intensity is a crucial aspect of electronic fetal monitoring, which focuses on measuring the strength or force of uterine contractions during labor. It allows the healthcare provider, particularly the Electronic Fetal Monitoring Specialist, to assess the effectiveness of the contractions and monitor the well-being of the fetus.

In the context of labor, intensity refers to the strength of contractions, commonly measured using an external tocodynamometer or an internal intrauterine pressure catheter. The tocodynamometer is a device that is placed on the mother's abdomen to detect and record uterine activity. It provides a graphical representation of the contractions, allowing the specialist to analyze their intensity. The intensity of contractions can be differentiated as either mild, moderate, or strong. Mild contractions are gentle and usually not accompanied by discomfort. They may be observed by a small increase in uterine activity on the monitor. Moderate contractions are stronger and may cause some discomfort for the mother. They appear as larger peaks on the monitoring strip. Strong contractions are the most intense, often resulting in significant discomfort for the mother. They are represented by even larger peaks on the monitor tracing.

Monitoring the intensity of contractions is crucial because it provides valuable information about the effectiveness of labor and the fetus's well-being. It helps determine if the contractions are sufficiently strong to aid in cervical dilation and if the uterine muscles are adequately oxygenating the fetus during labor. Weak or irregular contractions may indicate the need for medical intervention to induce or augment labor and prevent complications.

Furthermore, the intensity of contractions is closely associated with the duration of labor. Strong and effective contractions often lead to faster cervical dilation and efficient progress in labor. Monitoring the intensity allows the specialist to identify patterns or abnormalities that may require intervention, such as prolonged or stalling labor.

In addition to assessing the intensity of contractions, monitoring the frequency and duration of contractions is essential. The frequency refers to how often contractions occur, usually measured in minutes from the start of one contraction to the beginning of the next. The duration, on the other hand, refers to the length of each contraction, typically measured in seconds. Analyzing the frequency and duration in conjunction with the intensity provides a comprehensive picture of the uterine activity during labor.

By closely monitoring the intensity of contractions, the Electronic Fetal Monitoring Specialist plays a vital role in ensuring the well-being of both the mother and the fetus during labor. They are skilled in recognizing patterns of uterine activity and can intervene promptly if any abnormalities or complications arise. Ultimately, intensity monitoring allows for proactive care and better outcomes for both mother and baby.

4   FETAL ASSESSMENT METHODS:

Fetal assessment methods are techniques used to evaluate the health and well-being of the fetus during pregnancy. These methods help healthcare providers monitor the baby's growth, development, and **overall** condition to ensure a safe and healthy pregnancy. As an Electronic Fetal Monitoring Specialist, it is essential to have a comprehensive understanding of these assessment methods to accurately interpret fetal monitoring data and provide the necessary care.

One of the most common fetal assessment methods is ultrasound. Ultrasound uses high-frequency sound waves to create real-time images of the fetus on a screen. It is non-invasive and allows healthcare providers to assess fetal growth, monitor organ development, and detect any abnormalities or potential complications. Ultrasound is also used to determine the baby's position, the placenta's location, and the amount of amniotic fluid present.

Another important assessment method is fetal heart rate monitoring. This involves monitoring the baby's heart rate using electronic fetal monitors. There are two types of fetal heart rate monitoring: external and internal. External monitoring involves placing sensors on the mother's abdomen to record the baby's heart rate. Internal monitoring, on the other hand, involves placing a small electrode directly on the baby's scalp through the cervix. Fetal heart rate monitoring helps assess the baby's well-being, oxygen supply, and response to contractions during labor.

Additionally, fetal movement counting is used as a method for assessing fetal well-being. The mother is encouraged to monitor the baby's movements regularly and report any significant changes or decreases to her healthcare provider. A decrease in fetal movement could indicate potential problems and may require further evaluation or intervention. This method helps detect any signs of fetal distress or inadequate oxygen supply.

Another crucial assessment method is amniocentesis. This procedure involves the insertion of a thin needle through the mother's abdomen into the amniotic sac to collect a small sample of amniotic fluid. Amniocentesis is typically performed between 15 and 20 weeks of pregnancy and is used to diagnose genetic disorders, chromosomal abnormalities, and neural tube defects. It provides valuable information about the baby's health and helps parents and healthcare providers make informed decisions about their pregnancy.

Genetic screening and testing, such as non-invasive prenatal testing (NIPT) and chorionic villus sampling (CVS), are also important fetal assessment methods. NIPT is a blood test that analyzes the baby's DNA to screen for certain chromosomal abnormalities, such as Down syndrome. CVS, on the other hand, involves the removal of a small tissue sample from the placenta to test for genetic disorders. These tests help identify potential genetic issues early in pregnancy, allowing parents to make informed decisions about their baby's health and potential treatment options. Ultrasound, fetal heart rate monitoring, fetal movement counting, amniocentesis, and genetic screening/testing are all important techniques used by Electronic Fetal Monitoring Specialists to ensure the well-being of both the baby and the mother. It is vital for these specialists to have a thorough understanding of these methods to accurately interpret the data and provide the best possible care for the pregnant woman and her baby.

4.1   Auscultation:

Auscultation is an important method used in fetal assessment to monitor the well-being and health of the fetus during pregnancy. It involves listening to the sounds made by the fetus using a device called a Doppler ultrasound or a handheld ultrasound device. This non-invasive procedure allows healthcare professionals, such as Electronic Fetal Monitoring Specialists, to assess the fetal heart rate and detect any abnormalities or complications.

During auscultation, a gel is applied to the mother's abdomen to help transmit sound waves and enable better detection of the fetal heartbeat. The Doppler ultrasound device is then placed on the abdomen and moved around to locate the best position for obtaining clear sounds. The device emits high-frequency sound waves that bounce back off the fetal heartbeat, creating audio signals that can be heard through a speaker or headphones.

One of the main benefits of auscultation is that it can be performed quickly and easily in various settings, such as hospitals, clinics, or even at home. It is a safe and painless procedure that does not pose any risks to either the mother or the fetus. Furthermore, it does not require specialized training to perform, making it accessible to a wide range of healthcare professionals.

Auscultation provides valuable information about the fetal heart rate, which is a crucial indicator of fetal well-being and development. The normal fetal heart rate ranges from **120** to **160** beats per minute. Variations in the heart rate can indicate fetal distress or potential complications. For example, an unusually high or low heart rate may signify a lack of oxygen, fetal infection, or other issues that require further investigation or intervention.

Another aspect of auscultation is the ability to detect additional sounds known as fetal heart tones. These tones are different from the regular heartbeat and can provide valuable insights into the **overall** health and development of the fetus. Listening for the presence and quality of these sounds can help identify any abnormalities or irregularities that may require further prenatal care or medical interventions.

Auscultation is typically performed throughout pregnancy during routine prenatal check-ups. It allows healthcare providers to monitor the fetal heartbeat and assess the well-being of the fetus at different stages of development. Regular auscultation helps to establish a baseline for the fetal heart rate and detect any deviations from the norm. It also enables healthcare professionals to identify and address any potential complications or issues early on. It is a non-invasive, safe, and easily accessible procedure that provides valuable information about the well-being and development of the fetus. By listening to the sounds made by the fetus, healthcare providers can ensure the health and safety of both the mother and the baby throughout the pregnancy journey.

4.2   Fetal movement and stimulation:

Fetal movement and stimulation play a significant role in the assessment of the fetus during pregnancy. Monitoring the movement of the fetus is an essential part of assessing its well-being and development. Fetal movements are the first expressions of the baby's developing neuromuscular system, and they provide valuable insights into the central and peripheral nervous system integrity. These movements can be observed and recorded using various methods, including ultrasound imaging and maternal perception.

Ultrasound imaging is commonly used to assess fetal movements. This non-invasive method allows healthcare providers to visualize the fetus inside the womb and observe its movements in real-time. The ultrasound scan provides detailed information about the nature, frequency, and intensity of fetal movements. It also helps in identifying any abnormalities or potential problems. This imaging technique is safe for both the mother and the baby.

Maternal perception of fetal movements is another crucial aspect of fetal assessment. As the pregnancy progresses, the mother becomes increasingly aware of the movements of her baby. Maternal perception can be subjective, but it helps in providing additional information about the well-being of the fetus. The mother may use methods such as kick counting to monitor the frequency and strength of fetal movements. Counting the number of kicks or movements within a specific time frame can give an indication of the fetal well-being.

Fetal movement patterns vary throughout pregnancy. Initially, the movements may be sporadic and subtle, often described as flutters or bubbles. As the fetus grows and becomes more developed, the movements become more pronounced, and the mother can feel distinct kicks, rolls, or stretches. It is important for healthcare providers to educate expectant mothers about typical fetal movement patterns to help them recognize any changes or abnormalities.

Stimulation techniques can be used to assess fetal movement and responsiveness. These techniques are used when there are concerns about the well-being of the fetus or if additional information is needed. Stimulation can be achieved through various methods, including sound, light, or tactile stimulation. For example, a healthcare provider may use a device that emits a sound or vibration near the mother's abdomen to check the fetal response. The provider will then assess the quality and quantity of the fetal movements in response to the stimulation.

Fetal stimulation is generally safe and does not pose any risks to the mother or the baby. However, it is important for healthcare providers to follow proper guidelines and protocols while performing these techniques to ensure the well-being of both. The information obtained from fetal movement and stimulation assessments can help in identifying potential problems or abnormalities early on, allowing for timely interventions and appropriate management. Through ultrasound imaging and maternal perception, healthcare providers can monitor and evaluate the well-being and development of the fetus. Understanding the typical patterns of fetal movement and using stimulation techniques when necessary can provide valuable information about the fetal nervous system and **overall** health. These assessments contribute to the comprehensive care provided during pregnancy and ensure the best possible outcomes for both the mother and the baby.

4.3   Nonstress testing:

Nonstress testing is a common method used in the assessment of fetal well-being. It is a noninvasive procedure that helps monitor the fetal heart rate and the presence of any potential issues. This test is usually done during the later stages of pregnancy and is vital in ensuring the health and safety of the unborn baby.

During a nonstress test, the expectant mother is comfortably positioned, and sensors are attached to her abdomen. These sensors record the fetal heart rate and contractions. The mother will also be given a button to press whenever she feels the baby move. The test typically lasts for about **20** to **30** minutes, but it can be extended if necessary.

There are several goals of nonstress testing. One of these goals is to assess the **overall** health and well-being of the fetus. By measuring the heart rate, doctors can determine if the baby is receiving enough oxygen and nutrients. If the heart rate accelerates appropriately with fetal movement, it indicates that the baby is doing well. Conversely, a lack of accelerations may suggest potential issues.

Additionally, nonstress testing is useful in detecting any potential abnormalities in the baby's heart rate patterns. This can include signs of distress or potential complications. If the baby's heart rate does not react as expected during the test, it may indicate the need for further evaluation or intervention.

The nonstress test can also be used to evaluate the efficacy of certain medical interventions. For example, if the mother is given medication to stimulate fetal activity, the test can assess whether it is having the desired effect. This testing process can aid in identifying whether the intervention is effectively improving the **overall** health of the fetus.

There are certain factors that may affect the accuracy of a nonstress test. For instance, if the mother is obese, it may be more challenging to obtain clear readings. Similarly, if the mother is on certain medications, it can influence the interpretation of the test results. It is crucial for healthcare professionals to consider these factors and make appropriate adjustments when interpreting the data. It helps monitor the fetal heart rate, assesses **overall** well-being, detects abnormalities, evaluates interventions, and provides valuable information for the healthcare team. This noninvasive procedure plays a significant role in ensuring the safety and health of both the mother and the baby. It is crucial for healthcare professionals, especially electronic fetal monitoring specialists, to be well-versed in this testing method to provide accurate assessments and make informed decisions regarding fetal care.

4.4   Cord Blood Acid Base Testing:

Cord blood acid-base testing is a crucial method used in the assessment of a fetus during pregnancy. This test involves analyzing the pH and other parameters of the baby's blood obtained from the umbilical cord immediately after delivery. It provides valuable information about the baby's oxygen supply and acid-base balance, which can help determine the **overall** well-being of the newborn.

One important aspect of cord blood acid-base testing is its ability to assess the baby's oxygenation status. The pH value of the cord blood indicates the acidity or alkalinity of the baby's blood, providing insights into its oxygen levels. A low pH value reflects acidosis, which indicates poor oxygen supply to the baby during labor and delivery. On the other hand, a high pH value suggests alkalosis, which may occur when the baby is exposed to excessive stress or hyperventilation in the womb.

In addition to pH, cord blood acid-base testing also evaluates other parameters such as base excess and bicarbonate levels. Base excess indicates the amount of acid or base in the baby's blood and provides a deeper understanding of the acid-base balance. Abnormal base excess values can indicate respiratory or metabolic disturbances that may require immediate medical intervention. Bicarbonate levels, on the other hand, reflect the baby's ability to regulate acid-base balance and can provide further insight into any underlying issues.

Cord blood acid-base testing is particularly valuable in situations where the fetus is at risk of hypoxia. It helps identify conditions such as fetal distress, placental insufficiency, or umbilical cord abnormalities that can potentially compromise the baby's oxygen supply. This information can guide obstetricians and healthcare professionals in making timely decisions regarding delivery methods, such as emergency cesarean section or assisted vaginal delivery.

Furthermore, cord blood acid-base testing is performed when electronic fetal monitoring (EFM) shows worrisome signs, such as abnormal heart rate patterns. This helps in confirming the presence of fetal acidemia, a condition characterized by excessively low cord blood pH. Fetal acidemia is associated with an increased risk of neonatal complications, including hypoxic-ischemic encephalopathy (HIE) and cerebral palsy.

It is essential to note that cord blood acid-base testing should be interpreted in conjunction with other fetal assessment methods to obtain a comprehensive evaluation of the baby's well-being. These may include ultrasound scans, biophysical profiles, and the assessment of amniotic fluid volume. Combining these methods allows healthcare providers to make well-informed decisions for the mother and baby throughout pregnancy and delivery. It provides valuable information about fetal oxygenation, acid-base balance, and **overall** well-being. By analyzing pH, base excess, and bicarbonate levels, healthcare professionals can identify potential issues and make timely interventions to optimize the outcome for both mother and baby. When used in conjunction with other fetal assessment methods, cord blood acid-base testing enhances the accuracy and reliability of the **overall** fetal assessment process.

4.5   Biophysical profile:

The biophysical profile is a prenatal screening test that assesses the well-being and development of the fetus. It is a noninvasive procedure that combines various measurements and observations to provide an **overall** evaluation of the fetal health. This test is typically recommended for women with high-risk pregnancies or those who have certain medical conditions that may affect the baby's well-being.

The biophysical profile consists of five components: fetal heart rate monitoring, fetal movement, fetal breathing, fetal tone, and the amniotic fluid volume. Each component is assessed and given a score of either **0** or **2**, depending on the presence or absence of certain indicators. The individual scores are then added together to obtain the **overall** biophysical profile score.

Fetal heart rate monitoring is a crucial part of the biophysical profile. It involves measuring the baby's heart rate using ultrasound or electronic fetal monitoring. A normal heart rate indicates a healthy fetus, while abnormalities may suggest potential issues with the baby's oxygenation.

Fetal movement is another important aspect of the biophysical profile. The baby's movements are observed and recorded within a specific time frame. An active and responsive baby signifies good neurological function and **overall** well-being.

Fetal breathing is assessed by observing the presence of rhythmic breathing motions. The absence of breathing movements may indicate fetal distress or immaturity.

Fetal tone is evaluated by observing the baby's muscle tone and level of activity. A fetus with good muscle tone and active movements is considered healthy, while decreased or absent movements can be indicators of potential problems.

Amniotic fluid volume is measured using ultrasound. An adequate amount of amniotic fluid is essential for the baby's lung development and **overall** growth. Too little or too much fluid may suggest potential issues, such as placental dysfunction or fetal abnormalities.

In addition to the components mentioned above, the biophysical profile may also include a nonstress test, which measures the baby's heart rate in response to its own movements. This helps to further assess the baby's well-being and determine the need for immediate medical intervention.

The biophysical profile is a reliable and safe method for assessing fetal health. It provides valuable information to healthcare providers, allowing them to make informed decisions about the management of high-risk pregnancies. By detecting potential issues early on, the biophysical profile can help prevent complications and ensure the best possible outcome for both the mother and the baby. It combines various measurements and observations to provide a comprehensive evaluation of the baby's health. Through the evaluation of fetal heart rate, movement, breathing, tone, and amniotic fluid volume, healthcare providers can gather valuable information about the baby's development and **overall** health. The biophysical profile is a noninvasive and reliable method that helps in the early detection of potential issues, allowing for timely intervention and improved outcomes.

4.6   Fetal Acoustic Stimulation:

Fetal acoustic stimulation is a technique used in fetal assessment methods, specifically in electronic fetal monitoring. It involves applying sound waves to the mother's abdomen to stimulate the fetus and assess its well-being. This procedure is non-invasive and is typically performed during the third trimester of pregnancy.

The primary goal of fetal acoustic stimulation is to evaluate the responsiveness of the fetus to external stimuli. It provides valuable information about the fetal central nervous system and its **overall** health. By analyzing the fetal heart rate in response to acoustic stimulation, healthcare professionals can assess the fetal well-being and identify any potential issues that may require further investigation.

During the procedure, a specialized device called an acoustic stimulator is used. It emits a series of audible sounds or tones that are directed towards the mother's abdomen. These sounds, usually resembling a musical chime or bell-like tones, penetrate the uterus and stimulate the fetus. The fetal heart rate is then monitored and recorded to observe its response to the auditory stimulus.

Fetal acoustic stimulation can be performed using both external and internal methods. External stimulation involves placing the acoustic stimulator on the mother's abdomen, while internal stimulation requires inserting a small electrode through the cervix into the uterus. The choice of method depends on various factors, including the position of the fetus, the gestational age, and the specific needs of the healthcare provider.

The procedure itself is generally painless and safe for both the mother and the fetus. It does not pose any known risks or complications when performed by trained healthcare professionals. However, certain precautions may be taken, such as ensuring the mother's comfort and maintaining a sterile environment during internal stimulation.

Fetal acoustic stimulation provides valuable information about the fetal central nervous system and its **overall** health. It can help identify fetal distress, assess the reactivity of the fetal heart rate, and evaluate the well-being of the fetus. It is often used in conjunction with other fetal assessment methods, such as electronic fetal monitoring, to obtain a comprehensive understanding of the fetal condition.

One of the sub**topics** within fetal acoustic stimulation is the interpretation of the fetal heart rate response. Healthcare professionals analyze the fetal heart rate tracings to detect any abnormalities or variations that may indicate fetal distress. Changes in the heart rate pattern, such as acceleration or deceleration, can provide vital information about the fetal condition.

Another sub**topic** is the benefits and limitations of fetal acoustic stimulation. The procedure is a non-invasive and cost-effective method to assess fetal well-being. It allows for rapid screening and can be repeated multiple times if necessary. However, it is important to note that fetal acoustic stimulation is a complementary tool and should be used in conjunction with other fetal assessment methods to ensure accurate results. It involves applying sound waves to the mother's abdomen to stimulate the fetus and evaluate its responsiveness. This procedure provides valuable information about the fetal central nervous system and can help identify any potential issues. Fetal acoustic stimulation is a safe and effective method that is often used in combination with other assessment methods for a comprehensive evaluation of the fetal condition.

5   PROFESSIONAL ISSUES:

Professional issues are an important aspect of any profession, and this is particularly true for Electronic Fetal Monitoring (EFM) specialists. As EFM specialists, there are a number of professional issues that we must consider in order to provide effective and safe care to our patients.

First and foremost, confidentiality is a key professional issue that EFM specialists must adhere to. We are entrusted with sensitive and personal health information about our patients, and it is our professional responsibility to respect and protect their privacy. This means that we must take appropriate measures to ensure that patient information is kept confidential and only shared with authorized individuals.

Another professional issue to consider is the proper documentation of patient care. EFM specialists must maintain accurate and detailed records of their assessments, interventions, and observations. This documentation is essential for providing continuity of care, ensuring proper communication among healthcare providers, and for legal and reimbursement purposes.

Ethics is also a significant professional issue for EFM specialists. We must adhere to high ethical standards in our practice, including honesty, integrity, and respect for patient autonomy. This means that we must always act in the best interests of our patients and uphold their rights to informed consent and the right to refuse treatment.

Continuing education is another important aspect of professional issues for EFM specialists. Our field is constantly evolving, with new research and technologies emerging all the time. It is our professional responsibility to stay up-to-date with the latest evidence-based practice guidelines and to continually enhance our knowledge and skills through ongoing education and professional development.

In addition to these general professional issues, there are some specific professional issues that are unique to the field of Electronic Fetal Monitoring. One of these issues is the proper interpretation and application of fetal monitoring tracings. As EFM specialists, we must have a thorough understanding of the various types of tracings and be able to accurately interpret them in order to make informed decisions about patient care.

Effective communication is another crucial professional issue for EFM specialists. We work as part of a multidisciplinary team and must be able to communicate effectively with physicians, nurses, and other healthcare providers. This includes clearly conveying our findings and recommendations, as well as actively listening and collaborating with other team members.

Finally, patient advocacy is a key professional issue for EFM specialists. We must be strong advocates for our patients, ensuring that their voices are heard and their needs are met. This may involve advocating for appropriate monitoring and interventions, as well as empowering patients with information and support to make informed decisions about their care. From maintaining patient confidentiality and proper documentation to upholding ethical standards and advocating for our patients, there are many important considerations for us to navigate in our practice. By addressing these professional issues, we can ensure that we are providing the highest level of care to our patients and upholding the standards of our profession.

5.1   Legal:

Legal issues are a crucial aspect for Electronic Fetal Monitoring Specialists to consider in their professional practice. These legal considerations are meant to ensure the safety and well-being of both the healthcare provider and the patients. In the context of electronic fetal monitoring, there are several legal aspects that healthcare professionals need to be aware of.

One important legal aspect is informed consent. Before conducting any electronic fetal monitoring procedure, it is necessary to obtain the informed consent of the expectant mother or legal guardian. Informed consent means that the patient is fully informed about the procedure, its potential risks, benefits, and alternatives, and gives voluntary consent to undergo the procedure. It is the responsibility of the Electronic Fetal Monitoring Specialist to ensure that the patient understands the implications of the procedure and has the capacity to make informed decisions.

Another legal consideration is patient privacy and confidentiality. Electronic Fetal Monitoring Specialists have a duty to protect the privacy and confidentiality of their patients' medical information. This includes taking measures to secure electronic fetal monitoring data and only disclosing it to authorized individuals involved in the patient's care. Failure to uphold patient privacy and confidentiality can result in legal consequences, such as violating healthcare privacy laws or breaching patient confidentiality.

Electronic Fetal Monitoring Specialists should also be familiar with the applicable laws and regulations governing their practice. This includes understanding the scope of their professional practice, the limitations on their authority, and any specific legal requirements for electronic fetal monitoring procedures. It is essential to stay updated with changes in healthcare laws and regulations to ensure compliance and avoid legal issues.

Documentation is another critical legal aspect for Electronic Fetal Monitoring Specialists. Accurate and comprehensive documentation of electronic fetal monitoring procedures, observations, and any interventions is essential for legal and patient safety purposes. Complete and timely documentation can help protect healthcare professionals in case of a legal dispute and ensure continuity of care for the patient.

Furthermore, Electronic Fetal Monitoring Specialists must adhere to professional standards and guidelines. These guidelines are usually established by professional organizations to ensure quality care and patient safety. Familiarity with these standards and guidelines is crucial to meeting the professional expectations of the role and avoiding legal pitfalls.

In the unfortunate event of adverse outcomes or medical errors related to electronic fetal monitoring, legal issues may arise. Electronic Fetal Monitoring Specialists must be prepared to cooperate with any investigations or legal proceedings that may follow such incidents. They may be required to provide accurate and detailed accounts of the events leading to the adverse outcomes and participate in legal proceedings as necessary. Informed consent, patient privacy and confidentiality, knowledge of laws and regulations, proper documentation, adherence to professional standards, and preparedness for legal proceedings are all essential aspects of the legal framework surrounding electronic fetal monitoring. By being mindful of these legal aspects, Electronic Fetal Monitoring Specialists can ensure that they provide safe and lawful care to their patients.

5.2   Ethics:

Ethics is a crucial aspect of the professional role of an Electronic Fetal Monitoring (EFM) Specialist. It refers to the moral principles and values that guide their conduct and decision-making in the workplace.

One important aspect of ethics for EFM Specialists is ensuring patient confidentiality. They must maintain strict confidentiality regarding all patient information they come across while performing their duties. This includes not sharing any sensitive information with unauthorized individuals, protecting electronic data, and respecting the privacy of patients.

Another vital ethical consideration is respecting the autonomy and informed consent of pregnant women. EFM Specialists should provide accurate and understandable information about the fetal monitoring process, explaining its benefits and potential risks. They must obtain informed consent from pregnant women before conducting any monitoring procedures, ensuring that they fully understand the process and its implications.

EFM Specialists are also expected to prioritize the well-being and safety of both the mother and the fetus. This ethical commitment includes ensuring the accurate interpretation of fetal monitoring results, promptly reporting any abnormalities or concerns to the healthcare team, and advocating for appropriate interventions or changes in the monitoring approach when necessary.

Moreover, EFM Specialists should promote cultural competence and respect diversity when caring for patients. They must understand and appreciate the unique cultural backgrounds, beliefs, and practices of individuals they encounter, providing care that is sensitive to their needs and preferences.

Maintaining professional integrity is another ethical obligation for EFM Specialists. This involves being honest and transparent in their interactions with patients, colleagues, and other healthcare professionals. EFM Specialists should ensure accurate documentation of all procedures and findings, share information truthfully, and report any errors or discrepancies that may impact patient care.

Furthermore, ethical considerations expect EFM Specialists to continuously update their knowledge and skills, striving for professional growth and development. They should stay informed about the latest research and evidence-based practices in fetal monitoring and participate in relevant educational opportunities that enhance their **expert**ise.

In the event of ethical dilemmas, EFM Specialists should employ an ethical decision-making framework. This involves identifying the problem, considering all relevant ethical principles, exploring available options, evaluating the potential consequences, and making a well-justified decision that upholds the best interest of the patient.

Lastly, collaboration and teamwork play a vital role in ethical practice for EFM Specialists. They should work together with the healthcare team, respecting the **expert**ise and input of other professionals. By fostering open communication, mutual respect, and shared decision-making, EFM Specialists can ensure ethical care delivery and optimal outcomes for their patients. These include patient confidentiality, informed consent, prioritizing safety, promoting cultural competence, maintaining professional integrity, ongoing professional development, ethical decision-making, and collaboration. Adhering to ethical principles allows EFM Specialists to provide competent, compassionate, and patient-centered care while upholding the highest standards of professional conduct.

5.3   Patient safety:

Patient safety is a crucial aspect of healthcare, including the role of an Electronic Fetal Monitoring Specialist. It refers to the prevention of errors, injuries, accidents, and infections that can occur during medical care. Ensuring patient safety requires a collaborative effort from healthcare professionals, patients, and healthcare systems.

One important aspect of patient safety is the prevention of medical errors. This involves accurately identifying patients, administering the correct medications and dosages, and following proper protocols to minimize the risk of complications. As an Electronic Fetal Monitoring Specialist, it is essential to maintain a high level of accuracy in interpreting fetal heart rate tracings to avoid misdiagnosis that could lead to potential harm.

Another key aspect of patient safety is infection prevention. Healthcare-associated infections can be detrimental to patients' health and prolong hospital stays. Adhering to strict hygiene practices, such as handwashing and maintaining a clean work environment, can significantly reduce the risk of infections. As an Electronic Fetal Monitoring Specialist, maintaining a sterile and safe environment during fetal monitoring procedures is of utmost importance.

Additionally, communication plays a vital role in patient safety. Effective and clear communication between healthcare professionals can prevent misunderstandings and ensure that accurate information is relayed. This includes communicating critical information about fetal well-being and potential risks to other members of the healthcare team promptly.

Patient safety also involves the continuous monitoring of equipment and technology used in healthcare. Regular maintenance, calibration, and testing of electronic fetal monitoring equipment are essential to prevent malfunctions and ensure accurate readings. As an Electronic Fetal Monitoring Specialist, it is crucial to promptly report any equipment malfunction or discrepancies to the appropriate individuals to minimize risks.

Moreover, patient education is integral to maintaining patient safety. Providing clear instructions and information to patients and their families empowers them to actively participate in their own care. Educating expectant mothers about the importance of fetal monitoring and what to expect during the process promotes a safe and informed healthcare experience.

Furthermore, creating a culture of safety within healthcare organizations is paramount. This involves fostering an environment where all healthcare professionals feel comfortable reporting errors or near misses without fearing repercussions. Encouraging open communication and a non-punitive approach to error reporting allows for the identification of potential risks and the implementation of strategies to prevent future occurrences.

Lastly, staying abreast of current evidence-based practices is crucial to maintaining patient safety. As an Electronic Fetal Monitoring Specialist, it is essential to stay updated with the latest research, guidelines, and best practices in fetal monitoring. This ensures that the care provided aligns with current standards, minimizing potential risks to patients. As an Electronic Fetal Monitoring Specialist, prioritizing patient safety is essential to provide optimal care and minimize potential harm to both the mother and fetus.

5.4   Quality Improvement:

Quality improvement is an essential aspect of any profession, including that of an Electronic Fetal Monitoring Specialist. It refers to the systematic approach taken to identify and address areas of improvement in order to enhance the quality of care provided to patients.

In the context of an Electronic Fetal Monitoring Specialist's role, quality improvement involves assessing and improving the accuracy, reliability, and effectiveness of fetal monitoring techniques and practices. This is crucial as fetal monitoring plays a critical role in assessing the well-being of both the mother and the unborn baby during pregnancy and labor.

One important aspect of quality improvement is the evaluation of current practices and policies. This includes reviewing the electronic fetal monitoring procedures, protocols, and guidelines to ensure that they are up-to-date and based on the latest evidence-based practices. By staying abreast of the latest research and best practices, Electronic Fetal Monitoring Specialists can ensure that they provide the highest quality of care to their patients.

Another essential element of quality improvement is the ongoing monitoring and assessment of clinical outcomes. This involves regularly reviewing and analyzing the data collected during fetal monitoring, such as electronic tracings and other relevant measurements. By closely examining the data, Electronic Fetal Monitoring Specialists can identify any patterns or trends that may indicate areas for improvement. For example, they may notice a higher rate of false alarms or instances where interventions could have been avoided. By addressing these issues, they can improve patient safety and outcomes.

Collaboration and communication are also crucial aspects of quality improvement. Electronic Fetal Monitoring Specialists should work closely with other healthcare professionals, including obstetricians, nurses, and midwives, to ensure that there is a shared understanding of the best practices in fetal monitoring. This can involve regular meetings, case discussions, and educational initiatives to promote a culture of continuous learning and improvement.

In addition to clinical aspects, quality improvement also encompasses factors such as patient satisfaction and organizational efficiency. Electronic Fetal Monitoring Specialists should strive to provide patient-centered care, addressing the individual needs and preferences of each patient. This can be achieved through effective communication, empathy, and shared decision-making. Furthermore, quality improvement extends beyond individual practice and includes the broader healthcare system. Electronic Fetal Monitoring Specialists should actively engage in quality improvement initiatives at the organizational level, such as participating in audits, contributing to policy development, and implementing standardized processes.

Continuous learning and professional development are critical for quality improvement. Electronic Fetal Monitoring Specialists should stay informed about the latest advancements in fetal monitoring technology and attend relevant conferences, workshops, and training programs. By continuously expanding their knowledge and skills, they can provide the best possible care to their patients. By evaluating current practices, monitoring outcomes, collaborating with other healthcare professionals, and focusing on patient-centered care, Electronic Fetal Monitoring Specialists can continually enhance the quality of care they provide. Through ongoing learning and engagement in quality improvement initiatives, they can ensure that their practice remains up-to-date, efficient, and effective.

C-EFM

Exam

Practice

Questions

Question 1: Ms. Hernandez, a 25-year-old primigravida at 36 weeks of gestation, presents to the labor and delivery unit with sudden onset vaginal bleeding. On examination, the bleeding is painless and the fundus of the uterus is located above the umbilicus. Which of the following uteroplacental complications is most likely responsible for this presentation?
A) Placental abruption
B) Uterine rupture
C) Placenta previa
D) Placenta accreta

Question 2: Which of the following conditions can result in maternal hemorrhage during pregnancy or childbirth?
A) Hyperemesis gravidarum
B) Ectopic pregnancy
C) Amniotic fluid embolism
D) Gestational diabetes

Question 3: Mrs. Thompson, a 32-year-old primigravida, is in active labor. On electronic fetal monitoring, his baby's heart rate tracing shows recurrent late decelerations. The nurse performs an internal fetal heart rate monitoring and notices decreased beat-to-beat variability. What is the nurse's next appropriate action?
A) Administer oxygen via face mask
B) Begin continuous fetal monitoring
C) Start intravenous fluids rapidly
D) Prepare for an emergency cesarean section

Question 4: Which of the following can cause ectopic beats in a fetus?
A) Maternal anxiety
B) Umbilical cord compression
C) Fetal hypoxia
D) Fetal sleep pattern

Question 5: Which of the following is NOT a potential cause of tachycardia in fetal monitoring?
A) Maternal fever
B) Fetal hypoxia
C) Maternal hypoglycemia
D) Fetal Anemia

Question 6: Rachel, a 30-year-old pregnant woman at 42 weeks of gestation, is in active labor. Fetal monitoring shows a baseline fetal heart rate (FHR) of 110 bpm with minimal variability. Contractions are occurring every 2 minutes with a duration of 60 seconds. The nurse suspects tachysystole. Which nursing action is the priority?
A) Decreasing the maternal pushing efforts.
B) Assisting with intrauterine resuscitation.
C) Administering meperidine for pain relief.
D) Preparing for immediate delivery by vacuum extraction.

Question 7: Which of the following is an early deceleration pattern on the fetal heart rate monitoring strip?
A) Deceleration that occurs after a contraction
B) Deceleration that begins before the contraction peak and returns to baseline after the contraction ends
C) Deceleration that occurs randomly throughout labor
D) Deceleration that is prolonged and gradual in onset and recovery

Question 8: During a routine prenatal visit, the nurse notices that the fetal heart rate is consistently above 160 beats per minute. The mother denies any symptoms or concerns. What is the best course of action for the nurse to take?
A) Inform the obstetrician immediately
B) Schedule a non-stress test within the next 24 hours
C) Reassure the mother and continue with regular prenatal care
D) Recommend immediate hospitalization for further evaluation

Question 9: Ms. Johnson, at 36 weeks gestation, presents to the antenatal clinic. She complains of decreased fetal movements over the past 24 hours. You decide to perform external fetal monitoring to assess the well-being of the fetus. Which of the following parameters is measured during external fetal monitoring?
A) Fetal heart rate
B) Maternal blood pressure
C) Uterine contractions
D) Fetal breathing movements

Question 10: During a routine prenatal visit, your patient, Mrs. Thompson, mentions that she feels neglected and unheard by the healthcare professionals she has encountered throughout her pregnancy journey. What should be your ethical response to Mrs. Thompson's concerns?
A) Dismiss her concerns as common pregnancy-related emotions.
B) Offer her empathy and actively listen to her concerns.
C) Refer her to a mental health professional for further evaluation.
D) Avoid acknowledging her concerns to prevent a time-consuming conversation.

Question 11: Which fetal complication is characterized by a decrease in variability, repetitive late decelerations, and absence of accelerations?
A) Fetal bradycardia
B) Fetal tachycardia
C) Fetal distress
D) Fetal acidemia

Question 12: Which fetal complication is characterized by persistent late decelerations, decreased variability, and repetitive variable decelerations?
A) Fetal bradycardia
B) Fetal tachycardia
C) Fetal distress
D) Fetal acidemia

Question 13: In a monochorionic-diamniotic twin pregnancy, what is the most common type of placental vascular anastomosis?
A) Arteriovenous anastomosis
B) Arterioarterial anastomosis
C) Venovenous anastomosis
D) Venous-arterial anastomosis

Question 14: Mrs. Clark, a 35-year-old woman, is in active labor at 40 weeks gestation. The electronic fetal monitoring (EFM) reveals a sudden loss of fetal heart rate variability with repetitive decelerations. After ruling out maternal hypotension and cord compression, which of the following interventions should the nurse prioritize?
A) Increase intravenous fluids to the patient
B) Administer uterine relaxation medication

C) Prepare for an emergent forceps-assisted delivery
D) Administer oxygen to the pregnant woman

Question 15: Ms. Thompson, a 30-year-old G1P0, is admitted to the labor and delivery unit at 41 weeks gestation. Her prenatal course has been uncomplicated. During the assessment, her initial EFM tracing shows the following: Baseline rate: 170 bpm, variability: 30 bpm, and recurrent variable decelerations lasting 30 seconds. Which category does the EFM tracing belong to?
A) Category II
B) Category III
C) Category I
D) Category IV

Question 16: Which hormone is responsible for inducing uteroplacental vasodilation during pregnancy?
A) Progesterone
B) Estrogen
C) Oxytocin
D) Relaxin

Question 17: At 36 weeks gestation, Mrs. Rodriguez, a woman with gestational diabetes, is scheduled for an induction of labor. During the induction process, continuous fetal heart rate monitoring is initiated. What should the nurse be particularly vigilant about in this situation?
A) Fetal movement patterns
B) Uterine contractions
C) Blood glucose levels
D) Maternal blood pressure

Question 18: Mrs. Thompson, a 36-year-old gravida 3 para 2 at 28 weeks of gestation, presents with contractions and vaginal bleeding. Electronic fetal monitoring reveals regular, symmetrical FHR decelerations beginning at the onset of the contractions and persisting beyond their end. What is the most likely fetal dysrhythmia in this situation?
A) Late decelerations
B) Variable decelerations
C) Early decelerations
D) Prolonged decelerations

Question 19: Which fetal assessment method involves sampling and analysis of the fetal blood obtained from the umbilical cord?
A) Nonstress test (NST)
B) Biophysical profile (BPP)
C) Fetal blood sampling
D) Contraction stress test (CST)

Question 20: Emma, a 28-year-old primigravida, is in active labor and has an IUPC inserted. The nurse noticed a sudden decrease in the amplitude of uterine contractions on the monitor. Which of the following actions should the nurse take first?
A) Reposition the mother
B) Administer an IV fluid bolus
C) Administer oxygen to the mother
D) Call the obstetrician

Question 21: Which of the following is not a common cause of fetal bradycardia?
A) Maternal hypotension
B) Fetal anemia
C) Maternal hyperglycemia
D) Umbilical cord compression

Question 22: Which of the following is an effective method to minimize artifact in EFM?
A) Using adhesive electrodes
B) Ensuring tight electrode application
C) Providing clear instructions to the patient
D) All of the above

Question 23: How does gestational age influence fetal heart rate variability?
A) Variability decreases with increasing gestational age
B) Variability increases with increasing gestational age
C) Variability remains constant throughout gestational age
D) Variability is not influenced by gestational age

Question 24: Which of the following is a late deceleration pattern on the fetal heart rate monitoring strip?
A) Deceleration that occurs after a contraction
B) Deceleration that begins before the contraction peak and returns to baseline after the contraction ends
C) Deceleration that occurs randomly throughout labor
D) Deceleration that is prolonged and gradual in onset and recovery

Question 25: During anesthesia, which of the following factors has the greatest impact on fetal oxygenation?
A) Decreased maternal blood pressure
B) Increased maternal blood pressure
C) Decreased maternal heart rate
D) Increased maternal heart rate

Question 26: Which of the following is an abnormal biophysical profile score that suggests the need for further evaluation or intervention?
A) 8/10
B) 6/10
C) 4/8
D) 10/10

Question 27: When should an obstetrician be consulted for hypertonus during labor?
A) If the maternal blood pressure is elevated
B) If cervical dilation is less than 4 cm
C) If there is persistent fetal hypoxia
D) If the contractions are irregular

Question 28: Which type of diabetes is an autoimmune disease where the body's immune system mistakenly attacks and destroys the insulin-producing cells in the pancreas?
A) Type 1 diabetes
B) Type 2 diabetes
C) Gestational diabetes
D) None of the above

Question 29: In which situation would internal fetal heart rate monitoring be particularly useful?
A) When the mother is unable to tolerate external monitoring.
B) When the baby is in a breech position.
C) When the mother is in the early stage of labor.
D) When the caregiver wants to assess the maternal heart rate.

Question 30: Mrs. Rodriguez, a 29-year-old multiparous woman at 29 weeks gestation, presents with contractions every 2 minutes. During electronic fetal monitoring, there is a late deceleration noted in the fetal

heart rate (FHR) pattern. Which of the following is the most likely cause for this pattern?
A) Uterine hyperstimulation
B) Fetal hypoxemia
C) Maternal hypoglycemia
D) Fetal tachycardia

Question 31:   Mrs. Smith, a 34-year-old pregnant woman, is in her 30th week of pregnancy. She is scheduled for a biophysical profile (BPP) today. The BPP includes a fetal acoustic stimulation test. What is the purpose of including fetal acoustic stimulation in the BPP?
A) To assess fetal heart rate reactivity
B) To measure amniotic fluid volume
C) To evaluate fetal movements
D) To monitor fetal oxygenation

Question 32:   Which of the following statements about uterine activity is incorrect?
A) Uterine contractions help with cervical effacement and dilation.
B) The frequency of contractions is measured from the end of one contraction to the beginning of the next.
C) Intensity of contractions refers to the strength of the contraction.
D) Uterine activity has no impact on fetal heart rate.

Question 33:   Which of the following factors can affect uterine contraction intensity?
A) Maternal age
B) Fetal position
C) Uterine fibroids
D) Amniotic fluid volume

Question 34:   Liam, a 39-week gestation pregnant woman, is being monitored during labor. The fetal heart rate (FHR) pattern shows a smooth, wavelike motion with a uniform frequency of 2-4 cycles per minute. The FHR ranges between 110-150 beats per minute, and there are repetitive, prolonged decelerations after uterine contractions. What is the most likely interpretation of this FHR pattern?
A) Early decelerations
B) Variability
C) Variable decelerations
D) Sinusoidal pattern

Question 35:   Ms. Johnson, a 36-year-old woman at 38 weeks gestation, arrives at the labor and delivery unit. During her initial assessment, the nurse notes that the duration of her contractions is inconsistent. Which of the following information is correct about the duration of contractions?
A) Duration refers to the time from the beginning to the end of a contraction.
B) Duration should be less than 30 seconds for optimal uterine activity.
C) Duration is measured from the peak of one contraction to the peak of the next.
D) Duration is constant throughout labor stages.

Question 36:   Which of the following is NOT a possible cause of sinusoidal pattern in electronic fetal monitoring?
A) Fetal anemia
B) Maternal administration of opioids
C) Maternal hypotension
D) Acceleration in the fetal heart rate

Question 37:   Mrs. Johnson, a 28-year-old G2P1, presents to the labor and delivery unit at 39 weeks gestation. Her pregnancy is complicated by gestational diabetes, and she is currently on glyburide 10 mg daily. Her prenatal course has been uncomplicated, but she has a body mass index (BMI) of 32. Upon admission, her initial electronic fetal monitoring (EFM) shows the following tracing: Baseline rate: 140 bpm, variability: 7 bpm, and no decelerations. Which pattern is noted on the EFM tracing?
A) Category II
B) Category III
C) Category I
D) Category IV

Question 38:   Lisa, a 25-year-old pregnant woman, is being seen for a prenatal check-up at 36 weeks gestation. She asks her healthcare provider about the importance of fetal movement monitoring. Which of the following statements accurately explains the role of fetal movement monitoring?
A) Fetal movement monitoring is used to assess the fetal heart rate.
B) Fetal movement monitoring helps predict the due date.
C) Fetal movement monitoring provides an indirect measure of fetal well-being.
D) Fetal movement monitoring is not necessary during the third trimester.

Question 39:   What is the purpose of using an IUPC during labor?
A) To measure fetal heart rate
B) To assess maternal blood pressure
C) To evaluate cervical dilation
D) To monitor uterine contractions

Question 40:   Which maternal condition is associated with an increased risk of abnormal fetal heart rate patterns?
A) Gestational diabetes
B) Maternal smoking
C) Preeclampsia
D) Fetal hypoxia

Question 41:   Which uterine monitoring technique is used to measure the duration of contractions?
A) External monitoring
B) Internal monitoring
C) Toco transducer
D) Intrauterine pressure catheter

Question 42:   What is the role of uteroplacental circulation in drug transfer to the fetus?
A) Uteroplacental circulation actively transports drugs from the maternal circulation to the fetal circulation.
B) Uteroplacental circulation provides a barrier preventing drug transfer to the fetus.
C) Drug transfer to the fetus primarily occurs through the umbilical artery.
D) Uteroplacental circulation has no influence on drug transfer to the fetus.

Question 43:   A 34-year-old pregnant woman, Mrs. Smith, is in active labor at 41 weeks gestation. She has an epidural in place for pain management. The EFM tracing reveals persistent variable decelerations. Which of the following interventions should be implemented first?
A) Administer oxygen via facemask
B) Change the maternal position

C) Insert an intrauterine pressure catheter (IUPC)
D) Increase the rate of oxytocin infusion

Question 44: Which of the following measures should be taken to minimize the risk of patient harm during electronic fetal monitoring?
A) Ensuring the equipment is properly calibrated
B) Educating the patient about the procedure and any potential risks
C) Monitoring the maternal blood pressure regularly
D) Taking frequent breaks during the monitoring process

Question 45: Which of the following is the primary mechanism regulating blood flow to the placenta?
A) Oxygen tension,
B) Carbon dioxide tension,
C) Maternal blood pressure,
D) Fetal heart rate

Question 46: What is the optimal resting tone of the uterus between contractions during labor?
A) 0-5 mmHg
B) 6-10 mmHg
C) 11-15 mmHg
D) 16-20 mmHg

Question 47: Which of the following actions is essential for maintaining patient privacy during electronic fetal monitoring?
A) Using curtains or screens to create privacy during the procedure
B) Minimizing the number of healthcare providers present in the room
C) Avoiding unnecessary discussions about the patient in the presence of others
D) Allowing visitors to stay during the monitoring process

Question 48: Olivia, a 39-year-old pregnant woman, is receiving labor induction with oxytocin. She has an IUPC in place for monitoring uterine contractions. The nurse notices a sudden increase in the duration of contractions on the monitor. What should the nurse suspect as the most likely cause?
A) Uterine hyperstimulation
B) Fetal distress
C) Maternal fatigue
D) IUPC dislodgment

Question 49: Mr. and Mrs. Smith, a couple expecting their first child, arrive at the labor and delivery unit. Mrs. Smith is in labor, and the healthcare provider decides to perform external fetal monitoring. Which of the following is a potential limitation of external fetal monitoring?
A) Limited mobility for the mother during labor
B) Risk of infection to the fetus
C) Inaccuracy in assessing fetal heart rate
D) Inability to monitor uterine contractions

Question 50: Riley, a 38-week gestation pregnant woman, is being monitored during labor. The fetal heart rate (FHR) pattern shows a consistent smooth, wavelike motion with a uniform frequency of 3-5 cycles per minute. The FHR ranges between 120-160 beats per minute and there are no periodic changes. What is the most likely interpretation of this FHR pattern?
A) Early decelerations
B) Accelerations
C) Variable decelerations
D) Sinusoidal pattern

Question 51: Emma, a 26-year-old patient at 32 weeks of gestation, presents to the antepartum clinic for a routine check-up. Upon reviewing the EFM tracing, you notice a pattern of prolonged decelerations. Which of the following interventions is recommended for the management of prolonged decelerations?
A) Administering magnesium sulfate
B) Immediate delivery via cesarean section
C) Performing a fetal scalp blood sampling
D) Applying gentle fundal pressure

Question 52: Mr. Patel, a 35-year-old man, and his wife are planning to have a child. His wife has type 1 diabetes and is concerned about the risks during pregnancy. Which of the following statements is true regarding preconception counseling and diabetes?
A) Preconception counseling is not necessary for women with type 1 diabetes.
B) Glycemic control can be effectively achieved during pregnancy without preconception counseling.
C) Preconception counseling helps to optimize glycemic control before pregnancy.
D) Glycemic control during pregnancy has no impact on fetal outcomes.

Question 53: Sophie, a 30-year-old woman in her 39th week of pregnancy, arrives at the labor and delivery unit. She is experiencing regular contractions and her cervix is dilated at 4 cm. Fetal heart monitoring reveals a baseline heart rate of 130 bpm with episodic accelerations. Suddenly, a deceleration is noted that begins at the onset of a contraction and returns to baseline by the end of the contraction. Which of the following best describes this deceleration?
A) Early deceleration
B) Variable deceleration
C) Late deceleration
D) Prolonged deceleration

Question 54: A 28-year-old pregnant woman, Mrs. Smith, is in active labor. While monitoring her fetal heart rate, you notice baseline fluctuations accompanied by irregular oscillations in the tracing pattern. Upon further examination, you realize that these oscillations appear only on the paper printout and not on the monitor screen. What may cause this specific artifact?
A) Fetal movement
B) Maternal shivering
C) Power line interference
D) Mechanical transducer malfunction

Question 55: A pregnant patient has a BMI of 35, indicating obesity. Which maternal factor related to obesity can potentially impact fetal oxygenation?
A) Insulin resistance
B) Iron deficiency
C) Poor nutrition
D) Ovarian dysfunction

Question 56: Which maternal factor can potentially affect fetal oxygenation during labor?
A) Diabetes
B) Hypertension
C) Obesity
D) All of the above

Question 57: What is the purpose of uterine monitoring during pregnancy?
A) Assess uterine blood flow
B) Evaluate cervix dilation

C) Monitor fetal growth
D) Detect uterine contractions

Question 58: Which fetal presentation is most common in multiple gestations?
A) Vertex presentation
B) Breech presentation
C) Transverse presentation
D) Compound presentation

Question 59: Mrs. Johnson, a 32-year-old pregnant woman at 38 weeks gestation, comes to the antenatal clinic for a routine check-up. Her blood pressure is within normal limits, and there are no signs of preeclampsia. During the visit, Mrs. Johnson asks about the uteroplacental circulation. Which of the following statements accurately describes uteroplacental circulation?
A) Uteroplacental circulation begins at the umbilical cord and ends at the placenta.
B) Uteroplacental circulation is responsible for transporting oxygen and nutrients from the placenta to the fetus.
C) Uteroplacental circulation involves the flow of deoxygenated blood from the fetus to the placenta.
D) Uteroplacental circulation is primarily regulated by the maternal kidneys.

Question 60: Mrs. Thompson, a 32-year-old G2P1, is admitted to the labor and delivery unit. The external fetal heart rate tracing shows late decelerations. Which of the following actions should the nurse take first?
A) Administer oxygen to the mother
B) Reposition the mother
C) Increase the intravenous fluid rate
D) Perform a vaginal examination

Question 61: Olivia, a 36-year-old woman at 39 weeks of gestation, is in labor and receiving oxytocin augmentation. Her uterine contractions are frequent and intense, lasting longer than 90 seconds. On continuous fetal monitoring, the FHR tracing shows prolonged decelerations. Which of the following is the most likely cause of these decelerations?
A) Uteroplacental insufficiency
B) Maternal hypotension
C) Fetal head compression
D) Nuchal cord

Question 62: Which fetal assessment method provides continuous monitoring of fetal heart rate, uterine activity, and fetal movement?
A) Nonstress test (NST)
B) Biophysical profile (BPP)
C) Fetal blood sampling
D) Contraction stress test (CST)

Question 63: What is the management approach for high-frequency contractions during labor?
A) Administer tocolytic medications
B) Monitor fetal heart rate closely
C) Encourage maternal rest and hydration
D) Perform a vaginal examination

Question 64: Which fetal assessment method involves the measurement of the fetal heart rate in response to fetal movement?
A) Nonstress test (NST)
B) Biophysical profile (BPP)
C) Fetal blood sampling
D) Contraction stress test (CST)

Question 65: Sarah, a 32-year-old pregnant woman, is scheduled for a non-stress test to evaluate fetal well-being. What does a non-stress test involve?
A) Measurement of fetal heart rate variability
B) Visualization of the placental position
C) Assessment of fetal movements
D) Evaluation of amniotic fluid volume

Question 66: Which of the following is a potential complication for the neonate of a mother with poorly controlled diabetes during pregnancy?
A) Macrosomia
B) Premature rupture of membranes
C) Ectopic pregnancy
D) Gestational hypertension

Question 67: Which of the following placental factors can contribute to fetal hypoxia?
A) Maternal hypertension
B) Umbilical cord compression
C) Placental abruption
D) Placenta previa

Question 68: Which of the following refers to the variation in the fetal heart rate (FHR) over time?
A) Fetal heart rate variability
B) Fetal distress
C) Fetal bradycardia
D) Fetal tachycardia

Question 69: Mrs. Johnson, 32-year-old G2P1, presents to the labor and delivery unit at 38 weeks gestation with decreased fetal movements. On admission, the fetal heart rate (FHR) tracing reveals a baseline of 140 bpm, with minimal variability, infrequent accelerations, no decelerations, and no contractions. What is the most appropriate next step in management?
A) Begin continuous external fetal monitoring
B) Administer oxygen via face mask
C) Perform a contraction stress test
D) Order a biophysical profile score

Question 70: Which hormone, secreted by the placenta, is responsible for maintaining the corpus luteum during early pregnancy?
A) Human Chorionic Gonadotropin (hCG)
B) Estrogen
C) Progesterone
D) Follicle-Stimulating Hormone (FSH)

Question 71: Which factor is NOT associated with an increased risk of uterine rupture/scar dehiscence?
A) Previous cesarean section
B) Use of oxytocin for labor induction or augmentation
C) Maternal age over 35
D) Pregnancy with multiple gestations

Question 72: Mrs. Johnson, a 38-year-old G3P2 at 38 weeks of gestation, presents to the antenatal clinic with complaints of decreased fetal movements for the past 24 hours. Her last ultrasound was 4 weeks ago and showed no abnormalities. On fetal monitoring, you notice a persistent loss of beat-to-beat variability of the fetal heart rate below 5 bpm for more than 10 minutes. What is the most appropriate course of action?
A) Perform a biophysical profile (BPP) immediately
B) Administer intravenous fluids to the mother
C) Administer oxygen via a non-rebreather face mask
D) Schedule a follow-up appointment in 1 week

Question 73: Mrs. Smith, a 35-year-old pregnant woman, presents for a follow-up visit at 30 weeks gestation. She is pregnant with monoamniotic-monochorionic twins. What is the most important concern for this type of twin pregnancy?
A) Increased risk of preterm delivery
B) Increased risk of fetal anomalies
C) Increased risk of placental abruption
D) Increased risk of gestational diabetes

Question 74: Which of the following actions helps in preventing infection during electronic fetal monitoring?
A) Proper hand hygiene before and after the procedure
B) Using sterile gloves during the procedure
C) Administering antibiotics prophylactically to the patient
D) Avoiding the use of lubricating jelly

Question 75: Which of the following infections can be transmitted to the fetus through the placenta?
A) Urinary tract infection
B) Chlamydia
C) Syphilis
D) Influenza

Question 76: Miss Johnson, a 32-year-old primigravida at 38 weeks gestation, presents to the labor and delivery unit with contractions every 3 minutes. The fetal heart rate (FHR) is 150 beats per minute (bpm) with good variability and no decelerations. The nurse performs a scalp pH analysis, which reveals a pH of 7.24. What is the interpretation of the fetal scalp pH in this situation?
A) Acidemia
B) Normal pH
C) Alkalemia
D) Acidosis

Question 77: Which fetal complication is characterized by a sudden, transient increase in the fetal heart rate?
A) Fetal bradycardia
B) Fetal tachycardia
C) Fetal distress
D) Fetal acidemia

Question 78: Emma, a 30-year-old primigravida with chronic essential hypertension, is regularly monitored for her blood pressure throughout her pregnancy. At a routine antenatal visit, her blood pressure is measured as 140/90 mmHg. Which additional investigations should be considered for Emma?
A) Fasting blood glucose
B) Complete blood count (CBC)
C) Renal ultrasound
D) 24-hour urine protein collection

Question 79: Mrs. Patel, a 26-year-old pregnant woman at 40 weeks gestation with a previous cesarean delivery, presents to triage with lower abdominal pain and a feeling of "something tearing." On examination, the cervix is closed and the fetal heart rate tracing shows prolonged fetal bradycardia. An ultrasound reveals a retroplacental hematoma. What is the most likely diagnosis?
A) Placental abruption
B) Uterine rupture
C) Placenta previa
D) Vasa previa

Question 80: Amanda, a 35-year-old woman in her 40th week of pregnancy, is in active labor. Fetal heart monitoring reveals a baseline heart rate of 140 bpm with occasional decelerations. The decelerations are visually apparent, vary in duration and depth, and do not correlate with contractions. Which of the following best describes these decelerations?
A) Early deceleration
B) Variable deceleration
C) Late deceleration
D) Prolonged deceleration

Question 81: Mrs. Johnson, a 34-year-old pregnant woman with a history of gestational diabetes, presents for her routine antenatal check-up at 32 weeks gestation. Upon auscultation of the fetal heart rate (FHR), the nurse hears a continuous, high-pitched, musical sound superimposed on the maternal heart rate. This sound is most likely due to:
A) Fetal tachycardia
B) Fetal bradycardia
C) Fetal heart murmur
D) Maternal arterial bruit

Question 82: Ms. Johnson, a 40-year-old woman, is at 41 weeks gestation and is undergoing induction of labor due to post-term pregnancy. Her electronic fetal monitoring (EFM) shows sinusoidal fetal heart rate pattern persisting for more than 30 minutes. Which of the following should the nurse do first?
A) Administer intravenous fluids to the patient
B) Perform a vaginal examination to assess cervical dilatation
C) Initiate continuous electronic fetal monitoring
D) Notify the obstetrician for further evaluation

Question 83: Which maternal complication is commonly associated with postdates pregnancy?
A) Gestational diabetes
B) Preeclampsia
C) Postpartum hemorrhage
D) Placenta previa

Question 84: Which intervention is most effective in preventing preterm labor in women with a history of preterm birth?
A) Progesterone supplementation
B) Bed rest
C) Induction of labor
D) Increased fluid intake

Question 85: Mrs. Johnson, a 32-year-old pregnant woman, presents to the antenatal clinic for her routine check-up. Which of the following statements accurately describes the fetal circulation?
A) Oxygenated blood is carried from the placenta to the fetus through the umbilical artery.
B) The foramen ovale connects the right and left atria of the fetal heart.
C) The ductus arteriosus connects the pulmonary artery and the aorta in the fetal heart.
D) The umbilical vein carries oxygenated blood from the fetus to the placenta.

Question 86: Mrs. Adams, a 38-year-old pregnant woman, presents to the labor and delivery unit with decreased fetal movement. Upon examination, the fetal heart rate tracing reveals a baseline heart rate of 160 beats per minute with moderate variability, accelerations, and no decelerations. The nurse notifies

the physician who orders further monitoring. Which of the following statements is true regarding the legal implications of this scenario?
A) The nurse is responsible for notifying the physician promptly.
B) The physician is responsible for taking appropriate actions based on the nurse's notification.
C) Both the nurse and physician share the responsibility for the fetal monitoring process.
D) Only the physician is accountable for the monitoring process.

Question 87: Julia, a 36-year-old primigravida at 32 weeks gestation, presents to the antenatal clinic with concerns about decreased fetal movements. Upon fetal heart rate monitoring, you notice a variability pattern that is almost absent. Which of the following factors can contribute to decreased fetal heart rate variability?
A) Maternal diabetes
B) Fetal sleep cycle
C) Maternal smoking
D) Fetal anemia

Question 88: A 28-year-old woman at 39 weeks of gestation is in active labor. The nurse notices an irregular, unstable baseline fetal heart rate tracing with frequent signal dropouts. The fetal heart rate tracing becomes difficult to interpret due to signal ambiguity. What could be a potential cause of this signal ambiguity?
A) Fetal movement
B) Poor electrode connection
C) Maternal tachycardia
D) Electronic interference

Question 89: Mrs. Adams, at 38 weeks gestation, is in active labor. You decide to initiate continuous external fetal monitoring for accurate assessment of fetal well-being. Which device would you use for this purpose?
A) Fetal heart rate monitor
B) Doppler ultrasound
C) Electronic fetal monitor
D) Tocodynamometer

Question 90: Maternal obesity is associated with an increased risk of which of the following complications during pregnancy?
A) Gestational diabetes
B) Preterm birth
C) Shoulder dystocia
D) Preeclampsia

Question 91: In cases of fetal demise, which of the following findings is most likely to be observed on the fetal heart rate tracing?
A) Absent variability
B) Accelerations
C) Early decelerations
D) Fetal tachycardia

Question 92: Sarah, a 32-year-old pregnant woman at 28 weeks gestation, is admitted to the labor and delivery unit with signs of preterm labor. The nurse is preparing to monitor the uterine contractions using an internal uterine pressure catheter. Which of the following statements accurately describes the use of an internal uterine pressure catheter for uterine monitoring?
A) It is a non-invasive method of monitoring uterine contractions

B) It provides more accurate measurement of uterine contractions compared to an external tocodynamometer
C) It does not require rupture of the membranes
D) It is contraindicated in cases of placenta previa

Question 93: Emily, a 26-year-old pregnant woman at 40 weeks of gestation, is being monitored using electronic fetal monitoring. The fetal heart rate has a baseline variability of 4-6 bpm. What action should the healthcare provider take based on this finding?
A) Inform the patient that this is a normal finding.
B) Administer oxygen to the mother to improve fetal oxygenation.
C) Prepare for immediate delivery as this indicates fetal distress.
D) Increase intravenous fluid administration to improve fetal circulation.

Question 94: What is the typical frequency range for uterine contractions during the active phase of labor?
A) 1-3 contractions in 10 minutes
B) 4-7 contractions in 10 minutes
C) 8-10 contractions in 10 minutes
D) 11-15 contractions in 10 minutes

Question 95: Emma, a 30-year-old pregnant woman at 39 weeks of gestation, presents to the labor and delivery unit with a history of decreased fetal movement. The healthcare provider decides to perform an external fetal monitoring test to assess the well-being of the fetus. Which of the following findings would indicate a non-reassuring fetal status?
A) Fetal heart rate of 150 bpm
B) Absence of accelerations in the fetal heart rate
C) Reactive non-stress test
D) Uterine contractions lasting 60 seconds

Question 96: What is the primary risk associated with internal fetal heart rate monitoring?
A) Increased risk of infection.
B) Higher cost compared to external monitoring.
C) Limited mobility during labor.
D) Difficulty in obtaining a clear signal.

Question 97: Emma, a 38-year-old pregnant woman, is scheduled for a routine ultrasound at 20 weeks gestation. What information can be obtained from this fetal assessment method?
A) Fetal heart rate
B) Fetal movements
C) Placental position
D) Fetal weight

Question 98: What is the recommended management for uterine rupture/scar dehiscence?
A) Immediate vaginal delivery
B) Emergency cesarean section
C) Administration of tocolytic agents
D) Observation without intervention

Question 99: Lisa, a 35-year-old pregnant woman at 39 weeks' gestation, is admitted to the labor and delivery unit. The healthcare provider is monitoring her uterine activity and observes that the contractions last for 75 seconds from the start of one contraction to the start of the next contraction. What is the frequency of Lisa's contractions?
A) 1 contraction every 75 seconds
B) 1 contraction every 150 seconds
C) 1 contraction every 225 seconds

D) 2 contractions every 75 seconds

Question 100: Mrs. Smith, a 28-year-old primigravida at 38 weeks of gestation, is admitted to the labor and delivery unit in active labor. The electronic fetal monitoring (EFM) reveals repetitive late decelerations in the fetal heart rate (FHR) tracing. Which of the following interventions should be implemented immediately?
A) Administer intravenous fluids
B) Change the mother's position
C) Administer oxygen to the mother
D) Perform an episiotomy

Question 101: Mrs. Adams, a primigravida at 38 weeks of gestation, presents to the labor and delivery unit. The initial assessment indicates a normal fetal heart rate of 140 beats per minute, moderate variability, no accelerations or decelerations, and a resting uterine tone of 10 mmHg. What does this resting tone value indicate?
A) Hypertonic uterus
B) Hypotonic uterus
C) Normal uterine activity
D) Hyperstimulation

Question 102: What is a common cause of decreased fetal heart rate variability?
A) Maternal hypertension
B) Uterine contractions
C) Fetal head compression during labor
D) Fetal tachycardia

Question 103: Mr. Smith, a 26-year-old expectant father, rushes his wife into the emergency room at 38 weeks gestation. The nurse assesses the fetal heart rate at 100 bpm. The mother reports no history of medical complications during pregnancy. Upon further examination, the nurse notes no fetal movement, and variable decelerations are present on the fetal monitor strip. What is the most appropriate nursing action?
A) Administer a tocolytic medication to the mother
B) Administer oxygen to the mother
C) Perform a biophysical profile
D) Prepare for immediate delivery

Question 104: Which of the following is NOT a risk factor for gestational hypertension?
A) Obesity
B) Teenage pregnancy
C) History of preeclampsia in previous pregnancies
D) Multiple gestation

Question 105: Mrs. Thompson, a 30-year-old pregnant woman, is pregnant with dizygotic twins. What is the most common zygosity of twin pregnancies?
A) Dizygotic
B) Monozygotic
C) Triplet
D) Quadruplet

Question 106: Which of the following interventions is recommended for a pregnant woman with diabetes to reduce the risk of fetal complications?
A) Increased caffeine intake
B) Regular physical exercise
C) Smoking cessation
D) Heavy alcohol consumption

Question 107: What does the principle of justice entail in medical ethics?

A) Respecting the patient's right to autonomy and self-determination
B) Promoting equality in the distribution of healthcare resources
C) Upholding the confidentiality and privacy of patient information
D) Acting in the patient's best interest while ensuring no harm is done

Question 108: Which maternal condition is associated with an increased risk of preterm labor?
A) Gestational diabetes
B) Hypertension
C) Ovarian cysts
D) Thyroid disorders

Question 109: Emma, a 25-year-old pregnant woman at 20 weeks gestation, presents to the emergency department with fever, cough, and shortness of breath. Chest X-ray reveals bilateral pneumonia. Laboratory tests show lymphopenia and thrombocytopenia. Polymerase chain reaction (PCR) testing confirms the diagnosis of H1N1 influenza. What is the most appropriate management for this patient's condition?
A) Initiate antiviral treatment with oseltamivir within 48 hours of symptom onset
B) Prescribe an antibiotic course targeting atypical pathogens
C) Admit the patient to the intensive care unit for close monitoring
D) Recommend bed rest and symptomatic treatment only

Question 110: Which of the following statements regarding contractions is true?
A) Contractions in the active phase of labor are usually irregular.
B) Contractions in the latent phase of labor are usually intense and frequent.
C) Contractions in the active phase of labor are characterized by a shorter duration.
D) Contractions in the latent phase of labor are typically less painful.

Question 111: Which of the following hormones is responsible for initiating labor contractions?
A) Estrogen
B) Progesterone
C) Oxytocin
D) Prostaglandins

Question 112: The intensity of uterine contractions is measured in which unit?
A) Volts
B) Amps
C) Millimeters of Mercury (mmHg)
D) Montvield Units (MU)

Question 113: Which recreational drug is known to cause vasoconstriction and decrease uterine blood flow, potentially compromising fetal oxygenation?
A) Marijuana
B) Cocaine
C) Alcohol
D) LSD

Question 114: You are a certified EFM professional working in a hospital setting. On your shift, you notice a fellow healthcare professional mishandling the fetal monitoring equipment, resulting in inaccurate readings. What is your ethical responsibility in this situation?

A) Ignore the situation and assume someone else will address the issue.
B) Confront the healthcare professional and criticize their actions.
C) Report the incident to a supervisor or the appropriate authority.
D) Retrain the healthcare professional on the proper use of the equipment.

Question 115: What is the most common cause of cord compression during labor?
A) Maternal positioning
B) Uterine contraction
C) Umbilical cord prolapse
D) Fetal movement

Question 116: Emma, a 34-year-old multigravida at 38 weeks gestation, is in active labor and being monitored. During a vaginal examination, you observe meconium-stained amniotic fluid. Subsequently, you notice repetitive variable decelerations on the fetal heart rate monitor. What is the most appropriate management in this situation?
A) Perform a fetal scalp pH sampling
B) Administer oxygen to the mother
C) Prepare for immediate cesarean section
D) Continue monitoring while awaiting the second stage of labor

Question 117: A 39-year-old pregnant woman, Mrs. Anderson, is receiving oxytocin augmentation for labor induction. The EFM is displaying a high frequency of uterine activity on the tracing. Which of the following troubleshooting steps should the nurse take first?
A) Verify the accuracy of the tocodynamometer placement
B) Stop the oxytocin infusion
C) Change the mother's position
D) Assess the mother for signs of uterine hyperstimulation

Question 118: Sarah, a 65-year-old female patient, is admitted to the medical-surgical unit with a diagnosis of pneumonia. The healthcare provider prescribes levofloxacin 500 mg IV infusion every 24 hours. Before administering the medication, what is the nurse's priority action?
A) Assess the patient's vital signs and document the findings.
B) Verify the patient's allergy history and previous adverse reactions.
C) Review the patient's laboratory results, specifically renal function.
D) Teach the patient about potential side effects and adverse reactions.

Question 119: Mrs. Lewis, a 35-year-old woman at 32 weeks of gestation, presents to the hospital with decreased fetal movement. Electronic fetal monitoring shows a sinusoidal fetal heart rate pattern accompanied by decreased fetal movements. What condition is most likely associated with this finding?
A) Gestational diabetes
B) Fetal anemia
C) Preeclampsia
D) Fetal tachycardia

Question 120: Mrs. Thompson, a 33-year-old pregnant woman at 30 weeks of gestation, is diagnosed with a first-degree atrioventricular (AV) block in her fetus. What is the recommended management for this condition?
A) Immediate medical termination of the pregnancy.

B) Serial fetal echocardiography every week to assess progression.
C) Expectant management with no specific interventions.
D) Initiation of transplacental therapy with corticosteroids.

Question 121: Which of the following statements regarding tachysystole is correct?
A) Tachysystole is defined as less than five contractions in ten minutes.
B) Tachysystole is defined as more than two contractions in ten minutes.
C) Tachysystole is a normal variant in fetal heart rate.
D) Tachysystole is usually characterized by a decrease in uterine activity.

Question 122: Emily, a 32-year-old pregnant woman at 38 weeks of gestation, is admitted to the labor and delivery unit. During labor, the fetal heart rate (FHR) is continuously monitored. The nurse observes a FHR pattern with a baseline rate of 170 bpm, minimal variability, and repetitive late decelerations. The contractions are occurring every 1.5 minutes with a duration of 60 seconds. The nurse suspects tachysystole. Which intervention should the nurse prioritize?
A) Administer tocolytic medication to decrease contractions.
B) Facilitate a change in maternal position.
C) Administer oxygen via face mask at 10L/min.
D) Prepare for an emergency cesarean delivery.

Question 123: Which of the following best describes a prolonged deceleration pattern on the fetal heart rate tracing?
A) A deceleration lasting 10-15 seconds.
B) A deceleration lasting 30 seconds or longer.
C) A deceleration with a gradual onset and return to baseline.
D) A deceleration with a quick onset and rapid return to baseline.

Question 124: Which of the following is not a common cause of hypoxemia in the fetus?
A) Placental insufficiency
B) Maternal hypotension
C) Fetal anemia
D) Maternal hyperoxygenation

Question 125: What is the primary principle of medical ethics?
A) Autonomy
B) Beneficence
C) Non-maleficence
D) Justice

Question 126: Which of the following can cause artifact in electronic fetal monitoring (EFM)?
A) Maternal movement
B) Fetal movement
C) Loose electrodes
D) All of the above

Question 127: Which of the following statements is true regarding variable decelerations in fetal heart rate?
A) Variable decelerations are caused by umbilical cord compression.
B) Variable decelerations are characterized by a gradual decrease in FHR followed by an abrupt return to baseline.
C) Variable decelerations are classified as early decelerations.

D) Variable decelerations are usually associated with fetal head compression.

Question 128:   Which maternal factor can result in decreased fetal oxygenation due to reduced blood volume?
A) Maternal anemia
B) Gestational diabetes
C) Hypothyroidism
D) None of the above

Question 129:   During electronic fetal monitoring, the nurse observes a pattern of uterine contractions with a duration exceeding 90 seconds. Which of the following conditions is associated with prolonged uterine contractions?
A) Uterine tachysystole
B) Uterine hyperstimulation syndrome
C) Hypotonic uterine dysfunction
D) Hypertonic uterine dysfunction

Question 130:   Mrs. Thompson, a 37-year-old woman at 39 weeks of gestation, presents to the labor and delivery unit with bright red vaginal bleeding. On examination, the cervix appears closed. The fetal heart rate tracing shows minimal variability. Which placental factor is most likely responsible for this presentation?
A) Placental abruption
B) Placenta previa
C) Uterine rupture
D) Placental insufficiency

Question 131:   Which fetal surveillance test is recommended for postdates pregnancy?
A) Non-stress test (NST)
B) Biophysical profile (BPP)
C) Amniotic fluid index (AFI)
D) Doppler velocimetry

Question 132:   Which maternal position should be avoided to prevent cord compression?
A) Supine position
B) Lateral position
C) Semi-Fowler's position
D) Trendelenburg position

Question 133:   Ms. Thompson, a 19-year-old primigravida at 34 weeks of gestation, presents to the antenatal clinic for a routine check-up. On examination, her fundal height is lower than expected for her gestational age. Which of the following uteroplacental complications is most commonly associated with small-for-gestational-age fetuses?
A) Placental abruption
B) Uterine rupture
C) Placenta previa
D) Placenta accreta

Question 134:   Susan, a 28-year-old patient in her 32nd week of pregnancy, is scheduled for an emergency appendectomy under general anesthesia. The anesthetist administers an inhalation anesthetic agent. Which of the following effects is MOST likely to occur in the fetus?
A) Decreased fetal heart rate variability
B) Increased fetal movement
C) Elevated fetal arterial oxygen saturation
D) Increased uterine blood flow

Question 135:   During electronic fetal monitoring, the nurse notes that the intensity of the uterine contractions is within the normal range. Which of the following classifications would be appropriate for normal uterine contractions?
A) Less than 25mmHg
B) 50-60mmHg
C) 100-120mmHg
D) Greater than 150mmHg

Question 136:   Mrs. Wilson is a 30-year-old multigravida at 42 weeks gestation with postdates pregnancy. She is scheduled for induction of labor. Which one of the following is the most appropriate method for cervical ripening in this situation?
A) Prostaglandin E2 gel
B) Cervical Foley catheter
C) Oxytocin infusion
D) Amniotomy

Question 137:   Which pattern in electronic fetal monitoring represents a normal baseline heart rate variability?
A) Absence of variability
B) Minimal variability
C) Moderate variability
D) Marked variability

Question 138:   Mrs. Anderson, a 28-year-old pregnant woman at 41 weeks low transverse cesarean delivery, presents to the labor and delivery unit in active labor. She has a previous history of precipitous labor. During labor, she experiences sudden increased pain, fetal distress, and loss of contraction pattern. On examination, the fetal head is palpable above the symphysis pubis and there is bulging of the abdominal wall. What is the most likely diagnosis?
A) Uterine rupture
B) Amniotic fluid embolism
C) Placental abruption
D) Placenta previa

Question 139:   Sarah, a 26-year-old pregnant woman at 28 weeks of gestation, visits the antenatal clinic for a routine check-up. She reports experiencing irregular contractions. Which of the following terms best describes this pattern of uterine activity?
A) Contractions of labor
B) Prodromal labor
C) Hypertonic contractions
D) Hypotonic contractions

Question 140:   Which of the following is a correct procedure for applying the transducer during external fetal heart rate monitoring?
A) Placing the transducer over the umbilical cord
B) Applying excessive pressure to the transducer
C) Positioning the transducer close to the maternal back
D) Ensuring proper contact and alignment with the fetal heart

Question 141:   Which of the following factors can contribute to decreased blood flow to the fetus?
A) Maternal hypertension
B) Fetal tachycardia
C) Placental abruption
D) Maternal hyperglycemia

Question 142:   Which infection poses the highest risk to the fetus during pregnancy?

A) Urinary tract infection
B) Hepatitis B
C) Influenza
D) Rubella

Question 143: Which of the following is a potential uteroplacental complication during pregnancy?
A) Placenta previa
B) Polyhydramnios
C) Preeclampsia
D) Gestational diabetes

Question 144: Mr. Thompson's wife, a 32-year-old primigravida, is currently in labor. The nurse detects variable decelerations in the fetal heart rate (FHR) tracing. Which of the following would be the most appropriate initial action by the nurse?
A) Reassess the client's blood pressure
B) Administer oxygen via face mask to the client
C) Reposition the client
D) Prepare for a rapid delivery

Question 145: What is the normal frequency range of contractions during active labor?
A) 2 to 4 contractions in 10 minutes
B) 5 to 7 contractions in 10 minutes
C) 8 to 10 contractions in 10 minutes
D) 11 to 13 contractions in 10 minutes

Question 146: Sophia, a 25-year-old pregnant woman, is admitted to the labor and delivery unit. She has a history of previous cesarean delivery and is being monitored for uterine contractions. Which of the following statements is true regarding the use of electronic monitoring equipment for uterine contractions in this scenario?
A) Electronic monitoring equipment is not suitable for monitoring uterine contractions in women with a history of previous cesarean delivery.
B) External monitoring devices are more accurate than internal monitoring devices for assessing uterine contractions in this scenario.
C) Internal monitoring devices are preferred for accurate assessment of uterine contractions in women with a history of previous cesarean delivery.
D) Electronic monitoring equipment should only be used during the active phase of labor in this scenario.

Question 147: Mrs. Davis, a 28-year-old G1P0, is in active labor. The external fetal heart rate tracing shows variable decelerations. Which of the following interventions is appropriate for this situation?
A) Administer oxygen to the mother
B) Perform a fetal scalp blood sample
C) Initiate continuous fetal monitoring
D) Perform an amniotomy

Question 148: Which drug used for therapeutic purposes is known to potentially cause fetal respiratory depression?
A) Antihypertensive medications
B) Antibiotics
C) Analgesics
D) Antidiabetic medications

Question 149: Which pattern of fetal heart rate variability is characterized by a flat line with no discernible variability?
A) Moderate Variability
B) Marked Variability

C) Minimal Variability
D) Absent Variability

Question 150: A hospital implements a new electronic fetal monitoring (EFM) system to enhance the monitoring and assessment of fetal well-being. The staff undergo training on the new system, and clinical practice guidelines are updated accordingly. However, after a few weeks, it becomes evident that some healthcare providers are still struggling to use the system effectively. What is the most appropriate action to address this quality issue?
A) Ignore the issue as some healthcare providers may never fully adapt to the new system.
B) Provide additional training and support to the healthcare providers who are struggling.
C) Remove the new EFM system and revert to the old paper-based monitoring method.
D) Punish the healthcare providers who are struggling to use the new EFM system.

Question 151: What is the threshold blood pressure for diagnosing gestational hypertension?
A) Systolic ? 120 mm Hg or diastolic ? 80 mm Hg
B) Systolic ? 140 mm Hg or diastolic ? 90 mm Hg
C) Systolic ? 160 mm Hg or diastolic ? 100 mm Hg
D) Systolic ? 180 mm Hg or diastolic ? 110 mm Hg

Question 152: Tachycardia in fetal monitoring is defined as a baseline heart rate greater than:
A) 100 bpm
B) 110 bpm
C) 120 bpm
D) 130 bpm

Question 153: Which of the following is considered a normal range for fetal movements during a 60-minute period?
A) Less than 5 movements
B) 5 to 10 movements
C) 10 to 20 movements
D) More than 20 movements

Question 154: Which intervention is recommended for a fetus with bradycardia that persists despite maternal repositioning?
A) Amnioinfusion
B) Oxytocin augmentation
C) Fetal scalp stimulation
D) Epidural administration

Question 155: Sarah, a 28-year-old pregnant woman at 36 weeks' gestation, is in labor. The nurse is monitoring her uterine activity and notes that the contractions last for 45 seconds from the start of one contraction to the start of the next contraction. What is the frequency of Sarah's contractions?
A) 1 contraction every 30 seconds
B) 1 contraction every 45 seconds
C) 1 contraction every 90 seconds
D) 2 contractions every 45 seconds

Question 156: A fetal baseline heart rate above 160 bpm may indicate:
A) Fetal distress
B) Maternal distress
C) Normal variation
D) Positional change

Question 157:   Isabella, a 25-year-old pregnant woman, has an IUPC inserted for uterine monitoring during labor. The nurse notices irregular baseline fluctuations on the monitor that are not related to uterine contractions. What condition should the nurse suspect as the potential cause?
A) Fetal tachycardia
B) Uterine rupture
C) Chorioamnionitis
D) Cord compression

Question 158:   Which of the following is a characteristic pattern associated with tachycardia in fetal monitoring?
A) Sinusoidal pattern
B) Early decelerations
C) Variable decelerations
D) Accelerations

Question 159:   During a prenatal check-up, a pregnant patient reports smoking cigarettes regularly. Which maternal factor is likely to be affected by this behavior and influence fetal oxygenation?
A) Respiratory rate
B) Cardiac output
C) Blood pressure
D) Hemoglobin levels

Question 160:   Which condition is characterized by the premature separation of the placenta from the uterine wall?
A) Placenta Previa
B) Placental Abruption
C) Uterine Rupture
D) Cord Prolapse

Question 161:   Mrs. Thompson, a 28-year-old pregnant woman, at 36 weeks gestation is admitted to the labor and delivery unit with known preterm labor and ruptured membranes. Upon examination, the cervix is found to be 4cm dilated and 60% effaced. A fetal heart tracing shows late decelerations. What intervention would you prioritize?
A) Administer corticosteroids for fetal lung maturation
B) Prepare the patient for immediate delivery via cesarean section
C) Initiate magnesium sulfate therapy for fetal neuroprotection
D) Prepare the patient for vaginal delivery with continuous fetal monitoring

Question 162:   Laura, a 26-year-old patient, presents for an elective surgery under general anesthesia. Her obstetric history reveals that she had two previous cesarean sections. Which of the following factors related to previous cesarean section may increase the risk of complications during anesthesia?
A) Increased uterine blood flow
B) Formation of adhesions
C) Decreased risk of uterine rupture
D) Enhanced tolerance to anesthetic agents

Question 163:   True or False: Fetal heart rate accelerations are a reliable indicator of fetal acidemia.
A) True
B) False

Question 164:   A 28-year-old pregnant woman, Mrs. Wilson, at 39 weeks gestation presents for a nonstress test. The fetal heart rate baseline is 120 bpm, with absent variability. No accelerations or decelerations are seen during the 20-minute test. What is the interpretation of this nonstress test?
A) Reactive
B) Nonreactive
C) Equivocal
D) Abnormal

Question 165:   Which of the following is a risk factor for the development of gestational hypertension?
A) Obesity
B) Nulliparity
C) Young maternal age
D) Multiparity

Question 166:   Patient: Mrs. Smith, a 35-year-old pregnant woman at 36 weeks gestation, presents with right upper quadrant pain, malaise, and nausea. Her blood pressure is 150/90 mmHg. Laboratory results show elevated liver enzymes and normal platelet count. What is the most appropriate management for this patient?
A) Immediate delivery
B) Administer antihypertensive medication
C) Start prophylactic antibiotics
D) Encourage bed rest

Question 167:   Mrs. Smith, a 33-year-old multigravida at 37 weeks of gestation, presents with severe hypertension and proteinuria. Which of the following medications is contraindicated in the management of her condition?
A) Magnesium sulfate
B) Hydralazine
C) Labetalol
D) Nifedipine

Question 168:   Ms. Anderson, a 35-year-old G5P4, is in active labor. The external fetal heart rate tracing reveals prolonged decelerations. Which of the following interventions is appropriate for this situation?
A) Administer oxygen to the mother
B) Perform a fetal scalp blood sample
C) Apply pressure to the fetal head
D) Perform a Cesarean section

Question 169:   Beth, a 28-year-old patient at 38 weeks of gestation, comes to the antepartum unit for monitoring due to decreased fetal movement. On the electronic fetal monitoring (EFM), you observe a pattern of prolonged decelerations. What is the most appropriate intervention in this situation?
A) Administer oxygen via a face mask
B) Perform a scalp stimulation test
C) Place the patient in the Trendelenburg position
D) Start an IV infusion of oxytocin

Question 170:   Which of the following is a characteristic feature of preeclampsia-eclampsia?
A) Hypotension
B) Decreased proteinuria
C) Severe headaches
D) Normal fetal heart rate

Question 171:   Mrs. John, a 35-year-old patient, is scheduled for a cesarean section under regional anesthesia. The anesthetist administers a spinal block. Which of the following maternal physiologic changes is MOST likely to occur following the administration of spinal anesthesia?

A) Decreased cardiac output
B) Decreased uterine blood flow
C) Increased blood pressure
D) Increased respiratory rate

Question 172: In cases of chronic (essential) hypertension during pregnancy, close monitoring of which fetal parameter is crucial?
A) Fetal heart rate variability
B) Fetal movement count
C) Fetal growth rate
D) Fetal limb movements

Question 173: Lisa, a 30-year-old G4P3 woman at 32 weeks gestation, is found to have a positive screening test for hepatitis B surface antigen (HBsAg). What is the most appropriate management for this patient?
A) Administer a prophylactic dose of hepatitis B immune globulin (HBIG) and initiate hepatitis B vaccination to the newborn
B) Recommend hepatitis B vaccination to the newborn, but no need for HBIG administration
C) Delay HBIG administration until after delivery and then initiate hepatitis B vaccination to the newborn
D) There is no need for any intervention in pregnancy for HBsAg-positive mothers

Question 174: Which of the following is a characteristic of a reactive nonstress test (NST)?
A) Fetal heart rate accelerations of 10 bpm for at least 10 seconds, occurring twice in a 20-minute period
B) Fetal heart rate decelerations of 10 bpm for at least 10 seconds, occurring twice in a 20-minute period
C) Absence of fetal heart rate accelerations for the entire monitoring period
D) Fetal heart rate baseline variability greater than 10 bpm

Question 175: Mrs. Johnson, a 35-year-old pregnant woman with gestational diabetes, presents for a prenatal visit at 28 weeks gestation. Which of the following interventions is recommended to manage her glucose levels during pregnancy?
A) Avoiding exercise
B) Strict dietary restriction
C) Insulin therapy initiation
D) Frequent fasting during the day

Question 176: Which statement accurately describes a late deceleration pattern on the fetal heart rate tracing?
A) Late decelerations are characterized by a gradual onset, gradual recovery, and a duration of more than 2 minutes.
B) Late decelerations occur in response to fetal head compression during uterine contractions.
C) Late decelerations are often associated with umbilical cord compression and prolonged fetal hypoxia.
D) Late decelerations are considered benign and do not require any intervention.

Question 177: A 32-year-old pregnant woman, Mrs. Thompson, is undergoing electronic fetal monitoring. The fetal heart rate tracing shows sudden, brief accelerations every time the mother coughs or sneezes. What artifact is responsible for this pattern?
A) Maternal movement
B) Fetal scalp electrode
C) Uterine activity monitoring
D) Fetal acoustic stimulation

Question 178: What is the most common complication associated with the use of IUPC?

A) Fetal bradycardia
B) Premature rupture of membranes
C) Placental abruption
D) Uterine perforation

Question 179: Emma, a 28-year-old multipara at 39 weeks gestation, is being monitored after a prolonged induction of labor using oxytocin infusion. Fetal heart rate monitoring shows persistent fetal tachycardia with a baseline rate of 180 bpm. Which of the following factors is likely causing the increased demand on umbilical blood flow?
A) Maternal age
B) Fetal heart rate
C) Oxytocin infusion
D) Cervical dilation

Question 180: What is the abbreviation of IUPC?
A) Intrauterine pressure contraction
B) Interuterine pressure catheter
C) Intrapartum uterine preceptor
D) Interpartum uterine contraction

Question 181: Rebecca, a 29-year-old multigravida at 39 weeks gestation, is in active labor and being continuously monitored. During a contraction, you observe an abrupt and sustained decrease in fetal heart rate that returns to baseline after the contraction is over. Which of the following patterns is being observed?
A) Early deceleration
B) Late deceleration
C) Variable deceleration
D) Acceleration

Question 182: Which maternal condition is commonly associated with late decelerations?
A) Gestational diabetes
B) Chronic hypertension
C) Placenta previa
D) Oligohydramnios

Question 183: Which of the following is a potential uteroplacental complication in pregnancies complicated by chronic hypertension?
A) Preterm premature rupture of membranes
B) Polyhydramnios
C) Placental insufficiency
D) Gestational diabetes

Question 184: In the biophysical profile, which parameter measures the amount of fetal body movements?
A) Fetal breathing movements
B) Fetal tone
C) Amniotic fluid volume
D) Nonstress test

Question 185: What is the recommended management approach in cases of fetal demise?
A) Immediate cesarean delivery
B) Induction of labor
C) Expectant management
D) External cephalic version

Question 186: Laura, a 25-year-old gravida 2 para 1 at 39 weeks of gestation, presents to the labor and delivery unit with active labor. Electronic fetal monitoring is initiated, and it demonstrates a consistent acceleration of at least 15 beats per minute above the baseline FHR, lasting less than 2 minutes. What is the

most probable term used to describe this fetal dysrhythmia?
A) Sinus tachycardia
B) Prolonged decelerations
C) Accelerations
D) Early decelerations

Question 187:   Lisa, a pregnant patient at 37 weeks of gestation, is admitted to the labor and delivery unit with ruptured membranes. The nurse notes that the electronic fetal monitoring (EFM) is showing a baseline fetal heart rate of 155 bpm with moderate variability, no accelerations, and no decelerations. What is the nurse's most appropriate action?
A) Place the intrauterine pressure catheter (IUPC) to assess uterine contractions accurately.
B) Administer oxygen via a facemask to maintain adequate oxygenation.
C) Document the findings and continue to monitor the patient closely.
D) Prepare for an immediate cesarean delivery.

Question 188:   Which of the following statements regarding external uterine monitoring is correct?
A) It provides accurate information about the strength of contractions.
B) It requires an invasive procedure to insert the monitoring device.
C) It directly measures the fetal heart rate.
D) It is less convenient compared to internal uterine monitoring.

Question 189:   Patient: Mrs. Anderson, a 30-year-old pregnant woman at 26 weeks gestation, presents with epigastric pain, nausea, and vomiting. Her blood pressure is 140/100 mmHg. Laboratory results show normal liver enzymes and low platelet count. What is the most likely diagnosis for this patient?
A) Acute fatty liver of pregnancy
B) Cholecystitis
C) Gestational diabetes
D) HELLP syndrome

Question 190:   Which of the following interventions is recommended for managing maternal obesity during pregnancy?
A) Low-calorie diet
B) High-intensity aerobic exercise
C) Weight loss medications
D) Multidisciplinary approach

Question 191:   A nurse notices a colleague demonstrating unprofessional behavior, such as speaking rudely to a patient. What should the nurse do in this situation?
A) Confront the colleague immediately about their behavior
B) Ignore the situation and continue with own responsibilities
C) Report the incident to the nurse manager or supervisor
D) Join the colleague and engage in similar behavior towards the patient

Question 192:   Which of the following is NOT true regarding fetal heart rate accelerations?
A) They are brief increases in the fetal heart rate above the baseline.
B) They are considered a reassuring sign of fetal well-being.
C) They usually last for at least 30 seconds.
D) They can be induced by fetal movement.

Question 193:   Mrs. Johnson, a 34-year-old G3P2, is being continuously monitored due to decreased fetal movements. The external fetal heart rate tracing reveals a sudden deceleration in the heart rate, which is associated with the onset of maternal contractions. The contractions are regular and have a frequency of every 3 minutes. The baseline fetal heart rate is 140 beats per minute, with no significant variability. The fetal heart rate decelerations are symmetric, with an onset to nadir time of 20 seconds and a recovery time of 30 seconds. Which of the following is the most likely cause of these findings?
A) Cord compression
B) Fetal tachycardia
C) Late decelerations
D) Variable decelerations

Question 194:   In nonstress testing (NST), a reassuring result is obtained when:
A) The baseline fetal heart rate is 120 bpm.
B) The baseline fetal heart rate variability is <5 bpm.
C) There are no fetal heart rate accelerations.
D) There are decelerations in the fetal heart rate.

Question 195:   Which of the following is a uteroplacental complication associated with reduced placental perfusion?
A) Fetal growth restriction
B) Oligohydramnios
C) Preterm labor
D) Preterm premature rupture of membranes

Question 196:   Which of the following imaging techniques can be used to assess blood flow to the fetus?
A) Doppler ultrasound
B) Fetal blood sampling
C) Fetal scalp stimulation test
D) Electronic fetal heart rate monitoring

Question 197:   A 35-year-old pregnant woman, Mrs. Davis, at 37 weeks gestation presents for a nonstress test. The fetal heart rate baseline is 150 bpm, with increased variability. Fetal movements are noted, but no accelerations or decelerations are seen during the 20-minute test. What is the interpretation of this nonstress test?
A) Reactive
B) Nonreactive
C) Equivocal
D) Abnormal

Question 198:   Sarah, a 32-year-old patient at 40 weeks of gestation, presents to the labor and delivery unit in active labor. During the labor process, you observe a pattern of prolonged decelerations on the EFM tracing. What is the most appropriate intervention in this situation?
A) Administer tocolytic medications
B) Perform an amnioinfusion
C) Increase the rate of IV fluids
D) Change the patient's position

Question 199:   Sarah, a 28-year-old G2P1 woman at 39 weeks gestation, presents to the labor and delivery unit with preterm premature rupture of membranes (PPROM). She has a high vaginal swab that reveals group B streptococcus (GBS) colonization. What is the most appropriate management for this patient?

A) Administer intravenous ampicillin and continue prophylactic antibiotics until delivery
B) Start intravenous vancomycin and continue prophylactic antibiotics until delivery
C) Administer a single dose of intravenous cefazolin and continue prophylactic antibiotics until delivery
D) Delay prophylactic antibiotics until the onset of labor

Question 200: Which of the following injuries is characterized by the presence of scalp swelling due to the accumulation of blood beneath the periosteum?
A) Cephalohematoma
B) Intracranial hemorrhage
C) Spinal cord injury
D) Facial bruising

Question 201: Which of the following can help differentiate between true fetal heart rate (FHR) patterns and artifacts?
A) Increased baseline variability
B) Consistent accelerations
C) Absence of uterine contractions
D) All of the above

Question 202: Emily, 35 years old, is diagnosed with severe preeclampsia at 36 weeks of gestation. Which of the following is the most appropriate management option for her condition?
A) Immediate induction of labor
B) Administering corticosteroids for fetal lung maturity
C) Close monitoring of blood pressure and fetal well-being
D) Performing an emergency cesarean delivery

Question 203: Which infection is associated with the highest risk of neonatal sepsis?
A) Group B Streptococcus
B) Herpes simplex virus
C) Human immunodeficiency virus (HIV)
D) Chlamydia

Question 204: You are working in a fetal monitoring unit and you notice that the fetal heart rate tracing of a patient, Mr. Anderson, has a non-reassuring pattern. You decide to consult the obstetrician, Dr. Smith, to discuss your concerns. However, Dr. Smith dismisses your concerns and decides not to intervene. What should be your next course of action in this ethically challenging situation?
A) Follow Dr. Smith's decision and not intervene.
B) Document and communicate your concerns to the appropriate supervisor or authority.
C) Ignore the situation and continue monitoring the patient.
D) Communicate the concerns directly to the patient.

Question 205: Which type of diabetes is not associated with pregnancy and can occur at any age?
A) Type 1 diabetes
B) Type 2 diabetes
C) Gestational diabetes
D) None of the above

Question 206: Which intervention is appropriate for managing early decelerations during labor?
A) Administer oxygen to the mother.
B) Change the mother's position.
C) Perform a fetal scalp stimulation.
D) Prepare for an emergency cesarean section.

Question 207: A pregnant woman presents to the labor and delivery unit in active labor. She is currently taking a selective serotonin reuptake inhibitor (SSRI) for a diagnosed depressive disorder. Which of the following effects may be observed in the neonate due to this medication?
A) Hypoglycemia
B) Seizures
C) Decreased respiratory effort
D) Hyperbilirubinemia

Question 208: Which of the following statements about uterine contraction intensity is correct?
A) Intensity refers to the frequency of contractions.
B) Intensity is directly proportional to the duration of contractions.
C) Intensity is assessed by measuring the distance between contractions.
D) Intensity is a measure of the strength or power of contractions.

Question 209: Which professional organizations provide resources and guidelines for continuing education in electronic fetal monitoring (EFM)?
A) Society for Maternal-Fetal Medicine (SMFM)
B) Association of Women's Health, Obstetric and Neonatal Nurses (AWHONN)
C) National Association of Neonatal Nurses (NANN)
D) Both A and B

Question 210: Which of the following is an advantage of external uterine monitoring?
A) It allows for direct measurement of intrauterine pressure.
B) It provides continuous fetal heart rate monitoring.
C) It is less affected by maternal movement compared to internal monitoring.
D) It requires a less complex setup compared to internal monitoring.

Question 211: Which of the following statements regarding sinusoidal pattern in electronic fetal monitoring is correct?
A) Sinusoidal pattern is characterized by a regular, smooth, and continuous waveform with a baseline resembling a sine wave.
B) Sinusoidal pattern is a normal finding and does not require any intervention.
C) Sinusoidal pattern is commonly associated with fetal well-being and does not indicate any fetal distress.
D) Sinusoidal pattern is an irregular, jagged waveform with frequent fluctuations in the baseline.

Question 212: What is the role of the ductus venosus in umbilical blood flow?
A) It carries oxygenated blood from the placenta to the fetus.
B) It carries deoxygenated blood from the fetus to the placenta.
C) It bypasses the liver sinusoids, allowing oxygenated blood to enter the fetal systemic circulation.
D) It regulates blood flow to the fetal brain.

Question 213: Ms. Thompson is a 28-year-old primigravida at 40 weeks gestation who presents for a routine antenatal visit. On examination, her cervix is closed, firm, and posterior. Which one of the following is the most appropriate management in this situation?
A) Expectant management
B) Prostaglandin cervical ripening
C) Membrane sweep
D) Oxytocin induction of labor

Question 214: In the presence of tachycardia in fetal monitoring, which intervention is appropriate?
A) Administering oxygen to the mother
B) Performing a scalp stimulation test
C) Increasing intravenous fluids
D) Applying a fetal scalp electrode

Question 215: What is the primary source of oxygen supply to the fetus during intrauterine life?
A) Lungs
B) Placenta
C) Umbilical cord
D) Liver

Question 216: A healthcare facility notices an increase in medication errors related to wrong dosage administration. The quality improvement team is investigating the root cause of this issue. Which factor is most likely to contribute to this problem?
A) Adequate staffing and workload distribution.
B) Implementation of double-check systems during medication administration.
C) Lack of standardized medication labeling and packaging.
D) Efficient medication reconciliation processes during transitions of care.

Question 217: Which of the following is the correct interpretation of a prolonged deceleration in fetal heart rate?
A) A drop in heart rate lasting less than 30 seconds
B) A drop in heart rate lasting 30-60 seconds
C) A drop in heart rate lasting more than 2 minutes
D) A drop in heart rate with a variable duration

Question 218: Mrs. Thompson, a 35-year-old G3P2 at 28 weeks gestation, is admitted to the labor and delivery unit with vaginal bleeding and abdominal pain. On examination, her uterus is tender and she has a blood pressure of 90/50 mmHg and a heart rate of 110 bpm. Her electronic fetal monitoring (EFM) tracing shows absent variability with late decelerations. What is the most appropriate intervention in this situation?
A) Prepare the patient for immediate cesarean delivery
B) Administer oxytocin to augment labor
C) Administer intravenous fluids and stabilize the patient
D) Obtain an obstetric ultrasound and consult with a maternal-fetal medicine specialist

Question 219: Emily, a 30-year-old primigravida woman, presents to the triage unit at 41 weeks of gestation. She complains of decreased fetal movement over the past few hours. Upon examination, the nurse finds the fetal heart rate to be reassuring. However, uterine activity is minimal. Which of the following interventions would be most appropriate in this situation?
A) Administering oxytocin to stimulate uterine contractions
B) Placing the patient in the lithotomy position
C) Encouraging the patient to ambulate to increase uterine activity
D) Maintaining continuous fetal monitoring for further assessment

Question 220: Emily, a 28-year-old pregnant woman with gestational diabetes, attends her routine antenatal visit. Which of the following findings on a non-stress test (NST) would be considered abnormal for her gestational age?
A) Two accelerations in 20 minutes
B) Baseline heart rate of 150 bpm

C) Absence of fetal movements
D) Late decelerations during contractions

Question 221: Mrs. Johnson is a 42-year-old primigravida at 41 weeks gestation. She has been diagnosed with postdates pregnancy. Which one of the following monitoring techniques is most appropriate for assessing fetal well-being in this situation?
A) Non-stress test
B) Biophysical profile
C) Contraction stress test
D) Amniotic fluid index

Question 222: Ms. Anderson, a pregnant woman at 32 weeks gestation, is in labor. The electronic fetal monitoring (EFM) tracing shows a 20-second decrease in the fetal heart rate from the baseline lasting less than 2 minutes. What type of deceleration is this?
A) Early deceleration
B) Variable deceleration
C) Late deceleration
D) Prolonged deceleration

Question 223: Which of the following is a key component of quality improvement in healthcare?
A) Identifying problems and errors
B) Assessing current processes and outcomes
C) Implementing evidence-based practices
D) All of the above

Question 224: Ms. Rodriguez, a 28-year-old pregnant woman, is expecting triplets. The ultrasound shows a triangle sign, also known as the ? sign. Which condition is associated with this sign?
A) Twin-to-twin transfusion syndrome
B) Chorioamnionitis
C) Placenta previa
D) Aneuploidy

Question 225: Which of the following is a characteristic feature of supraventricular tachycardia (SVT) in a fetus?
A) Heart rate of less than 100 beats per minute (bpm)
B) Absence of P waves on the electrocardiogram (ECG)
C) Regular, well-defined QRS complexes on the ECG
D) Occurrence only during fetal sleep periods

Question 226: Ms. Johnson is a 28-year-old pregnant woman at 28 weeks of gestation. She has a history of systemic lupus erythematosus (SLE) and is on hydroxychloroquine. She undergoes an obstetric ultrasound which reveals a fetal heart rate of 54 bpm with a consistent 3:1 atrioventricular (AV) block. What is the most appropriate management for this condition?
A) Immediate medical termination of pregnancy.
B) Initiation of dexamethasone to improve fetal heart rate.
C) Serial fetal echocardiography to assess for further progression of the AV block.
D) Expectant management with close monitoring of fetal heart rate.

Question 227: Which maternal factor can increase the risk of uterine rupture during labor?
A) Previous cesarean section
B) Multiple gestation
C) Intrauterine growth restriction (IUGR)
D) All of the above

Question 228: Which intervention is recommended for the management of twin pregnancies after 32 weeks gestation?
A) Non-stress test (NST) twice weekly
B) Biophysical profile (BPP) weekly
C) Ultrasound examination every 4 weeks
D) Fetal fibronectin (fFN) testing every 2 weeks

Question 229: Which condition can impair placental blood flow and decrease fetal oxygen supply?
A) Gestational diabetes
B) Intrauterine growth restriction (IUGR)
C) Preterm labor
D) Polyhydramnios

Question 230: Mrs. Wilson, a 26-year-old multigravida, is in active labor at 39 weeks of gestation. The electronic fetal monitoring (EFM) tracing shows prolonged decelerations, which are persistent, lasting more than two minutes. Which intervention should the nurse implement first?
A) Perform a sterile vaginal examination
B) Administer oxygen via face mask at 10 L/min
C) Reposition the patient onto her left side
D) Prepare for an emergency cesarean delivery

Question 231: What is the most common symptom of uterine rupture/scar dehiscence?
A) Severe abdominal pain
B) Vaginal bleeding
C) Fetal distress
D) Maternal hypotension

Question 232: Mrs. Patel, a 32-year-old G2P1 at 41 weeks of gestation, is in active labor. On fetal monitoring, you notice the presence of late decelerations. Which of the following interventions is most appropriate in this situation?
A) Administer terbutaline
B) Administer magnesium sulfate
C) Administer oxygen via a face mask
D) Perform a fetal scalp blood sampling

Question 233: Which of the following is a possible complication of supraventricular tachycardia (SVT) in a fetus?
A) Ventricular septal defect
B) Hypoglycemia
C) Fetal hydrops
D) Umbilical cord prolapse

Question 234: Samantha, a 28-year-old pregnant woman at 36 weeks of gestation, is undergoing electronic fetal monitoring. The fetal heart rate has a baseline variability of less than 5 bpm. What does this suggest?
A) It indicates normal fetal oxygenation.
B) It is within the normal range for baseline variability.
C) It is an abnormal finding requiring further evaluation.
D) It suggests increased fetal well-being.

Question 235: Chronic (essential) hypertension during pregnancy may increase the risk of which of the following complications?
A) Preeclampsia
B) Gestational diabetes
C) Ectopic pregnancy
D) Preterm labor

Question 236: What is the advantage of using internal uterine monitoring compared to external monitoring?
A) Noninvasive
B) Provides continuous and accurate measurement
C) Allows mobility during labor
D) Less expensive

Question 237: Mr. and Mrs. Wilson are anxiously awaiting the birth of their baby. Mrs. Wilson has systemic lupus erythematosus (SLE) and is concerned about the possible development of a heart block in the fetus. Which of the following antibodies is most strongly associated with congenital heart block in infants of mothers with SLE?
A) Anti-Ro (SSA) antibodies
B) Anti-La (SSB) antibodies
C) Anti-double-stranded DNA antibodies
D) Anti-Smith antibodies

Question 238: Which condition involves an abnormal implantation of the placenta?
A) Placental abruption
B) Placenta previa
C) Placental calcification
D) Placental insufficiency

Question 239: Which of the following is a potential long-term complication of congenital heart block?
A) Neonatal jaundice
B) Pulmonary hypertension
C) Gastroschisis
D) Anencephaly

Question 240: What is the primary goal of managing hypertonus during labor?
A) Restoring normal fetal heart rate patterns
B) Reducing the risk of postpartum hemorrhage
C) Promoting active labor progression
D) Improving fetal oxygenation

Question 241: Anna, a 32-year-old pregnant woman at 38 weeks' gestation, is experiencing contractions. On monitoring her uterine activity, the contractions last for 60 seconds from the start of one contraction to the start of the next contraction. What is the frequency of Anna's contractions?
A) 1 contraction every 60 seconds
B) 1 contraction every 30 seconds
C) 2 contractions every 60 seconds
D) 2 contractions every 30 seconds

Question 242: What is the normal uterine contraction pattern during labor?
A) Contractions lasting less than 20 seconds with a frequency of 1 every 5 minutes.
B) Contractions lasting more than 60 seconds with a frequency of 4 every 20 minutes.
C) Contractions lasting 40-60 seconds with a frequency of 2-3 every 10 minutes.
D) Contractions lasting more than 80 seconds with a frequency of 1 every 15 minutes.

Question 243: During a non-stress test, Mrs. Carter, a G2P1 woman at 41 weeks of gestation, is found to have a resting uterine tone of 0 mmHg. What does this resting tone value represent?
A) Hypertonic uterus
B) Hypotonic uterus
C) Normal uterine activity
D) Hyperstimulation

Question 244: Which fetal complication is characterized by an abnormal pH value in the fetal blood?
A) Fetal bradycardia
B) Fetal tachycardia
C) Fetal distress
D) Fetal acidemia

Question 245: A 34-year-old woman at 41 weeks of gestation is undergoing continuous electronic fetal monitoring. The nurse notices intermittent signal loss on the tocodynamometer and fetal heart rate tracing. What can be a potential cause of this signal ambiguity?
A) Maternal obesity
B) Fetal artifact
C) Equipment calibration error
D) Inadequate gel application

Question 246: Which of the following is true regarding uterine activity?
A) It refers to the frequency, duration, and intensity of contractions.
B) It is not associated with changes in fetal oxygenation.
C) It is primarily influenced by maternal heart rate.
D) It does not play a role in cervical dilation.

Question 247: Which of the following maternal factors can influence fetal movement perception?
A) Maternal age
B) Number of previous pregnancies
C) Gestational age
D) Maternal body mass index (BMI)

Question 248: Maggie, a 35-year-old patient at 41 weeks of gestation, is admitted to the labor and delivery unit for induction of labor. During the induction process, you notice a pattern of prolonged decelerations on the EFM tracing. Which of the following would be the most appropriate action to take?
A) Administer terbutaline to the patient
B) Perform a biophysical profile evaluation
C) Prepare the patient for an emergency cesarean section
D) Place the patient in a knee-to-chest position

Question 249: Mrs. Roberts, a 25-year-old G4P3, presents to the labor and delivery unit at 38 weeks gestation. She has a history of two previous cesarean sections and is admitted for a vaginal birth after cesarean (VBAC) attempt. During the assessment, her initial EFM tracing shows the following: Baseline rate: 135 bpm, variability: 10 bpm, recurrent late decelerations. Which category does the EFM tracing belong to?
A) Category II
B) Category III
C) Category I
D) Category IV

Question 250: Which complication is more commonly seen in monochorionic twin pregnancies compared to dichorionic twin pregnancies?
A) Twin-to-twin transfusion syndrome
B) Twin reversed arterial perfusion sequence
C) Preterm premature rupture of membranes
D) Gestational hypertension

Question 251: Which of the following is a common clinical manifestation of hypertensive disorders in pregnancy?

A) Headache
B) Vaginal bleeding
C) Excessive fetal movement
D) Palpitations

Question 252: Mrs. Davis, a 31-year-old pregnant woman at 35 weeks gestation, presents to the labor and delivery unit with contractions and suspected preterm labor. During the cervical examination, the obstetrician notes fetal hypoxemia and acidemia. Which of the following interventions is the most appropriate to improve fetal oxygenation?
A) Administer tocolytic medication
B) Perform an emergency cesarean section
C) Administer corticosteroids for fetal lung maturity
D) Administer oxygen to the mother via face mask

Question 253: In a normal labor pattern, how should uterine contractions progress?
A) The frequency and intensity increase gradually over time.
B) The duration and intensity decrease toward the end of labor.
C) The frequency and duration decrease as labor progresses.
D) The intensity remains constant throughout labor.

Question 254: Which of the following is a quality improvement tool used to analyze and understand existing processes?
A) Flowchart
B) Histogram
C) Pareto chart
D) Scatter plot

Question 255: A pregnant woman is on long-term therapy for asthma. She is currently taking a selective beta-2 agonist for bronchodilation. Which of the following side effects is associated with this medication and may affect fetal oxygenation?
A) Increased uterine blood flow
B) Maternal tachycardia
C) Decreased maternal blood pressure
D) Decreased fetal heart rate variability

Question 256: Sarah, a 25-year-old woman at 36 weeks of gestation, is in active labor. Fetal monitoring shows a baseline fetal heart rate (FHR) of 150 bpm with minimal variability. The nurse observes contractions occurring every 3 minutes with a duration of 90 seconds. The nurse suspects tachysystole. Which medication should the nurse anticipate administering if conservative measures fail to correct the tachysystole?
A) Oxytocin
B) Nifedipine
C) Terbutaline
D) Methylergonovine

Question 257: Which of the following interventions is NOT recommended for the management of gestational hypertension?
A) Bed rest
B) Antihypertensive medications
C) Regular monitoring of blood pressure
D) Induction of labor

Question 258: Which of the following injuries is associated with damage to the spinal cord resulting in motor and sensory deficits?
A) Cephalohematoma
B) Intracranial hemorrhage

C) Spinal cord injury
D) Facial bruising

Question 259: Which of the following statements regarding uteroplacental circulation is correct?
A) Oxygenated blood flows from the placenta to the fetus through the umbilical vein.
B) The chorionic villi are responsible for oxygen and carbon dioxide exchange in the placenta.
C) Uterine artery carries deoxygenated blood to the placenta.
D) The intervillous space contains deoxygenated maternal blood.

Question 260: Ms. Anderson, a 39-year-old pregnant woman at 42 weeks gestation, is in active labor. During an internal examination, the midwife notes contractions that are lasting for 90 seconds and occurring every 2 minutes. What action should be taken based on these contractions?
A) Obtain a fetal heart rate tracing
B) Administer tocolytic medications
C) Prepare for a cesarean section
D) Encourage the mother to push

Question 261: Which of the following is considered a non-reassuring fetal heart rate pattern?
A) Variability of 1-5 beats per minute
B) Accelerations on the fetal heart rate strip
C) Early decelerations during labor
D) Late decelerations during labor

Question 262: Ava, a 35-year-old pregnant woman at 38 weeks gestation, presents to the labor and delivery unit reporting decreased fetal movements. On examination, the fetal heart rate is within normal limits. What is the appropriate action for the healthcare provider?
A) Recommend Ava to perform vigorous physical activity and monitor fetal movements.
B) Order a biophysical profile (BPP) to assess fetal well-being.
C) Suggest Ava to consume caffeine and monitor fetal movements.
D) Schedule an immediate cesarean section.

Question 263: Sarah, a 25-year-old primigravida at 36 weeks gestation, presents to the antenatal clinic with concerns of decreased fetal movements. Fetal heart rate monitoring shows repetitive late decelerations. Which of the following factors is likely causing the compromised umbilical blood flow?
A) Maternal age
B) Fetal heart rate
C) Decreased fetal movements
D) Uterine contractions

Question 264: In a legal context, which of the following is essential when documenting electronic fetal monitoring (EFM) findings?
A) Ensuring the accuracy of the recorded data.
B) Including the interpretation of the EFM tracings.
C) Timely notification of abnormal findings to the healthcare team.
D) All of the above.

Question 265: A pregnant woman in her third trimester is admitted to the hospital with a fever. On assessment, her fetal heart rate is consistently above 160 beats per minute, with the baseline at 170 bpm. The maternal temperature is elevated at 101.2℉ (38.4℃). What is the most likely cause of the tachycardia?
A) Fetal distress
B) Maternal dehydration
C) Maternal infection
D) Uteroplacental insufficiency

Question 266: Ms. Rodriguez, a 29-year-old pregnant woman at 28 weeks gestation, presents to the antepartum unit with complaints of decreased fetal movement. Upon assessment, the nurse notes a fetal heart rate of 80 bpm. The mother denies any medical complications during the pregnancy. The nurse should take which immediate action?
A) Administer oxygen to the mother
B) Administer a tocolytic medication to the mother
C) Prepare for immediate delivery
D) Reassure the mother and continue monitoring

Question 267: Mrs. Smith, a 32-year-old primigravida at 41 weeks of gestation, is admitted to the labor and delivery unit in spontaneous labor. Electronic fetal monitoring reveals severe variable decelerations lasting more than 60 seconds associated with a slow return to baseline. Maternal oxygenation is administered via face mask but does not improve the fetal heart rate pattern. The cervix is dilated to 4cm. What is the most appropriate next step in managing this situation?
A) Administer terbutaline
B) Perform an amnioinfusion
C) Prepare for immediate operative vaginal delivery
D) Prepare for immediate cesarean delivery

Question 268: Which of the following is a characteristic feature of external fetal heart rate monitoring?
A) Invasive procedure involving electrode insertion
B) Utilization of a catheter to measure fetal heart rate
C) Placement of a transducer on the mother's abdomen
D) Continuous monitoring of uterine contractions

Question 269: Which diagnostic tool is commonly used to confirm uterine rupture/scar dehiscence?
A) Ultrasound
B) Fetal heart rate monitoring
C) Magnetic resonance imaging (MRI)
D) Maternal blood tests

Question 270: Which of the following legal principles governs the use of electronic fetal monitoring (EFM) in healthcare?
A) Confidentiality
B) Informed consent
C) Standard of care
D) Right to refuse treatment

Question 271: Mrs. Thompson, a 36-year-old multi gravida, is in her 39th week of gestation and is admitted to the labor and delivery unit in active labor. Upon electronic fetal monitoring, ectopic beats are noted on the fetal heart rate strip. What is the priority nursing intervention in this situation?
A) Administer oxygen to the mother.
B) Increase the rate of intravenous fluid administration to the mother.
C) Document the finding and continue monitoring the fetal heart rate.
D) Perform a vaginal examination to assess cervical dilation.

Question 272:   Which of the following anesthesia agents is considered the safest during pregnancy?
A) Sevoflurane
B) Propofol
C) Nitrous oxide
D) Ketamine

Question 273:   Mrs. Johnson is a 32-year-old primigravida at 34 weeks of gestation. She has a history of chronic hypertension. On fetal monitoring, the nurse observes prolonged deceleration in the fetal heart rate tracing. This finding is most likely related to which of the following placental factors?
A) Decreased intervillous space
B) Placental infarction
C) Placental previa
D) Placental abruption

Question 274:   Hypoxemia refers to:
A) Decreased oxygen content in the blood
B) Increased oxygen content in the blood
C) Decreased carbon dioxide content in the blood
D) Increased carbon dioxide content in the blood

Question 275:   Which of the following is a characteristic of a successful quality improvement initiative?
A) Clear goals and objectives
B) Inadequate data collection
C) Lack of stakeholder involvement
D) Reactive approach to problem-solving

Question 276:   Sarah, a 28-year-old pregnant woman at 36 weeks of gestation, is admitted to the labor and delivery unit in active labor. The healthcare provider decides to monitor the fetus externally using an electronic fetal monitor. Which of the following parameters can be assessed using external fetal monitoring?
A) Fetal heart rate variability
B) Uterine contractions intensity
C) Fetal scalp pH
D) Fetal oxygen saturation

Question 277:   Which factors can influence the fetal baseline heart rate?
A) Maternal age
B) Fetal position
C) Maternal emotions
D) All of the above

Question 278:   What is the normal range for fetal baseline heart rate?
A) 100-120 bpm
B) 120-160 bpm
C) 160-200 bpm
D) 200-240 bpm

Question 279:   During labor, a contraction has a duration of 45-50 seconds. What should the healthcare provider interpret from this duration?
A) Normal uterine activity
B) Inadequate contractions
C) Tachysystole
D) Preterm labor

Question 280:   What is the typical duration of early decelerations?
A) Less than 30 seconds.

B) 30 seconds to 2 minutes.
C) 2 to 5 minutes.
D) More than 5 minutes.

Question 281:   Which of the following factors can affect uterine activity?
A) Maternal hydration level.
B) Fetal position.
C) Administration of oxytocin.
D) Maternal age.

Question 282:   Mrs. Davis, a 35-year-old G3P2, presents to the labor and delivery unit at 40 weeks gestation. Her previous pregnancies have been uneventful. During the admission assessment, her initial EFM tracing shows the following: Baseline rate: 135 bpm, variability: 2 bpm, early decelerations. Which category does the EFM tracing belong to?
A) Category II
B) Category III
C) Category I
D) Category IV

Question 283:   Sarah, a 29-year-old pregnant woman at 28 weeks gestation, undergoes a routine prenatal ultrasound. The fetal heart rate is noted to be irregular with periodic abrupt accelerations and decelerations. The baseline fetal heart rate is normal. Which of the following is the most likely diagnosis based on this fetal heart rate pattern?
A) Sinus tachycardia
B) Ventricular tachycardia
C) Fetal atrial flutter
D) Supraventricular tachycardia

Question 284:   Which of the following medications is commonly used for the management of chronic (essential) hypertension during pregnancy?
A) Angiotensin-converting enzyme (ACE) inhibitors
B) Calcium channel blockers
C) Diuretics
D) Nonsteroidal anti-inflammatory drugs (NSAIDs)

Question 285:   When managing a patient with late decelerations, which intervention would be the most appropriate?
A) Administering oxygen to the mother
B) Administering terbutaline to reduce uterine contractions
C) Performing a vaginal examination to assess cervical dilation
D) Applying fundal pressure during uterine contractions

Question 286:   Mrs. Adams, a 28-year-old multigravida, is in labor and her fetal heart rate tracing shows late decelerations. What nursing intervention should be implemented based on this finding?
A) Increase the rate of oxytocin infusion
B) Administer a tocolytic medication
C) Place the mother in a side-lying position
D) Administer a fluid bolus

Question 287:   Which maternal factor can contribute to reduced fetal oxygenation by impairing placental blood flow?
A) Maternal smoking
B) Maternal diabetes
C) Maternal anxiety
D) Maternal hypothyroidism

Question 288: Which of the following statements regarding fetal circulation is correct?
A) Oxygenated blood in the umbilical vein returns to the placenta
B) The foramen ovale connects the right and left ventricles of the fetal heart
C) The ductus arteriosus connects the aorta to the pulmonary artery in the fetus
D) The umbilical arteries carry oxygenated blood back to the fetus

Question 289: Sue, a 32-year-old pregnant woman at 38 weeks of gestation, is being monitored using electronic fetal monitoring. The fetal heart rate has a baseline variability of 8-10 bpm. Which statement accurately reflects the significance of this variability?
A) A baseline variability of 8-10 bpm is within the normal range.
B) A baseline variability of 8-10 bpm is indicative of fetal distress.
C) A baseline variability of 8-10 bpm is considered mild compared to normal variability.
D) A baseline variability of 8-10 bpm is abnormal and requires immediate intervention.

Question 290: You are performing external fetal monitoring on Ms. Lewis, who is at 32 weeks gestation. While listening to the fetal heart rate, you notice an irregular pattern with frequent accelerations. Which of the following conditions is associated with this finding?
A) Fetal distress
B) Fetal tachycardia
C) Fetal arrhythmia
D) Normal fetal heart rate pattern

Question 291: What is the most common cause of electronic fetal monitor failure in clinical settings?
A) Power outage
B) Loose connection
C) Software malfunction
D) Water damage

Question 292: Mrs. Anderson, a 28-year-old pregnant woman, is in her 41st week of pregnancy. She is scheduled for a contraction stress test (CST) today. During the CST, the nurse performs fetal acoustic stimulation. What is the purpose of fetal acoustic stimulation in the CST?
A) To determine the presence of uterine contractions
B) To assess fetal heart rate response to contractions
C) To evaluate amniotic fluid index
D) To monitor fetal heart rate variability

Question 293: Which of the following is an advantage of auscultation as a fetal assessment method?
A) It requires expensive equipment.
B) It is not influenced by maternal factors.
C) It provides continuous monitoring of fetal well-being.
D) It requires specialized training for healthcare providers.

Question 294: Which of the following factors can affect the resting tone during electronic fetal monitoring?
A) Fetal heart rate patterns
B) Maternal position
C) Uterine contractions
D) All of the above

Question 295: During auscultation, the normal fetal heart rate range is:

A) 80-100 beats per minute.
B) 120-160 beats per minute.
C) 180-200 beats per minute.
D) 220-240 beats per minute.

Question 296: Sophia, a 34-year-old G2P1 at 35 weeks of gestation, presents to the clinic with complaints of persistent abdominal pain and contractions. On fetal monitoring, you notice the presence of variable decelerations in the fetal heart rate. What is the most appropriate intervention in this situation?
A) Administer tocolytic therapy
B) Perform a cord blood gas analysis
C) Administer fluid bolus
D) Administer betamethasone for fetal lung maturity

Question 297: Mrs. Johnson, a 32-year-old pregnant woman, presents for an ultrasound at 20 weeks gestation. The ultrasound reveals a dichorionic-diamniotic twin pregnancy. What does this finding indicate?
A) Two separate placentas and two amniotic sacs
B) Two separate placentas and one amniotic sac
C) One placenta and two amniotic sacs
D) One placenta and one amniotic sac

Question 298: Amelia, a 28-year-old primigravida at 30 weeks gestation, is diagnosed with chronic essential hypertension. She asks about the potential complications associated with her condition. Which of the following maternal complications is commonly associated with chronic essential hypertension during pregnancy?
A) Gestational diabetes
B) Preterm labor
C) Placenta previa
D) HELLP syndrome

Question 299: In a labor and delivery unit, a nurse overhears a conversation between two colleagues discussing a patient's medical condition. Which action should the nurse take?
A) Join the conversation and offer input based on personal experience
B) Report the incident to the unit manager or supervisor
C) Ignore the conversation and continue working
D) Assume the conversation is confidential and do nothing

Question 300: During a routine ultrasound examination, it is found that the fetus has a congenital heart defect involving the atria. Which of the following structures would be impacted by this defect?
A) Foramen ovale
B) Ductus arteriosus
C) Umbilical artery
D) Pulmonary artery

Question 301: What is the most common presenting sign of fetal demise during labor?
A) Absence of fetal movements
B) Meconium-stained amniotic fluid
C) Prolonged decelerations
D) Foul-smelling vaginal discharge

Question 302: Mrs. Wilson, a primigravida at 39 weeks of gestation, presents to the labor and delivery unit. The initial assessment reveals a resting uterine tone of 35 mmHg. What does this resting tone value indicate?

A) Hypertonic uterus
B) Hypotonic uterus
C) Normal uterine activity
D) Hyperstimulation

Question 303:   Mrs. Johnson, a 35-year-old pregnant woman at 38 weeks of gestation presents to the antenatal clinic for a routine check-up. She has a history of gestational diabetes and is currently on insulin therapy. The doctor orders a non-stress test to assess fetal well-being. Which of the following methods is commonly used for external fetal monitoring during a non-stress test?
A) Invasive monitoring using fetal scalp electrode
B) Electronic fetal monitoring using a handheld Doppler device
C) Real-time ultrasound monitoring of fetal heart rate
D) Monitoring uterine contractions using a tocometer

Question 304:   Mrs. Johnson, a 29-year-old primigravida, is at 41 weeks of gestation and in active labor. The electronic fetal monitoring (EFM) tracing shows recurrent variable decelerations with a slow return to baseline. Which intervention should the nurse implement to address this pattern?
A) Administer a tocolytic medication
B) Increase intravenous fluid rate
C) Perform a sterile vaginal examination
D) Reposition the patient onto her hands and knees

Question 305:   Which factor is unlikely to cause variability in fetal heart rate?
A) Maternal hypotension
B) Fetal movements
C) Fetal sleep cycles
D) Fetal head compression during labor

Question 306:   Which of the following is a characteristic of accelerations in fetal heart rate?
A) Gradual onset and offset
B) Associated with uterine contractions
C) Sudden increase in heart rate
D) Variable duration

Question 307:   Mrs. Johnson, a 35-year-old pregnant woman, is admitted to the labor and delivery unit. The electronic fetal monitor (EFM) is displaying a flat line on the fetal heart rate (FHR) tracing. Which of the following troubleshooting steps should the nurse take first?
A) Check the maternal vital signs and position
B) Reattach the FHR transducer to the mother's abdomen
C) Determine if the EFM is set to the correct mode
D) Assess the mother for any signs of distress

Question 308:   Mrs. Johnson, a 32-year-old primigravida, presents to the antenatal clinic at 30 weeks gestation. Her blood pressure reading is consistently above 140/90 mmHg, and she complains of headaches and swelling in her hands and feet. She has no past medical history of hypertension. What is the most appropriate diagnosis for Mrs. Johnson?
A) Preeclampsia
B) Chronic hypertension
C) Gestational hypertension
D) Essential hypertension

Question 309:   Which pattern of fetal heart rate variability is characterized by a variance of 5-25 beats per minute?
A) Moderate Variability

B) Absent Variability
C) Marked Variability
D) Minimal Variability

Question 310:   Which of the following is not a typical characteristic of fetal dysrhythmias?
A) Irregular fetal heart rate patterns
B) Prolonged decelerations
C) Accelerated fetal heart rate
D) Absence of beat-to-beat variability

Question 311:   Sarah, a 30-year-old pregnant woman at 36 weeks gestation, presents to the clinic concerned about decreased fetal movements over the past 24 hours. On examination, the fetal heart rate is within normal limits. What is the appropriate action for the healthcare provider?
A) Advise the patient to continue monitoring fetal movements and return if they do not improve.
B) Order a non-stress test (NST) to assess fetal well-being.
C) Schedule an immediate induction of labor.
D) Prescribe a tocolytic agent to stimulate fetal movement.

Question 312:   Ms. Johnson, a primigravida at 30 weeks of gestation, presents to the antepartum unit with complaints of decreased fetal movements. Upon electronic fetal monitoring, ectopic beats are noted on the fetal heart rate strip. What is the appropriate nursing intervention in this situation?
A) Notify the healthcare provider immediately.
B) Administer a tocolytic medication to the mother.
C) Increase the rate of intravenous fluid administration to the mother.
D) Perform a nonstress test to assess fetal well-being.

Question 313:   Mrs. Anderson is a 35-year-old multiparous woman at 42 weeks gestation. She presents for a routine antenatal visit, and a biophysical profile is performed. The amniotic fluid index is found to be 4 cm. What is the most appropriate management in this situation?
A) Induction of labor
B) Repeat biophysical profile in 24 hours
C) Cesarean section
D) Observation with daily fetal movement counts

Question 314:   Which of the following interventions is commonly recommended for persistent fetal dysrhythmias?
A) Fetal scalp stimulation
B) Administration of tocolytic medications
C) Maternal position change
D) Epidural anesthesia

Question 315:   Which of the following is a recommended troubleshooting step for resolving issues with electronic fetal monitoring equipment?
A) Replace the entire equipment
B) Ignore the issue if it does not affect the data
C) Consult the user manual
D) Call technical support immediately

Question 316:   Mrs. Johnson, a 28-year-old primigravida at 39 weeks of gestation, presents to the labor and delivery unit in active labor. Continuous electronic fetal monitoring (EFM) reveals a non-reassuring fetal heart rate pattern, and a decision is made to proceed with an emergent cesarean delivery. Cord blood gases are collected at delivery and reveal a

pH of 7.1. Which acid-base imbalance is most likely present in the newborn?
A) Respiratory acidosis
B) Respiratory alkalosis
C) Metabolic acidosis
D) Metabolic alkalosis

Question 317: A 37-year-old gravida 4 para 3 woman presents with bright red painless vaginal bleeding at 26 weeks gestation. On examination, her uterus is non-tender, and the fundus is at the level of the xiphoid process. Fetal heart rate monitoring shows a reassuring pattern. Which of the following is the most likely diagnosis in this patient?
A) Placenta previa
B) Placental abruption
C) Uterine rupture
D) Vasa previa

Question 318: What is the fetal heart rate criterion for defining bradycardia during labor?
A) Less than 120 beats per minute
B) Less than 80 beats per minute
C) Less than 100 beats per minute
D) Less than 60 beats per minute

Question 319: Which of the following is a potential limitation of external fetal heart rate monitoring?
A) Limited mobility for the mother
B) Inability to detect contractions accurately
C) Risk of infection due to invasive procedures
D) Difficulty in assessing fetal heart rate variability

Question 320: Mrs. Anderson is a 36-year-old woman who is at 41 weeks gestation. She presents to the antepartum unit for a non-stress test. On electronic fetal monitoring, you note a baseline fetal heart rate of 130 bpm with absent variability. There are no accelerations or decelerations present. Which of the following is the most likely cause of this fetal heart rate pattern?
A) Fetal acidemia
B) Fetal hypoxemia
C) Fetal anemia
D) Fetal sleep cycle

Question 321: Which pattern of fetal heart rate variability is characterized by a sinusoidal pattern with a frequency of 2-5 cycles per minute?
A) Moderate Variability
B) Minimal Variability
C) Marked Variability
D) Absent Variability

Question 322: Ms. Johnson, a 35-year-old G3P2, is in active labor at 39 weeks gestation. During the electronic fetal monitoring (EFM), the nurse observes the uterine contractions. The nurse measures the intensity of the contractions and determines that they are mild, with a peak intensity of less than 25mmHg. How would you classify this intensity of uterine contractions?
A) Moderate
B) Strong
C) Weak
D) Hyperstimulation

Question 323: During electronic fetal monitoring, the nurse notices a pattern in the uterine contractions where the resting tone between contractions is elevated. Which of the following conditions is associated with this finding?

A) Hypertonic uterine dysfunction
B) Hypotonic uterine dysfunction
C) Uterine tachysystole
D) Uterine hyperstimulation syndrome

Question 324: Mrs. Johnson, a 32-year-old pregnant woman at 28 weeks gestation, arrives at the labor and delivery unit with signs of preterm labor. The nurse notifies you, the healthcare provider, and upon assessment, you determine that contractions are occurring every 3 minutes and lasting for 45 seconds. The tocodynamometer shows a resting tone of 15mmHg. What intervention would you prioritize?
A) Administer betamethasone to enhance fetal lung maturity
B) Begin tocolytic therapy with indomethacin
C) Administer magnesium sulfate to prevent cerebral palsy
D) Prepare the patient for immediate delivery via cesarean section

Question 325: Mrs. Ramirez, a 25-year-old pregnant woman at 34 weeks gestation, presents to the labor and delivery unit reporting contractions. On examination, her cervix is closed, and the contractions are irregular and non-progressive. What is the most likely cause of these contractions?
A) Braxton Hicks contractions
B) Preterm labor contractions
C) Dehydration
D) False labor contractions

Question 326: Mrs. Rodriguez, a 38-year-old multigravida, is at 36 weeks gestation. She has a history of chronic hypertension and is currently on antihypertensive medication. Her blood pressure readings have been well-controlled throughout her pregnancy. During a routine antenatal visit, her blood pressure is noted to be significantly elevated (160/100 mmHg) on two consecutive occasions, with no symptoms. What is the most appropriate management for Mrs. Rodriguez?
A) Increase the dose of the current antihypertensive medication
B) Administer antihypertensive medication not used during pregnancy
C) Admit for immediate induction of labor
D) Monitor closely and repeat blood pressure measurements

Question 327: Mrs. Thompson is a 32-year-old gravida 3, para 2 at 38 weeks of gestation. She presents to the labor and delivery unit in active labor. Continuous electronic fetal monitoring (EFM) reveals a non-reassuring fetal heart rate pattern, and a decision is made to proceed with an emergent cesarean delivery. Cord blood gases are collected at delivery and reveal a base deficit of -8 mmol/L. What does this base deficit value suggest?
A) Normal acid-base balance
B) Mild metabolic alkalosis
C) Mild metabolic acidosis
D) Severe metabolic acidosis

Question 328: Maria, a 32-year-old pregnant woman at 36 weeks gestation, presents with a rapid fetal heart rate during a prenatal visit. The fetal heart rate pattern is regular, with a rate ranging from 180 to 220 beats per minute. The maternal heart rate is normal. Which of the following is the most likely diagnosis for this fetal heart rate pattern?
A) Ventricular tachycardia
B) Atrial flutter

C) Sinus tachycardia
D) Supraventricular tachycardia

Question 329: Which hormone is responsible for initiating uteroplacental circulation?
A) Estrogen,
B) Progesterone,
C) Human Chorionic Gonadotropin (hCG),
D) Human Placental Lactogen (hPL)

Question 330: Mrs. Johnson, a 28-year-old gravida 3 para 1 woman, presents to the emergency department at 36 weeks gestation complaining of sudden onset abdominal pain and dark vaginal bleeding. On examination, there is uterine tenderness and a rigid abdomen. Fetal heart rate monitoring shows late decelerations. Which of the following is the most likely diagnosis in this patient?
A) Placenta previa
B) Placental abruption
C) Uterine rupture
D) Uterine leiomyoma

Question 331: A 32-year-old pregnant woman, Ms. Smith, presents to the labor and delivery unit with complaints of intense uterine contractions. She is currently at 37 weeks of gestation and is expecting her first child. Electronic Fetal Monitoring (EFM) reveals late decelerations coinciding with the uterine contractions. Which intervention should the nurse initiate immediately?
A) Reposition the patient on her left side
B) Administer oxygen via face mask at 10 L/min
C) Perform a vaginal examination to assess for cervical dilation
D) Increase intravenous fluid rate to optimize maternal blood volume

Question 332: Emily, a 25-year-old pregnant woman at 40 weeks gestation, is in labor and undergoing electronic fetal monitoring. The fetal heart rate tracing shows an absence of fetal heart rate accelerations. What action would you take based on this finding?
A) Administer tocolytic medication to reduce contractions.
B) Initiate immediate emergency cesarean section.
C) Perform an ultrasound to assess amniotic fluid volume.
D) Continue labor management and reassess fetal heart rate periodically.

Question 333: Which of the following best describes cable movement artifact in EFM?
A) Irregular baseline fluctuations caused by electrode displacement
B) Sawtooth-like waveforms resulting from electrode contact issues
C) Loss of signal due to inadequate ultrasound transmission
D) Distorted tracings caused by maternal/fetal movement or loose cables

Question 334: What is signal ambiguity in electronic fetal monitoring equipment?
A) It refers to a situation where the fetal heart rate signal is unclear and cannot be properly interpreted.
B) It refers to a malfunction in the electronic fetal monitoring equipment that causes the loss of the fetal heart rate signal.
C) It refers to the interference of external electrical signals that disrupt the accuracy of the fetal heart rate signal.
D) It refers to the inability of the healthcare provider to accurately place the ultrasound transducer on the mother's abdomen, resulting in a weak fetal heart rate signal.

Question 335: When assessing fetal heart rate accelerations, which of the following criteria must be met?
A) Increase in heart rate of at least 15 bpm above the baseline.
B) The acceleration must last for at least 10 seconds.
C) The duration of accelerations must be between 15-60 seconds.
D) The acceleration must coincide with fetal movement.

Question 336: Sarah, 29 years old, is pregnant and has been diagnosed with severe preeclampsia. She presents to the hospital with complaints of severe headache and blurred vision. On examination, her blood pressure is 160/100 mmHg and she has edema in her face and hands. Which of the following is the most appropriate initial step in the management of this patient?
A) Administering oral antihypertensive medications
B) Initiating magnesium sulfate infusion
C) Ordering a complete blood count and liver function tests
D) Scheduling an urgent cesarean delivery

Question 337: A 36-year-old woman at 38 weeks of gestation is being monitored for an abnormal fetal heart rate tracing. The nurse notices that the fetal heart rate tracing appears distorted and exhibits frequent signal interference. What could be a potential cause of this signal ambiguity?
A) Uterine hyperstimulation
B) Cross-talk interference
C) Dysfunctional fetal monitor
D) Poor transducer placement

Question 338: Ms. Thompson, a 30-year-old pregnant woman with a BMI of 38, is diagnosed with gestational diabetes mellitus (GDM). Which of the following fetal heart rate patterns is commonly seen in pregnant women with maternal obesity and GDM?
A) Early decelerations
B) Sinusoidal pattern
C) Accelerations
D) Variable decelerations

Question 339: Miss Thompson, a 32-year-old pregnant woman at 32 weeks gestation, is admitted to the labor and delivery unit for close monitoring due to gestational diabetes. Upon assessment, the nurse notes a fetal heart rate of 110 bpm, which abruptly drops to 60 bpm and remains there for 5 minutes. The nurse should take which immediate action?
A) Administer a tocolytic medication to the mother
B) Administer oxygen to the mother
C) Prepare for immediate delivery
D) Reassure the mother and continue monitoring

Question 340: Which of the following is not typically associated with a prolonged deceleration pattern?
A) Umbilical cord compression.
B) Fetal head compression.
C) Maternal hypotension.
D) Uterine hyperstimulation.

Question 341: Mrs. Adams, a 26-year-old gravida 2 para 1 woman, presents to the antenatal clinic at 34 weeks gestation. She reports painless vaginal bleeding that started earlier in the day. On examination, her uterus is non-tender and the fundus is above the umbilicus. Fetal heart rate monitoring shows a

reassuring pattern. Which of the following is the most likely diagnosis in this patient?
A) Placenta previa
B) Placental abruption
C) Uterine rupture
D) Cervical polyp

Question 342: Mrs. Smith, a 35-year-old pregnant woman at 30 weeks gestation, is admitted to the labor and delivery unit with suspected preterm labor. After assessment, the cervix is found to be closed. She is experiencing painful contractions every 10 minutes. The tocometer shows a resting tone of 30mmHg. What intervention would you recommend?
A) Administer tocolytic therapy with terbutaline
B) Begin a course of antibiotics for possible infection
C) Prepare the patient for immediate delivery via cesarean section
D) Administer magnesium sulfate for fetal neuroprotection

Question 343: Which of the following is an example of a professional issue related to electronic fetal monitoring (EFM)?
A) Ethical considerations in disclosing confidential EFM information
B) Proper positioning of the fetal monitor transducer on the mother's abdomen
C) Technique for sterile vaginal examinations during labor
D) Guidelines for cesarean section in cases of non-reassuring fetal heart rate patterns

Question 344: What is the role of the placenta in fetal oxygenation?
A) It produces fetal red blood cells
B) It filters waste products from the fetal bloodstream
C) It exchanges oxygen and nutrients between the maternal and fetal bloodstreams
D) It maintains the fetal heart rate
.

Question 345: Which of the following interventions can promote fetal heart rate variability?
A) Maternal position change
B) Amnioinfusion
C) Administration of oxygen to the mother
D) All of the above

Question 346: Which component in cord blood gases indicates the presence of fetal hypoxemia?
A) pH
B) Base excess
C) Partial pressure of carbon dioxide (pCO2)
D) Base deficit

Question 347: Which nursing action is appropriate for managing late decelerations during labor?
A) Assisting with amnioinfusion
B) Encouraging the mother to bear down during contractions
C) Monitoring maternal vital signs every 2 hours
D) Administering an epidural analgesia

Question 348: Which of the following interventions is appropriate for managing severe preeclampsia-eclampsia?
A) Increasing physical activity
B) Administering magnesium sulfate
C) Encouraging fluid restriction
D) Discontinuing antihypertensive medications

Question 349: What is the hallmark pattern associated with an early fetal heart rate deceleration?
A) Rapid onset and return to baseline.
B) Gradual onset and return to baseline.
C) Abrupt onset and return to baseline.
D) No changes in the baseline fetal heart rate.

Question 350: Mrs. Johnson, a 32-year-old pregnant woman at 37 weeks gestation, presents to the antenatal clinic complaining of regular contractions that are lasting for 70 seconds and occurring every 4 minutes. On examination, her cervix is dilated 3 cm. What is the correct description of these contractions?
A) Braxton Hicks contractions
B) False labor contractions
C) Preterm labor contractions
D) True labor contractions

Question 351: What is the duration of a typical contraction during the latent phase of labor?
A) 15-20 seconds
B) 30-45 seconds
C) 60-90 seconds
D) 120-180 seconds

Question 352: Which of the following statements best represents the principle of beneficence in medical ethics?
A) Acting in the patient's best interest while ensuring no harm is done
B) Respecting and promoting the rights of patients
C) Distributing healthcare resources fairly and equally
D) Maintaining patient confidentiality and privacy

Question 353: What is the normal range of uterine contraction intensity during active labor?
A) 5-20 Montvield Units (MU)
B) 20-40 Montvield Units (MU)
C) 40-100 Montvield Units (MU)
D) 100-200 Montvield Units (MU)

Question 354: What potential risks are associated with signal ambiguity in electronic fetal monitoring?
A) Delay in appropriate interventions
B) Incorrect interpretation of fetal heart rate pattern
C) Increased risk of adverse perinatal outcomes
D) All of the above

Question 355: During an antenatal visit, Mrs. Anderson, a 35-year-old pregnant woman at 28 weeks gestation, expresses concern about the absence of fetal movements. The fetal heart rate monitoring reveals the presence of fetal heart rate accelerations. Which of the following statements regarding the absence of fetal movements and the presence of fetal heart rate accelerations is true?
A) Absence of fetal movements is an expected finding during the third trimester.
B) Fetal heart rate accelerations are a compensatory response to reduced fetal movements.
C) Absence of fetal movements and fetal heart rate accelerations indicate fetal distress.
D) Fetal heart rate accelerations are an early sign of impending fetal demise.

Question 356: Which pattern in electronic fetal monitoring indicates early decelerations?
A) Variable decelerations
B) Late decelerations
C) Prolonged decelerations

D) Mirrored decelerations

Question 357: Which maternal factor is associated with an increased risk of placental abruption?
A) Smoking
B) Advanced maternal age
C) Substance abuse
D) All of the above

Question 358: Mr. Jones, a 35-year-old male, presents to the obstetric clinic with his pregnant wife who is at 36 weeks of gestation. During the routine antenatal check-up, the fetal heart rate (FHR) tracing reveals a prolonged deceleration of more than 3 minutes. Which of the following is the most appropriate intervention in this case?
A) Immediate cesarean section
B) Administer oxygen to the mother
C) Administer tocolytic therapy to the mother
D) Perform a vaginal examination

Question 359: Which of the following structures allows gas exchange between the fetal and maternal circulations?
A) Placenta
B) Umbilical cord
C) Amniotic fluid
D) Decidua

Question 360: Jamie, a 29-year-old pregnant woman, is at 30 weeks gestation. She is concerned about the well-being of her baby and wants to monitor the fetal heart rate at home. Which of the following fetal assessment methods would be appropriate for Jamie to use?
A) Blood tests
B) Amniocentesis
C) Electronic fetal monitoring (EFM)
D) Ultrasound

Question 361: Mrs. Thompson, a 34-year-old primigravida at 32 weeks gestation, presents to the labor and delivery unit with the complaint of painless vaginal bleeding. On examination, her uterus is non-tender, and the fundus is at the level of the umbilicus. The cervical os is closed on digital examination. Fetal heart rate monitoring reveals a non-reassuring pattern, with decelerations occurring during contractions. Which of the following is the most likely diagnosis in this patient?
A) Placenta previa
B) Placental abruption
C) Uterine rupture
D) Vasa previa

Question 362: Which of the following is a non-pharmacological intervention for hypertonus during labor?
A) Administering magnesium sulfate
B) Administering terbutaline
C) Applying warm compresses
D) Increasing intravenous fluids

Question 363: Ms. Lee, a 29-year-old primigravida at 32 weeks of gestation, is diagnosed with severe preeclampsia. Which of the following laboratory findings would you expect when assessing her condition?
A) Decreased platelet count
B) Decreased liver enzymes
C) Decreased urinary protein
D) Decreased blood glucose levels

Question 364: Which of the following fetal heart rate patterns is commonly seen in hypoxemic fetuses?
A) Sinusoidal pattern
B) Accelerations
C) Early decelerations
D) Variable decelerations

Question 365: Which statement about umbilical artery blood flow is correct?
A) Umbilical artery carries oxygenated blood from the placenta to the fetus.
B) Umbilical artery blood flow decreases during fetal hypoxia.
C) Umbilical artery carries deoxygenated blood from the fetus to the placenta.
D) Umbilical artery resistance increases in response to maternal hypertension.

Question 366: Which recreational drug, when used during pregnancy, can cause various adverse effects in the fetus, including low birth weight, developmental delays, and behavioral problems?
A) Heroin
B) Methamphetamine
C) Ecstasy
D) Ketamine

Question 367: Mrs. Roberts, a 29-year-old G1P0, is admitted to the labor and delivery unit at term. The nurse is assessing the intensity of her uterine contractions using an external tocodynamometer. The nurse notices that the intensity of the contractions is increasing and measures it to be 70mmHg at its peak. How would you classify this intensity of uterine contractions?
A) Weak
B) Moderate
C) Strong
D) Hyperstimulation

Question 368: Olivia, 25 years old, presents to the hospital at 34 weeks of gestation with complaints of upper abdominal pain, nausea, and vomiting. On examination, she has hypertension (blood pressure 150/100 mmHg) and epigastric tenderness. Laboratory investigations reveal elevated liver enzymes and low platelet count. What is the most likely diagnosis?
A) Severe preeclampsia
B) Gestational hypertension
C) Hemolysis, elevated liver enzymes, and low platelet count (HELLP) syndrome
D) Eclampsia

Question 369: Mrs. Johnson, a 36-year-old primigravida at 38 weeks gestation, presents to the antenatal clinic complaining of decreased fetal movement over the past 24 hours. On examination, the fetal heart rate is found to be normal, but minimal fetal movement is noted. What is the most appropriate next step?
A) Immediate induction of labor
B) Initiation of non-stress test (NST)
C) Ultrasonography for fetal biophysical profile (BPP)
D) Observation for 48 hours

Question 370: Which of the following factors can affect fetal heart rate variability?
A) Gestational age
B) Maternal position

C) Fetal sleep cycles
D) All of the above

Question 371: What is the most appropriate initial intervention for a fetus with supraventricular tachycardia (SVT)?
A) Administering intravenous adenosine
B) Administering oxygen to the mother
C) Performing fetal echocardiography
D) Applying fetal scalp electrodes

Question 372: Which of the following is an example of an appropriate fetal movement assessment method?
A) External cephalic version
B) Doppler ultrasound
C) Contraction stress test
D) Biophysical profile

Question 373: Which of the following is an indication for cord blood acid base testing?
A) Normal fetal heart rate pattern
B) Early decelerations
C) Variable decelerations
D) Late decelerations

Question 374: Mrs.John is a 28-year-old pregnant woman who has been diagnosed with gestational diabetes. She is in his third trimester and requires close monitoring of the fetal heart rate. Which of the following statements regarding the use of electronic monitoring equipment for fetal assessment in this scenario is correct?
A) Electronic monitoring equipment may not accurately assess the fetal heart rate in women with gestational diabetes.
B) Electronic monitoring equipment is of no use in women with gestational diabetes.
C) External monitoring devices are sufficient for accurate fetal assessment in women with gestational diabetes.
D) Internal monitoring devices are recommended for accurate fetal assessment in women with gestational diabetes.

Question 375: Which intervention is appropriate for managing cord compression during labor?
A) Administer terbutaline
B) Apply fetal scalp electrode
C) Administer oxygen to the mother
D) Perform immediate cesarean section

Question 376: Which of the following is a characteristic of normal fetal heart rate variability?
A) Minimal fluctuations
B) Absence of accelerations
C) Irregular rhythm
D) Smooth baseline

Question 377: Mrs. Johnson, a 26-year-old primigravida, is currently in labor at 42 weeks gestation. During electronic fetal monitoring, there is a sustained baseline fetal heart rate (FHR) greater than 160 bpm noted for an extended period of time. Which of the following is the most likely cause for this pattern?
A) Fetal tachycardia
B) Maternal fever
C) Fetal arrhythmia
D) Maternal anxiety

Question 378: Which of the following fetal heart rate patterns is commonly seen during supraventricular tachycardia (SVT)?
A) Sinusoidal pattern
B) Accelerations
C) Variable decelerations
D) Early decelerations

Question 379: A 25-year-old pregnant woman, Mrs. Smith, at 41 weeks gestation presents for a nonstress test. The fetal heart rate baseline is 110 bpm, with minimal variability. No accelerations or decelerations are seen during the 20-minute test. What is the interpretation of this nonstress test?
A) Reactive
B) Nonreactive
C) Equivocal
D) Abnormal

Question 380: Mrs. Johnson is a 34-year-old primigravida who is currently 38 weeks pregnant. She presents to the labor and delivery unit in early labor. Upon admission, the nurse evaluates her uterine activity. Which of the following is characteristic of normal uterine activity during early labor?
A) Contractions lasting 60 seconds or longer
B) Contractions occurring more than five minutes apart
C) Contractions palpable only on one side of the abdomen
D) Contractions causing severe pain and discomfort

Question 381: Which statement describes the variability of fetal heart rate during early decelerations?
A) Absent or minimal variability.
B) Moderate to marked variability.
C) Non-reassuring variability.
D) Unpredictable variability.

Question 382: In cases of prolonged decelerations, what additional intervention may be considered by the healthcare provider?
A) Increasing intravenous fluids.
B) Administering oxygen to the fetus.
C) Performing a cesarean section.
D) Administering tocolytic drugs.

Question 383: Which of the following statements about fetal dysrhythmias is true?
A) Fetal dysrhythmias are always a cause for concern and require immediate intervention.
B) Fetal dysrhythmias occur as a result of increased fetal heart rate variability.
C) Fetal dysrhythmias are benign and do not require any intervention.
D) Fetal dysrhythmias are characterized by a regular rhythm in the fetal heart rate.

Question 384: In a monochorionic-diamniotic twin pregnancy, what is the most common type of placental vascular anastomosis?
A) Arteriovenous anastomosis
B) Arterioarterial anastomosis
C) Venovenous anastomosis
D) Venous-arterial anastomosis

Question 385: Mrs. Thompson, a 42-year-old woman, presents with excessive sweating, palpitations, and weight loss despite increased appetite. Laboratory results reveal an increased level of thyroid-stimulating hormone (TSH) and decreased levels of free thyroxine (T4) and free triiodothyronine (T3). Which of the

following physiological mechanisms is primarily responsible for these findings?
A) Decreased hypothalamic thyrotropin-releasing hormone (TRH) production
B) Decreased pituitary thyroid-stimulating hormone (TSH) production
C) Increased thyroid hormone synthesis and release
D) Autoimmune destruction of thyroid tissue

Question 386:   What is the management approach for postdates pregnancy?
A) Induction of labor
B) Cesarean section
C) Expectant management
D) Maternal-fetal surveillance only

Question 387:   What is the purpose of the FHR baseline in electronic monitoring?
A) To determine the fetal heart rate variability
B) To assess the fetal well-being
C) To identify decelerations
D) To calculate the fetal heart rate acceleration

Question 388:   Ms. Garcia is a 36-year-old primigravida at 41 weeks of gestation, in active labor. Cord blood gas analysis is a useful tool for assessing fetal well-being at delivery. Which of the following parameters would be measured in cord blood gas analysis?
A) Fetal hemoglobin level
B) Placental oxygen saturation
C) Umbilical artery pH
D) Maternal arterial pH

Question 389:   Patient: Mrs. Johnson, a 28-year-old pregnant woman at 34 weeks gestation, presents with right upper quadrant pain, headache, and visual disturbances. Her blood pressure is 160/100 mmHg. Laboratory results show elevated liver enzymes and low platelet count. What is the most likely diagnosis for this patient?
A) Pre-eclampsia
B) Gestational diabetes
C) Placenta previa
D) Intrahepatic cholestasis of pregnancy

Question 390:   A pregnant woman with hypertension is prescribed a calcium channel blocker to control her blood pressure. Which of the following effects can be expected on the fetal heart rate tracing?
A) Decreased baseline rate
B) Increased variability
C) Early decelerations
D) Variable decelerations

Question 391:   During a fetal monitoring session, the EFM is displaying a loss of signal from the FHR monitor. Which of the following troubleshooting steps should the nurse take first?
A) Check the connection between the transducer and the monitor
B) Change the position of the mother
C) Increase the volume on the monitor
D) Restart the EFM system

Question 392:   Which of the following factors can influence umbilical blood flow?
A) Maternal hypotension
B) Fetal hypoxia
C) Umbilical cord compression
D) All of the above

Question 393:   Which infection is associated with the development of fetal hydrocephalus?
A) Toxoplasmosis
B) Urinary tract infection
C) Hepatitis C
D) Influenza

Question 394:   Ms. Thompson, a 35-year-old pregnant woman, is at 28 weeks of gestation and is admitted to the antepartum unit with hypertonic contractions. The electronic fetal monitoring (EFM) tracing reveals decreased variability. Which intervention should the nurse prioritize for this patient?
A) Administer intravenous tocolytic therapy
B) Administer an analgesic medication
C) Assess for signs of placental abruption
D) Perform an ultrasound to assess fetal well-being

Question 395:   Olivia, a 40-week gestation pregnant woman, is in active labor. The fetal heart rate (FHR) monitoring reveals a consistent pattern of smooth, wavelike motion with a uniform frequency of 3-4 cycles per minute. The FHR ranges between 130-150 beats per minute, and there are no decelerations or accelerations. What is the most appropriate action for the healthcare provider?
A) Perform fetal scalp stimulation
B) Prepare for an immediate emergency cesarean section
C) Monitor the mother's vital signs
D) Apply a uterine tocodynamometer to measure contractions

Question 396:   A pregnant woman with diabetes is at an increased risk of which of the following maternal complications?
A) Preterm labor
B) Gestational hypertension
C) Placenta previa
D) Ectopic pregnancy

Question 397:   Emily, a 30-year-old patient, is scheduled for an appendectomy under local anesthesia with intravenous sedation. Which of the following medications is commonly used for intravenous sedation during local anesthesia in a pregnant patient?
A) Propofol
B) Ketamine
C) Nitrous oxide
D) Midazolam

Question 398:   Mrs. Johnson, a 27-year-old pregnant woman at 36 weeks gestation, presents to the antenatal clinic for a routine check-up. The nurse is preparing to assess her uterine activity. Which of the following methods is commonly used to monitor the uterine contractions electronically during labor?
A) Leopold maneuvers
B) Auscultation with a Pinard stethoscope
C) External tocodynamometer
D) Vaginal examination

Question 399:   Mrs. Rodriguez, 28-year-old G4P2 at 36 weeks gestation with type 1 diabetes, presents to the labor and delivery unit for scheduled induction of labor. On admission, the fetal heart rate (FHR) tracing reveals a baseline of 160 bpm, with absent variability, no accelerations, and no decelerations. What would be the most appropriate initial intervention?
A) Administer a bolus of intravenous fluids

B) Administer oxygen via face mask
C) Change maternal position
D) Perform a scalp stimulation test

Question 400:   A 26-year-old patient, Emily, arrives at the antenatal clinic for her routine check-up during her second trimester. The nurse notices that Emily's medical records are missing key information, such as her blood type and previous medical history. What is the best approach to address this quality issue?
A) Ignore the missing information as it is not relevant to Emily's current visit.
B) Document the missing information in a temporary file and update Emily's medical record later.
C) Continue with the check-up without addressing the missing information.
D) Notify the healthcare provider in charge and assist in updating Emily's medical record immediately.

Question 401:   Which hormone stimulates the development of milk-producing glands in the breasts?
A) Estrogen
B) Progesterone
C) Oxytocin
D) Prolactin

Question 402:   Sarah, a 38-year-old pregnant woman, is in her third trimester of pregnancy. She reports frequent episodes of dizziness and shortness of breath. The healthcare provider suspects maternal hypotension as a potential factor affecting fetal oxygenation. Which of the following interventions is most appropriate to improve maternal blood pressure and fetal oxygenation in this situation?
A) Administering oxygen to the mother
B) Encouraging the mother to lie on her left side
C) Increasing maternal fluid intake
D) Administering beta-blockers to the mother

Question 403:   How can signal ambiguity in electronic fetal monitoring be resolved?
A) Repositioning the mother to eliminate external interference.
B) Adjusting the placement of the ultrasound transducer on the mother's abdomen.
C) Reducing maternal movement during monitoring.
D) All of the above.

Question 404:   Emma, 32 years old, is currently pregnant with her first baby. She is in her third trimester and has been diagnosed with preeclampsia. Which of the following is a characteristic finding in preeclampsia?
A) Hypotension
B) Edema of the lower extremities
C) Proteinuria
D) Bradycardia

Question 405:   Mrs. Davis, a 29-year-old multiparous woman at 37 weeks gestation, is in active labor. The fetal heart rate (FHR) shows a prolonged deceleration followed by a slow return to baseline with reduced variability. The obstetrician decides to perform a cord blood gas analysis, which reveals a pH of 7.39. What is the significance of this pH value?
A) Acidemia
B) Normal pH
C) Alkalemia
D) Acidosis

Question 406:   What is the primary vessel responsible for carrying oxygenated blood to the fetus?
A) Ductus arteriosus
B) Umbilical artery
C) Ductus venosus
D) Umbilical vein

Question 407:   Which of the following is a potential complication of HELLP syndrome?
A) Placental abruption
B) Polyhydramnios
C) Gestational diabetes
D) Preeclampsia

Question 408:   Mrs. Thompson, a 28-year-old pregnant woman at 40 weeks gestation, presents to the antenatal clinic complaining of contractions that stop when she changes position or ambulates. What is the most likely cause of these contractions?
A) Preterm labor contractions
B) True labor contractions
C) False labor contractions
D) Intestinal gas contractions

Question 409:   Mrs. Smith, a 32-year-old pregnant woman with Type 2 diabetes, is admitted to the labor and delivery unit at 38 weeks gestation. Which of the following interventions is appropriate for the management of her diabetes during labor and delivery?
A) Continuation of oral hypoglycemic agents
B) Insulin therapy began at the onset of labor
C) Discontinuation of all antidiabetic medications
D) Monitoring blood glucose levels every 8 hours

Question 410:   Sofia, a 32-year-old primigravida, is at 38 weeks of gestation and presents to the labor and delivery unit with decreased fetal movements. On examination, the fetal heart rate (FHR) tracing demonstrates decreased variability, late decelerations, and a baseline heart rate of 140 bpm. Which of the following is the most likely cause?
A) Fetal hypoxia
B) Uteroplacental insufficiency
C) Fetal structural abnormalities
D) Medication side effects

Question 411:   Ms. Smith, a 32-year-old pregnant woman at 39 weeks gestation, presents to the labor and delivery unit with decreased fetal movement. Upon electronic fetal monitoring, there is a prolonged deceleration noted in the fetal heart rate (FHR) lasting more than 3 minutes with a slow return to baseline. Which of the following is the most likely cause for this pattern?
A) Uteroplacental insufficiency
B) Fetal sleep state
C) Umbilical cord compression
D) Maternal hypotension

Question 412:   Mrs. Johnson, a 36-year-old multiparous woman at 38 weeks of gestation, presents to the antenatal clinic with reduced fetal movements and is diagnosed with suspected fetal growth restriction. Which of the following uteroplacental complications is most commonly associated with fetal growth restriction?
A) Placental abruption
B) Uterine rupture
C) Placenta previa
D) Placenta accreta

Question 413: Mrs. Thompson, a 35-year-old pregnant woman at 36 weeks gestation, presents with vaginal bleeding. Upon electronic fetal monitoring, there is persistent variable deceleration in the fetal heart rate (FHR) with rapid return to baseline. Which of the following is the most likely cause for this pattern?
A) Cord prolapse
B) Maternal hypertension
C) Fetal bradycardia
D) Premature rupture of membranes

Question 414: Which of the following best describes an advantage of internal fetal heart rate monitoring during labor?
A) It allows for continuous monitoring of the fetal heart rate.
B) It is less invasive compared to external monitoring.
C) It provides information about the strength of uterine contractions.
D) It can be easily applied by healthcare providers.

Question 415: A pregnant woman is prescribed an opioid pain medication for severe chronic back pain. Which of the following effects is associated with opioid use during pregnancy and may affect fetal oxygenation?
A) Increased uterine blood flow
B) Fetal tachycardia
C) Maternal hypotension
D) Decreased fetal respiratory movements

Question 416: Mrs. Anderson, a 32-year-old woman, presents to the labor and delivery unit at 38 weeks gestation with decreased fetal movement for the past 12 hours. Upon assessment, the electronic fetal monitoring (EFM) reveals absent fetal heart rate variability with recurrent late decelerations. Which of the following is the correct intervention in this situation?
A) Continue monitoring the fetal heart rate for another hour
B) Administer oxygen by face mask at 10 liters per minute
C) Notify the obstetrician for further evaluation
D) Initiate immediate delivery by emergency cesarean section

Question 417: Which of the following interventions is appropriate for managing tachysystole?
A) Increasing oxytocin infusion rate.
B) Encouraging maternal position changes.
C) Administering a tocolytic medication.
D) Administering a medication to stimulate contractions.

Question 418: Mrs. Johnson, a 35-year-old gravida 4, para 3 woman, is admitted to the labor and delivery unit for induction of labor at term. She has a medical history significant for gestational diabetes mellitus (GDM). Fetal heart rate monitoring reveals variable decelerations with slow return to baseline. Which of the following factors is most likely contributing to the compromised umbilical blood flow?
A) Maternal age
B) GDM
C) Fetal heart rate
D) Uterine contractions

Question 419: What is the term used to describe contractions that occur less frequently than normal during labor?
A) Tachysystole
B) Hypotonic contractions
C) Montevideo units
D) Uterine atony

Question 420: Emily, a 28-year-old pregnant woman, is advised to maintain good hydration during her pregnancy. Which of the following is the primary rationale for ensuring adequate maternal fluid intake to optimize fetal oxygenation?
A) Promotion of fetal lung development
B) Prevention of preterm labor
C) Maintenance of adequate blood volume
D) Enhancement of fetal hemoglobin production

Question 421: Which of the following is a common symptom of preterm labor?
A) Decreased fetal movements
B) Vaginal bleeding
C) Swollen ankles
D) Constipation

Question 422: What is considered a normal resting tone during electronic fetal monitoring?
A) 10-20 mmHg
B) 25-35 mmHg
C) 40-50 mmHg
D) 55-65 mmHg

Question 423: Which of the following is a characteristic feature of congenital heart block?
A) Decreased fetal heart rate variability
B) Intermittent acceleration of the fetal heart rate
C) Fetal bradycardia
D) U-shaped decelerations in the fetal heart rate

Question 424: Mrs. Garcia is a 28-year-old pregnant woman with a BMI of 40. She is now in her third trimester and complains of shortness of breath while lying flat. Which of the following interventions is recommended for managing maternal obesity-related dyspnea?
A) Encouraging the patient to sleep in a supine position
B) Referring the patient for a sleep study
C) Recommending left lateral positioning during sleep
D) Prescribing bronchodilator medication

Question 425: Mr. Brown, a 28-year-old man, accompanies his wife to the antenatal clinic at 37 weeks gestation. The electronic fetal monitoring (EFM) shows a prolonged fetal heart rate deceleration of more than 2 minutes. Which of the following is the most appropriate action for the nurse to take?
A) Administer oxygen to the pregnant woman
B) Change the maternal position to a lateral tilt
C) Apply a fetal scalp electrode for better monitoring
D) Prepare for an immediate emergency cesarean section

Question 426: Ms. Johnson, a 32-year-old primigravida at 34 weeks gestation, presents to the antepartum unit with a tender, swollen left leg. She has a history of smoking and is obese. The nurse suspects deep vein thrombosis (DVT). On electronic fetal monitoring (EFM), the tracing shows normal baseline variability, accelerations, and no decelerations. What would be the most appropriate action in this situation?
A) Initiate immediate thrombolytic therapy
B) Administer nonsteroidal anti-inflammatory drugs (NSAIDs)
C) Encourage bed rest
D) Notify the healthcare provider

Question 427: Miss Thompson, a 28-year-old primigravida at 39 weeks gestation, is in active labor. During a vaginal examination, the obstetric provider

notices a visible cord prolapse. What is the most appropriate immediate action?
A) Administer oxygen via face mask
B) Perform a sterile vaginal exam
C) Elevate the presenting fetal part
D) Prepare for immediate cesarean delivery

Question 428: Mr. Wilson is a 30-year-old expectant father who asks about the significance of cord blood acid-base testing during childbirth. How would you explain the importance of cord blood acid-base testing to him?
A) It assesses the newborn's lung maturity
B) It evaluates the adequacy of placental perfusion
C) It measures the newborn's cardiac function
D) It determines the newborn's blood type

Question 429: Which of the following is true regarding fetal oxygenation?
A) Fetal hemoglobin has a higher affinity for oxygen compared to adult hemoglobin
B) Fetal oxygen saturation is lower than maternal oxygen saturation
C) Fetal oxygenation primarily occurs through diffusion across the placenta
D) Fetal oxygen supply is dependent on maternal carbon dioxide levels

Question 430: A fetal baseline heart rate below 120 bpm for a prolonged period may indicate:
A) Fetal distress
B) Maternal distress
C) Normal variation
D) Positional change

Question 431: Mr. Johnson, an expectant father, Questions the healthcare provider about the potential legal implications of electronic fetal monitoring. Which of the following statements accurately reflects the legal considerations in this context?
A) Electronic fetal monitoring is solely the responsibility of the healthcare provider.
B) The expectant father has no legal rights or involvement in the fetal monitoring process.
C) Legal implications arise from the interpretation and actions taken based on the fetal monitoring findings.
D) The healthcare provider bears no legal accountability for the fetal monitoring process.

Question 432: Which of the following factors can contribute to decreased variability in fetal heart rate?
A) Fetal sleep cycles
B) Maternal infections
C) Fetal movement
D) Placental abruption

Question 433: During labor, Mrs. Johnson, a 30-year-old gravida 2 para 1, experiences a sudden decrease in the fetal heart rate (FHR) tracing and the loss of fetal movements. On assessment, the cervix is dilated at 8 cm. Which of the following is the most appropriate immediate action?
A) Perform a fetal scalp stimulation test
B) Perform an emergency cesarean section
C) Administer oxytocin augmentation
D) Change the mother's position

Question 434: Emma, a 28-year-old woman at 36 weeks of gestation, presents with pregnancy-induced hypertension. She is concerned about the well-being of

her baby. Which of the following non-stress test (NST) findings would suggest uteroplacental insufficiency?
A) Absence of fetal movements during the NST
B) Non-reactive NST with persistent absence of accelerations
C) Presence of early decelerations during the NST
D) Reactive NST with the presence of late decelerations

Question 435: Which of the following is an example of a professional issue related to technological advancements in electronic fetal monitoring (EFM)?
A) Understanding fetal heart rate patterns and their significance
B) Interpreting uterine activity on the tocodynamometer
C) Assessing the accuracy and reliability of new EFM devices
D) Collaborating with the obstetrician to make informed decisions during labor

Question 436: How is the position of an IUPC verified after insertion?
A) By measuring cervical dilation
B) By assessing the strength of uterine contractions
C) By visual inspection during a vaginal examination
D) By monitoring maternal blood pressure

Question 437: Jessica, a 26-year-old pregnant woman with Type 1 diabetes, is scheduled for an induction of labor at 39 weeks gestation. Which of the following medications should be administered to prevent neonatal hypoglycemia after birth?
A) Fentanyl
B) Oxytocin
C) Betamethasone
D) Glucose gel or solution

Question 438: A nurse is assessing a pregnant patient with a history of diabetes. Which maternal factor can potentially affect fetal oxygenation in this patient?
A) Hypertension
B) Hyperthyroidism
C) Hypoglycemia
D) Polycystic Ovary Syndrome (PCOS)

Question 439: Maternal complications such as placental abruption can result in which of the following fetal heart rate patterns?
A) Tachycardia
B) Bradycardia
C) Late decelerations
D) Variable decelerations

Question 440: Which of the following interventions is appropriate in a case of suspected decreased blood flow to the fetus?
A) Administering tocolytic agents
B) Increasing the maternal oxygenation
C) Encouraging maternal hydration
D) Facilitating immediate delivery

Question 441: Which of the following maternal complications can result in preterm birth?
A) Preeclampsia
B) Gestational diabetes
C) Placenta previa
D) Urinary tract infection

Question 442: Mrs. Smith, a 36-year-old pregnant woman at 39 weeks of gestation, is admitted to the labor and delivery unit in active labor. The nurse is assessing

her uterine activity using an external tocodynamometer. What is the primary advantage of using an external tocodynamometer for monitoring uterine activity?
A) It provides accurate measurement of intrauterine pressure.
B) It allows for continuous monitoring of fetal heart rate.
C) It is non-invasive and does not require cervical dilation.
D) It provides real-time visualization of uterine contractions.

Question 443: Mrs. Anderson, a 28-year-old multigravida, is at 36 weeks gestation. She has a history of gestational hypertension during her previous pregnancy. Today, her blood pressure is consistently above 140/90 mmHg, but she has no symptoms. What is the appropriate management for Mrs. Anderson?
A) Prescribe antihypertensive medication and schedule frequent follow-up visits
B) Admit for immediate induction of labor
C) Monitor closely and repeat blood pressure measurements
D) Request a 24-hour urine collection for protein quantification

Question 444: What is the normal baseline fetal heart rate range during labor?
A) 80-100 beats per minute
B) 110-130 beats per minute
C) 140-160 beats per minute
D) 170-190 beats per minute

Question 445: Which condition is associated with a higher risk of uterine rupture during labor?
A) Placenta Previa
B) Placental Abruption
C) Uterine Fibroids
D) Previous cesarean delivery

Question 446: Mrs. Thompson, a 32-year-old G3P2 at 41 weeks gestation, presents to the labor and delivery unit for a routine antenatal check-up. The obstetrician notes a fundal height consistent with gestational age, normal maternal vital signs, and a reactive non-stress test. What is the next appropriate step to further assess fetal well-being?
A) Fetal kick count
B) Amniotic fluid index (AFI) measurement
C) Fetal biophysical profile (BPP)
D) Doppler velocimetry of umbilical artery

Question 447: Amanda, a 30-year-old pregnant woman at 36 weeks of gestation, undergoes a non-stress test (NST) to evaluate fetal well-being. The nurse explains that the CTG tracing will record uterine activity in addition to the fetal heart rate. Which of the following types of uterine activity is commonly seen on the CTG tracing?
A) Uterine tachysystole
B) Uterine hypertonus
C) Uterine contractions with relaxation in-between
D) Uterine retraction

Question 448: Which fetal heart rate pattern is commonly associated with cord compression?
A) Early decelerations
B) Accelerations
C) Variable decelerations
D) Late decelerations

Question 449: A 28-year-old pregnant woman, Mrs. Anderson, is admitted to the labor and delivery unit at 32 weeks gestation with preterm labor. In monitoring the fetal heart rate, you observe persistent late decelerations. Which of the following interventions should be initiated first?
A) Administer tocolytic medication
B) Perform a vaginal examination to assess cervical dilation
C) Administer steroids for fetal lung maturation
D) Place a scalp electrode for continuous monitoring

Question 450: Which of the following maternal complications can significantly impact fetal well-being during labor and birth?
A) Gestational diabetes
B) Placenta previa
C) Preeclampsia
D) Urinary tract infection

Question 451: Sarah, a 25-year-old G2P1 at 32 weeks gestation, presents to the emergency department with decreased fetal movements and vaginal bleeding. On examination, the fetal heart rate tracing is reactive, but contractions are noted on tocodynamometry. What is the most appropriate next step?
A) Immediate cesarean section
B) Fetal kick count for 2 hours
C) Ultrasonography for fetal biophysical profile (BPP)
D) Evaluation for abruptio placentae

Question 452: Which maternal position is preferred during anesthesia to optimize fetal oxygenation?
A) Supine position
B) Trendelenburg position
C) Left lateral tilt position
D) Prone position

Question 453: Which of the following analgesic techniques is considered safe during labor anesthesia for optimal fetal oxygenation?
A) Intrathecal opioids
B) Epidural analgesia
C) Systemic opioids
D) Intravenous ketamine

Question 454: Laura, a 35-year-old multigravida with chronic essential hypertension, presents at 38 weeks gestation complaining of decreased fetal movements. On examination, the fetal heart rate tracing shows variable decelerations. What is the most appropriate intervention in this situation?
A) Administration of intravenous (IV) fluids
B) Immediate delivery by cesarean section
C) Expectant management with close fetal monitoring
D) Initiation of magnesium sulfate for fetal neuroprotection

Question 455: Maternal obesity is defined by which of the following criteria?
A) Body Mass Index (BMI) 30 kg/m
B) Body Mass Index (BMI) 25 kg/m
C) Body Mass Index (BMI) 35 kg/m
D) Body Mass Index (BMI) 20 kg/m

Question 456: Which pattern of fetal heart rate variability is characterized by an amplitude of less than 5 beats per minute?
A) Absent Variability
B) Marked Variability
C) Minimal Variability
D) Moderate Variability

Question 457: A 32-year-old pregnant woman, Mrs. Johnson, presents to the labor and delivery unit at 38

weeks gestation. Her medical history is unremarkable, and this is her first pregnancy. During the electronic fetal monitoring (EFM), you notice repetitive late decelerations. Which of the following is the most appropriate initial intervention?
A) Administer oxygen via facemask
B) Perform a vaginal examination to assess cervical dilation
C) Apply a fetal scalp electrode
D) Discontinue oxytocin infusion

Question 458: What is one of the key risk factors for preterm labor?
A) Smoking during pregnancy
B) Advanced maternal age
C) Multiparity (having multiple pregnancies)
D) Obesity

Question 459: Glycemic control in pregnant women with diabetes is achieved through which of the following measures?
A) Monitoring fetal heart rate
B) Frequent blood glucose monitoring
C) Administration of corticosteroids
D) Increasing carbohydrate intake

Question 460: Which type of monitoring system is considered a noninvasive method?
A) External monitoring
B) Internal monitoring
C) Wireless monitoring
D) Doppler monitoring

Question 461: Mary, a labor and delivery nurse, notices that a fetal heart rate (FHR) monitor shows a prolonged deceleration. What should be her next action?
A) Ignore it and continue monitoring
B) Document the finding and inform the primary care provider
C) Administer oxygen to the mother
D) Increase the rate of Pitocin infusion

Question 462: Mrs. Davis, a 36-year-old pregnant woman with a BMI of 37, is scheduled for a cesarean delivery. Which of the following maternal complications is associated with maternal obesity and can increase the risk of surgical site infection?
A) Postpartum hemorrhage
B) Deep vein thrombosis
C) Endometritis
D) Preterm labor

Question 463: Sarah, a 28-year-old primigravida at 36 weeks gestation, arrives at the labor and delivery unit in active labor. Continuous electronic fetal monitoring is initiated, and you notice fetal heart rate accelerations during contractions. What action would you take?
A) Administer tocolytic medication to reduce contractions.
B) Perform a fetal scalp pH sampling to assess fetal acid-base status.
C) Continue to monitor the patient and observe the fetal heart rate pattern.
D) Prepare the patient for an immediate emergency cesarean section.

Question 464: Which of the following clinical findings may be observed during tachysystole?
A) Fetal bradycardia.
B) Decreased uterine activity.
C) Maternal hypotension.

D) Prolonged intercontraction intervals.

Question 465: Which of the following is associated with an abnormal variability pattern in fetal heart rate?
A) Accelerations
B) Decelerations
C) Transient tachycardia
D) Sinusoidal pattern

Question 466: Sophia, a 35-year-old pregnant woman, is admitted to the labor and delivery ward in active labor. An intrauterine pressure catheter (IUPC) is inserted for monitoring uterine contractions. What is the primary purpose of using an IUPC in this situation?
A) To measure cervical dilation
B) To monitor fetal heart rate
C) To assess fetal movement
D) To measure uterine contractions

Question 467: What is the characteristic feature of ectopic beats in fetal monitoring?
A) Regular rhythm
B) Increase in fetal heart rate
C) Decrease in fetal heart rate
D) Irregular rhythm

Question 468: Mrs. Smith, a 27-year-old G2P1 at 28 weeks gestation, presents to the labor and delivery unit with severe headaches, visual disturbances, and epigastric pain. On assessment, her blood pressure is 160/110 mmHg and she has +3 proteinuria. Which intervention should be prioritized?
A) Administer intravenous magnesium sulfate
B) Initiate continuous electronic fetal monitoring (EFM)
C) Consult the anesthesiologist for an epidural
D) Administer an antihypertensive medication

Question 469: Ms. Johnson, a 36-year-old primigravida, is in active labor. The electronic fetal monitoring strip shows recurrent late decelerations. What is the most appropriate immediate action in this situation?
A) Administer oxytocin to augment labor
B) Place the patient in the Trendelenburg position
C) Administer oxygen via a non-rebreather mask
D) Proceed with a vaginal examination

Question 470: Which pattern in electronic fetal monitoring is associated with umbilical cord compression?
A) Variable decelerations
B) Early decelerations
C) Late decelerations
D) Prolonged decelerations

Question 471: Which of the following can cause signal ambiguity in electronic fetal monitoring?
A) Maternal obesity
B) Placental position
C) External electrical interference
D) All of the above

Question 472: How long should nonstress testing (NST) typically be performed for?
A) 10 minutes
B) 20 minutes
C) 30 minutes
D) 1 hour

Question 473:   Patient: Mrs. Thompson, a 42-year-old pregnant woman at 38 weeks gestation, presents with right upper quadrant pain, headache, and peripheral edema. Her blood pressure is 160/100 mmHg. Laboratory results show normal liver enzymes and normal platelet count. What is the most appropriate management for this patient?
A) Administer magnesium sulfate
B) Initiate antihypertensive therapy
C) Perform a liver biopsy
D) Induce labor

Question 474:   A decrease in fetal heart rate variability is commonly associated with which type of injury?
A) Cephalohematoma
B) Intracranial hemorrhage
C) Spinal cord injury
D) Facial bruising

Question 475:   What is a potential cause of late decelerations in the fetal heart rate?
A) Cord compression
B) Fetal movement
C) Fetal tachycardia
D) Placental abruption

Question 476:   Mrs. Johnson, a 26-year-old primigravida at 34 weeks of gestation, is diagnosed with gestational hypertension. Which of the following findings would you expect when monitoring her fetal heart rate (FHR) patterns?
A) Accelerations
B) Early decelerations
C) Variable decelerations
D) Late decelerations

Question 477:   Mr. and Mrs. Smith are expecting their first child. During their antenatal visit, they ask about the fetal circulation. Which of the following statements correctly describes the fetal circulation?
A) The placenta delivers oxygenated blood to the fetus through the umbilical artery.
B) The ductus arteriosus connects the aorta and the pulmonary artery in the fetal heart.
C) Oxygenated blood from the placenta enters the right atrium through the umbilical vein.
D) The foramen ovale connects the left ventricle to the aorta in the fetal heart.

Question 478:   What intervention is recommended for ectopic beats in fetal monitoring?
A) Immediate delivery
B) Administration of tocolytic agents
C) Maternal repositioning
D) Continuous fetal monitoring

Question 479:   Ms. Hernandez, a 30-year-old pregnant woman at 34 weeks gestation, presents with symptoms indicative of preterm labor. After assessing the patient, the nurse notes that the cervix is dilated 3cm and effaced 50%. The fetal heart tracing shows occasional early decelerations. What intervention would you recommend?
A) Administer tocolytic therapy with nifedipine
B) Place an intrauterine pressure catheter
C) Prepare the patient for immediate cesarean section
D) Administer magnesium sulfate for fetal neuroprotection

Question 480:   Mrs. Johnson, a 34-year-old pregnant woman, has a BMI of 35. During her regular prenatal visit, the nurse notes that her blood pressure is elevated. Which of the following fetal heart rate patterns is associated with maternal obesity?
A) Early decelerations
B) Variable decelerations
C) Late decelerations
D) Accelerations

Question 481:   Which of the following is the correct duration for a normal uterine contraction during the active phase of labor?
A) 10 seconds
B) 30 seconds
C) 60 seconds
D) 90 seconds

Question 482:   Mrs.Thomas, a 32-year-old pregnant woman, presents to the antenatal clinic for a routine check-up. During the assessment, the healthcare provider suspects maternal smoking to be affecting fetal oxygenation. Which of the following effects on the fetus is most commonly associated with maternal smoking?
A) Decreased fetal hemoglobin production
B) Increased fetal cardiac output
C) Decreased fetal respiratory rate
D) Increased fetal oxygen saturation

Question 483:   What is the purpose of external fetal heart rate monitoring during labor?
A) To assess the mother's blood pressure
B) To monitor the strength of uterine contractions
C) To evaluate the progress of cervical dilation
D) To assess the well-being of the fetus

Question 484:   Maria, a 25-year-old pregnant woman, is admitted to the labor and delivery unit. She is currently in the active phase of labor. The nurse notes a decrease in fetal heart rate variability on the electronic fetal monitoring (EFM) strip. Which of the following factors is most likely to contribute to this finding?
A) Maternal hyperglycemia
B) Uterine contractions
C) Fetal anemia
D) Maternal hypertension

Question 485:   Which type of uterine monitoring technique is non-invasive and measures the frequency, duration, and intensity of contractions?
A) Intrauterine pressure catheter (IUPC)
B) Tocodynamometer
C) Fetal scalp electrode (FSE)
D) Phonocardiography (PCG)

Question 486:   Which of the following factors can affect uteroplacental blood flow?
A) Hypertension
B) Maternal position
C) Maternal smoking
D) All of the above

Question 487:   Which medication, commonly used to treat hypertension in pregnant women, is known to improve placental blood flow and enhance fetal oxygenation?
A) Diuretics
B) Beta blockers
C) ACE inhibitors
D) Calcium channel blockers

Question 488: Which of the following actions can contribute to ensuring patient safety in electronic fetal monitoring?
A) Regularly monitoring the patient's vital signs
B) Documenting all interventions and observations accurately
C) Checking for proper placement of the fetal monitor
D) Administering medication without proper documentation

Question 489: Which of the following is true regarding auscultation during fetal assessment?
A) It involves the use of a stethoscope to listen to fetal heart sounds.
B) It is a non-invasive technique used to evaluate fetal well-being.
C) It can help detect abnormal heart rates or rhythm abnormalities in the fetus.
D) All of the above.

Question 490: When should cord blood acid base testing be performed during labor?
A) Only in high-risk pregnancies
B) Only in low-risk pregnancies
C) In all pregnancies regardless of risk
D) Only if fetal distress is suspected

Question 491: Which acid-base parameter in cord blood acid base testing indicates metabolic alkalosis?
A) pH less than 7.2
B) pH greater than 7.4
C) Bicarbonate (HCO3-) level less than 20 mmol/L
D) Base excess (BE) less than -8 mEq/L

Question 492: A pregnant woman in labor is experiencing variable decelerations on the electronic fetal monitoring (EFM) tracing. The nurse applies oxygen via a face mask to the mother. What is the rationale behind this intervention?
A) To increase fetal oxygenation
B) To increase maternal oxygenation
C) To alleviate maternal anxiety
D) To relieve uterine contractions

Question 493: Ms. Johnson, a multiparous woman at 28 weeks of gestation, is admitted to the antepartum unit for preterm contractions. The initial assessment shows a resting uterine tone of 25 mmHg. What does this resting tone value signify?
A) Hypertonic uterus
B) Hypotonic uterus
C) Normal uterine activity
D) Hyperstimulation

Question 494: Mrs. Rodriguez, a 42-year-old multigravida, is in labor. Her fetal heart rate tracing shows occasional late decelerations that resolve after the end of contractions. What is the nurse's most appropriate action in this situation?
A) Place the patient in the Trendelenburg position
B) Administer terbutaline as a tocolytic
C) Encourage the patient to push during contractions
D) Monitor the fetal heart rate closely

Question 495: Emma, a 25-year-old pregnant woman at 30 weeks gestation, is concerned about decreased fetal movements. On examination, the fetal heart rate is within normal limits. What is the appropriate advice for the healthcare provider to give Emma regarding fetal movement monitoring?
A) Instruct Emma to count fetal movements every hour.

B) Advise Emma to count fetal movements three times a day.
C) Recommend Emma to count fetal movements after meals only.
D) Encourage Emma to count fetal movements at the same time each day.

Question 496: How does a decreased resting tone affect uterine contractions during electronic fetal monitoring?
A) Increases contraction frequency
B) Decreases contraction strength
C) Reduces contraction duration
D) None of the above

Question 497: Mrs. Johnson, who is 38 weeks pregnant, is admitted to the labor and delivery unit complaining of contractions. Upon assessment, her fetal heart rate is found to be consistently above 160 beats per minute for the past 30 minutes. The baseline is at 180 bpm. What is the most likely cause of this finding?
A) Maternal fever
B) Fetal anomalies
C) Fetal hypoxia
D) Maternal anxiety

Question 498: Mrs. Garcia is a 29-year-old gravida 2, para 1-0-0-1 at 28 weeks of gestation. During a routine NST (non-stress test), the nurse identifies accelerations in the fetal heart rate (FHR) tracing that last less than 10 seconds. What is the appropriate interpretation of this finding?
A) FHR accelerations are normal and reassuring
B) FHR accelerations are abnormal and indicative of fetal distress
C) FHR accelerations should be monitored for at least 30 minutes
D) FHR accelerations suggest uteroplacental insufficiency

Question 499: Mrs. Smith is a 28-year-old pregnant woman who has been on continuous electronic fetal monitoring. Suddenly, the EFM tracing shows excessive baseline fetal movement artifacts. Which of the following troubleshooting steps should the nurse take first?
A) Reposition the mother to relieve pressure on the abdomen
B) Assess the mother's perception of fetal movement
C) Check the attachment of the transducer to the mother's abdomen
D) Decrease the sensitivity setting on the EFM

Question 500: Mrs. Thompson is a pregnant woman with preexisting type 2 diabetes. She asks her healthcare provider about the risk of congenital abnormalities in her baby. Which of the following congenital abnormalities is associated with maternal diabetes?
A) Ventricular septal defect
B) Down syndrome
C) Neural tube defects
D) Cleft lip and palate

Question 501: Which of the following is a potential complication of preeclampsia-eclampsia?
A) Hyperglycemia
B) Maternal hemorrhage
C) Fetal macrosomia
D) Reduced risk of preterm birth

Question 502:   Mrs. Rodriguez, a 37-year-old multigravida at 39 weeks of gestation, has chronic hypertension. Which of the following interventions is most appropriate to manage her hypertension during labor?
A) Administering oxytocin to increase uterine contractions
B) Encouraging the client to ambulate frequently
C) Maintaining a semi-fowler's position
D) Administering antihypertensive medication as ordered

Question 503:   Which of the following factors is associated with an increased risk of fetal dysrhythmias?
A) Maternal diabetes
B) Advanced maternal age
C) Low maternal body mass index
D) Maternal smoking

Question 504:   What does an elevated resting tone during electronic fetal monitoring indicate?
A) Uterine hypotonia
B) Normal uterine activity
C) Uterine hypertonia
D) Fetal distress

Question 505:   Fetal heart rate accelerations are associated with which of the following?
A) Umbilical cord compression.
B) Fetal hypoxemia.
C) Maternal fever.
D) Fetal sleep cycles.

Question 506:   Mrs. Martinez, a 32-year-old pregnant woman, is in her 36th week of pregnancy. She is scheduled for an amniotic fluid assessment today. As part of the assessment, fetal acoustic stimulation is performed. What is the purpose of fetal acoustic stimulation in an amniotic fluid assessment?
A) To estimate amniotic fluid volume
B) To assess fetal heart rate response to sound stimulus
C) To evaluate fetal movements
D) To determine the presence of meconium in the amniotic fluid

Question 507:   Which acid-base disorder is characterized by low pH and low bicarbonate (HCO3-) levels in cord blood gases?
A) Respiratory acidosis
B) Respiratory alkalosis
C) Metabolic acidosis
D) Metabolic alkalosis

Question 508:   Which of the following is considered an adequate variability in fetal heart rate?
A) Absent variability
B) Minimal variability
C) Moderate variability
D) Marked variability

Question 509:   Mrs. Johnson, a 30-year-old pregnant woman, is in her 39th week of pregnancy. She is scheduled for a non-stress test (NST) today. During the NST, the nurse performs fetal acoustic stimulation. Which of the following is the correct statement regarding fetal acoustic stimulation?
A) Fetal acoustic stimulation involves the use of sound to stimulate fetal activity.
B) Fetal acoustic stimulation is performed by applying pressure to the mother's abdomen.
C) Fetal acoustic stimulation is contraindicated after 32 weeks of gestation.

D) Fetal acoustic stimulation is a non-invasive method to assess fetal well-being.

Question 510:   Mrs. Thompson, a 28-year-old primigravida at 39 weeks gestation, is in active labor. The fetal heart rate (FHR) shows late decelerations, reduced variability, and tachycardia. The obstetrician decides to perform a cord blood gas analysis, which reveals a pH of 7.34 and a base excess of -5. What does this base excess value indicate?
A) Metabolic acidosis
B) Metabolic alkalosis
C) Respiratory acidosis
D) Respiratory alkalosis

Question 511:   Which component in electronic monitoring equipment is used to measure fetal heart rate?
A) Toco transducer
B) Ultrasound transducer
C) Pressure transducer
D) Intrauterine pressure catheter

Question 512:   Mr. Patel's partner is in labor, and you are monitoring the external fetal heart rate pattern. You notice late decelerations on the fetal heart rate tracing. What is the most appropriate action to take in this situation?
A) Administer oxygen to the mother
B) Encourage the mother to change positions
C) Increase intravenous fluid rate for the mother
D) Administer terbutaline to the mother

Question 513:   Which type of transducer is used to measure uterine contractions in electronic monitoring equipment?
A) Toco transducer
B) Ultrasound transducer
C) Pressure transducer
D) Intrauterine pressure catheter

Question 514:   Mrs. Johnson, a 32-year-old pregnant woman at 38 weeks of gestation, is admitted to the labor and delivery unit. The nurse is monitoring her uterine activity using an internal uterine pressure catheter (IUPC). Which of the following statements regarding uterine activity is correct?
A) Uterine contractions are typically strongest at the fundus.
B) Uterine contractions are primarily responsible for cervical dilation.
C) Uterine contractions initiate fetal descent during labor.
D) Uterine contractions increase blood flow to the placenta.

Question 515:   What is the average duration of a uterine contraction during the active phase of labor?
A) 15-25 seconds
B) 30-45 seconds
C) 50-60 seconds
D) 1-2 minutes

Question 516:   Which of the following is a strategy to sustain a quality improvement initiative?
A) Regular monitoring and evaluation
B) Resistance to change
C) Ignoring feedback from stakeholders
D) Compromising patient safety

Question 517:   Which of the following legal issues can arise due to improper use of electronic fetal monitoring (EFM) tracings?

A) Failure to detect fetal distress.
B) False-positive interpretations leading to unnecessary interventions.
C) Failure to implement timely interventions.
D) All of the above.

Question 518: A 32-year-old woman at 37 weeks of gestation is being monitored for an abnormal fetal heart rate tracing. The nurse notices that the baseline fetal heart rate has suddenly decreased from 140 bpm to 80 bpm with no signs of fetal distress. The nurse quickly checks the equipment and finds that the tocodynamometer is not picking up contractions. What is the most likely cause of this signal ambiguity?
A) Fetal scalp electrode malfunction
B) Poor electrode placement
C) Tocodynamometer probe displacement
D) Maternal movement causing artifact

Question 519: Which of the following is an effect of maternal hypotension on fetal heart rate?
A) Increased variability
B) Decreased variability
C) Accelerations
D) Early decelerations

Question 520: Mrs. Thompson, a 25-year-old primigravida, presents at 34 weeks gestation with a blood pressure reading of 150/100 mmHg. She has a urinary protein dipstick positive for 1+. Her laboratory investigations reveal thrombocytopenia, elevated liver enzymes, and decreased platelet count. What is the most appropriate next step in the management of Mrs. Thompson?
A) Admit for immediate induction of labor
B) Administer antihypertensive medication and recheck blood pressure in 24 hours
C) Perform a 24-hour urine collection for protein quantification
D) Begin fetal heart rate monitoring and schedule a follow-up visit

Question 521: Which of the following is the first-line antihypertensive medication recommended for the treatment of severe hypertension in pregnancy?
A) Methyldopa
B) Nifedipine
C) Labetalol
D) Hydralazine

Question 522: How are ectopic beats detected during fetal monitoring?
A) Absence of fetal movement
B) Decreased variability in fetal heart rate
C) Using ultrasound imaging
D) Palpation of the maternal abdomen

Question 523: Mrs. Johnson, a 32-year-old with a history of gestational diabetes, is currently at 38 weeks of gestation. During a routine antenatal visit, she reports decreased fetal activity. Electronic fetal monitoring is initiated and reveals a regular fetal heart rate (FHR) of 150 bpm, with occasional accelerations and decelerations. Which fetal dysrhythmia best describes this pattern?
A) Sinus tachycardia
B) Fetal bradycardia
C) Variable decelerations
D) Early decelerations

Question 524: Which of the following is NOT a potential effect of maternal obesity on fetal well-being?
A) Increased risk of neural tube defects
B) Increased risk of macrosomia
C) Increased risk of stillbirth
D) Increased risk of congenital anomalies

Question 525: A pregnant patient presents with a decreased oxygen supply to the fetus. Which condition is likely to affect the fetal oxygenation greatly?
A) Maternal hypotension
B) Decreased fetal heart rate
C) Umbilical cord compression
D) Maternal hyperglycemia

Question 526: In the context of medical ethics, what is the meaning of non-maleficence?
A) Respecting the patient's right to privacy and confidentiality
B) Promoting fairness and equality in healthcare delivery
C) Avoiding harm and minimizing risks to the patient
D) Upholding the patient's right to make autonomous decisions

Question 527: Ms. Johnson, a 35-year-old pregnant woman at 39 weeks gestation with a previous cesarean delivery, presents to the labor and delivery unit with severe abdominal pain, vaginal bleeding, and a nonreassuring fetal heart rate pattern. On examination, the fetal heart rate decelerations are variable and deep, with minimal spontaneous recovery. The uterus is tense and tender. What is the most likely diagnosis?
A) Placental abruption
B) Uterine rupture
C) Placenta previa
D) Cord prolapse

Question 528: Mrs. Roberts, a 37-year-old woman at 41 weeks gestation, is being monitored due to post-term pregnancy. During antenatal testing, the nurse observes late decelerations in the fetal heart rate (FHR) tracing. Which intervention should the nurse prioritize?
A) Administer oxygen via face mask to the client
B) Begin a continuous pitocin infusion
C) Notify the healthcare provider immediately
D) Perform a pelvic examination

Question 529: Mrs. Johnson, a 38-year-old pregnant woman at 34 weeks gestation, presents to the labor and delivery unit with decreased fetal movement. Upon assessment, the nurse notes a fetal heart rate of 90 bpm. Variable decelerations are present on the fetal monitor strip. The nurse should take which immediate action?
A) Administer oxygen to the mother
B) Administer a tocolytic medication to the mother
C) Prepare for immediate delivery
D) Reassure the mother and continue monitoring

Question 530: Which of the following factors can impair uteroplacental circulation?
A) Maternal hypertension,
B) Fetal growth restriction,
C) Placental abnormalities,
D) All of the above

Question 531: A 26-year-old pregnant woman, Mrs. Lee, presents with decreased fetal movement at 36 weeks gestation. Upon examination, you find the following EFM tracing pattern. Which of the following interventions would be most appropriate?
A) Perform a biophysical profile

B) Administer tocolytic medication
C) Apply continuous fetal scalp stimulation
D) Order a nonstress test

Question 532: Mr. and Mrs. Smith are expecting their first child. On admission to the labor and delivery unit, the fetal heart rate is consistently above 170 beats per minute. The nurse notices a regular pattern with accelerations. What is the most appropriate action for the nurse to take?
A) Administer oxygen to the mother
B) Encourage the mother to change positions
C) Prepare for an emergency cesarean section
D) Document the finding and continue monitoring

Question 533: A pregnant woman presents with symptoms of decreased fetal movement. Which of the following structures in fetal circulation is responsible for carrying deoxygenated blood away from the fetus?
A) Umbilical vein
B) Ductus arteriosus
C) Pulmonary artery
D) Umbilical artery

Question 534: A pregnant woman at 40 weeks of gestation presents with decreased fetal movements and late decelerations noted on the electronic fetal monitoring (EFM). On palpation, the uterine contractions are frequent and strong. Which of the following interventions is the most appropriate in managing this situation?
A) Start intravenous magnesium sulfate
B) Perform a non-stress test
C) Administer tocolytic therapy
D) Prepare for an immediate delivery

Question 535: Which of the following is a potential complication of gestational hypertension?
A) Preterm labor
B) Placental abruption
C) Fetal growth restriction
D) All of the above

Question 536: Ms. Thompson, a 25-year-old G2P1, is admitted to the antenatal ward for monitoring. During her electronic fetal monitoring, the nurse measures the intensity of the uterine contractions and classifies them as hyperstimulation. What characteristic would the nurse observe in hyperstimulation?
A) Peak intensity above 50mmHg
B) Peak intensity between 25-50mmHg
C) Intensity fluctuating between 70-90mmHg
D) Inconsistent intensity with frequent uterine relaxation

Question 537: What is the most common clinical manifestation associated with severe bradycardia in the fetus?
A) Meconium-stained amniotic fluid
B) Accelerations of the fetal heart rate
C) Uterine hyperstimulation
D) Fetal tachycardia

Question 538: Which of the following is a characteristic of early decelerations in fetal heart rate?
A) Gradual onset and offset
B) Associated with contractions
C) Sudden drop in heart rate
D) Variable duration

Question 539: Which acid-base parameter is primarily used to assess fetal well-being in cord blood acid base testing?
A) pH
B) Bicarbonate (HCO3-)
C) Base excess (BE)
D) Partial pressure of carbon dioxide (pCO2)

Question 540: Emma, a 29-year-old G1P0 at 37 weeks of gestation, is admitted to the labor and delivery unit with a diagnosis of decreased fetal blood flow. On fetal monitoring, you notice a sinusoidal fetal heart rate pattern. Which of the following interventions is most appropriate?
A) Administer tocolytic therapy
B) Perform an immediate emergency cesarean section
C) Apply a fetal scalp electrode
D) Encourage maternal position change

Question 541: What should be done if an electronic fetal monitoring equipment malfunctions during a clinical situation?
A) Continue using the equipment despite the malfunction
B) Immediately replace the equipment with a new one
C) Inform the appropriate personnel and document the issue
D) Attempt to fix the equipment yourself

Question 542: When monitoring a patient with tachysystole, which fetal heart rate pattern should be considered concerning?
A) Early decelerations.
B) Variable decelerations.
C) Accelerations.
D) Late decelerations.

Question 543: Mrs. Thompson is a 40-year-old multigravid woman who is at 36 weeks gestation. She presents to the antepartum unit for a non-stress test. On electronic fetal monitoring, you note a baseline fetal heart rate of 170 bpm with absent variability. There are recurrent late decelerations present. What is the most appropriate management of this fetal heart rate pattern?
A) Increase IV fluids
B) Administer oxygen by face mask
C) Perform a biophysical profile
D) Prepare for an emergency cesarean section

Question 544: Mr. Davis, a 28-year-old expectant father, accompanies his wife for her routine prenatal visit. The healthcare provider explains the process of auscultating the fetal heart rate (FHR) using a Doppler device. Mr. Davis asks why they don't use a traditional stethoscope instead. Which of the following is the most appropriate response?
A) "A Doppler device allows us to amplify and detect the fetal heart sounds more clearly."
B) "A traditional stethoscope is not capable of detecting the high-frequency sounds of the fetal heart."
C) "A Doppler device is more comfortable for the pregnant woman during the auscultation process."
D) "A traditional stethoscope is prone to interference from maternal heart sounds."

Question 545: Which of the following interventions may be necessary if contractions are too frequent and intense during labor?
A) Oxytocin infusion to strengthen contractions.
B) Administration of tocolytic medications to decrease contractions.
C) Epidural anesthesia to provide pain relief.

D) Continuous fetal monitoring to assess fetal well-being.

Question 546: Ms. Johnson is a 34-year-old primigravida who is 38 weeks pregnant. During a routine antenatal visit, the nurse noticed a decreased variability in the fetal heart rate (FHR) tracing. The FHR baseline is normal, with occasional decelerations. Which of the following interventions should the nurse initiate?
A) Administer oxygen via face mask
B) Apply an internal fetal scalp electrode
C) Increase intravenous fluid rate
D) Assist the client to change positions

Question 547: Emma, a 30-year-old pregnant woman at 37 weeks' gestation, is in labor. The nurse is monitoring her uterine activity and observes that the contractions last for 90 seconds from the start of one contraction to the start of the next contraction. What is the frequency of Emma's contractions?
A) 1 contraction every 30 seconds
B) 1 contraction every 45 seconds
C) 1 contraction every 90 seconds
D) 2 contractions every 45 seconds

Question 548: Which pattern in electronic fetal monitoring requires immediate intervention?
A) Abrupt baseline change
B) Minimal variability
C) Sinusoidal pattern
D) Prolonged decelerations

Question 549: During a labor induction, a pregnant patient refuses a procedure recommended by the healthcare provider. What is the nurse's responsibility in this situation?
A) Respect the patient's decision and document the refusal
B) Convince the patient to reconsider the recommendation
C) Continuously advocate for the procedure
D) Proceed with the procedure without the patient's consent

Question 550: Which of the following factors can influence the intensity of uterine contractions during labor?
A) Maternal age
B) Fetal position
C) Uterine fibroids
D) All of the above

Question 551: Which laboratory finding is considered indicative of severe HELLP syndrome?
A) Platelet count >150,000/mm^3
B) Serum LDH level within normal range
C) Elevated AST and ALT levels
D) Normal bilirubin level

Question 552: Which fetal heart rate pattern is most commonly associated with an abnormal biophysical profile?
A) Sinusoidal pattern
B) Accelerations
C) Early decelerations
D) Variable decelerations

Question 553: Which condition is characterized by the abnormal implantation of the placenta in the lower uterine segment, partially or completely covering the internal cervical os?
A) Placenta Previa
B) Placental Abruption
C) Uterine Rupture

D) Cord Prolapse

Question 554: Mrs. Johnson, a 32-year-old primigravida at 37 weeks gestation, presents to the labor and delivery unit with contractions and decreased fetal movement. Upon assessment, the fetal heart rate baseline is noted to be 160 bpm. Which of the following best describes this finding?
A) The fetal baseline heart rate is within the normal range.
B) The fetal baseline heart rate is mildly tachycardic.
C) The fetal baseline heart rate is mildly bradycardic.
D) The fetal baseline heart rate is significantly abnormal.

Question 555: Sophia is a 34-year-old primigravida at 38 weeks gestation who presents to the labor and delivery unit in active labor. On admission, her vital signs are stable, and fetal heart rate monitoring shows a baseline rate of 130 bpm with moderate variability. The nurse performs a vaginal examination and finds that the cervix is dilated 6 cm. Based on this scenario, which of the following factors is likely to affect the umbilical blood flow?
A) Uterine contractions
B) Maternal age
C) Fetal heart rate
D) Fetal position

Question 556: Ms. Rodriguez is a 28-year-old woman who presents to the labor and delivery unit in active labor at 39 weeks gestation. On electronic fetal monitoring, you note a baseline fetal heart rate of 160 bpm with minimal variability. There are frequent early decelerations present during contractions. What is the most appropriate interpretation of this fetal heart rate pattern?
A) Normal fetal heart rate pattern
B) Fetal heart rate tachycardia
C) Late decelerations
D) Abnormal fetal heart rate pattern

Question 557: Which type of diabetes is characterized by insulin resistance and impaired insulin production?
A) Type 1 diabetes
B) Type 2 diabetes
C) Gestational diabetes
D) None of the above

Question 558: Which of the following is an appropriate method to stimulate fetal activity during a non-reactive fetal heart rate tracing?
A) Administering intravenous fluids
B) Applying a cold compress to the abdomen
C) Placing the mother in a supine position
D) Decreasing maternal oxygen supplementation

Question 559: What is the normal range for pH in cord blood gases?
A) 6.8-7.2
B) 7.2-7.6
C) 7.4-7.8
D) 7.8-8.2

Question 560: Fetal Acoustic Stimulation is performed to assess fetal well-being and evaluate its response to external stimuli. Which of the following statements about Fetal Acoustic Stimulation is correct?
A) Fetal Acoustic Stimulation involves exposing the fetus to loud music to assess its heart rate.
B) Fetal Acoustic Stimulation involves using a Doppler ultrasound device to measure the fetal heart rate.

C) Fetal Acoustic Stimulation involves using sound waves to elicit a response from the fetus.
D) Fetal Acoustic Stimulation involves measuring the fetal blood pressure using an invasive technique.

Question 561:   Which of the following professional organizations sets standards for electronic fetal monitoring (EFM) education and certification?
A) American Heart Association (AHA)
B) American Association of Critical-Care Nurses (AACN)
C) American College of Obstetricians and Gynecologists (ACOG)
D) American Nurses Association (ANA)

Question 562:   A pregnant woman in labor is experiencing variable decelerations on the electronic fetal monitoring (EFM) tracing. The nurse decides to change the mother's position to alleviate cord compression. Which position is most likely to relieve cord compression?
A) Supine position
B) Left lateral position
C) Right lateral position
D) Trendelenburg position

Question 563:   Mr. Perez brings his 32-week-old pregnant wife to the clinic due to concerns about the baby's heart rate. Upon examination, it is found that the fetus has a complete heart block with bradycardia and an irregular rhythm. What should be the next step in management?
A) Administration of atropine to improve fetal heart rate.
B) Immediate delivery via emergency cesarean section.
C) Monitoring fetal heart rate during labor.
D) Referral to a fetal cardiologist for further evaluation and management.

Question 564:   During a routine prenatal visit, the nurse is performing auscultation of the fetal heart rate (FHR) in a 28-year-old primigravida at 16 weeks gestation. The nurse is unable to detect the fetal heart sounds using a Doppler device. Which of the following actions would be most appropriate?
A) Inform the pregnant woman that it is normal not to hear the fetal heart sounds at this gestational age.
B) Re-position the Doppler device and attempt to locate the fetal heart sounds again.
C) Proceed with an ultrasound examination to confirm the presence of fetal cardiac activity.
D) Inform the healthcare provider about the inability to detect the fetal heart sounds.

Question 565:   Mrs.James, a 35-year-old pregnant woman at 32 weeks gestation, arrives at the labor and delivery unit with complaints of palpitations and anxiety. The fetal heart rate pattern shows a rapid and irregular heart rate between 200-240 beats per minute. The maternal heart rate is normal. Which of the following is the most likely diagnosis for this fetal heart rate pattern?
A) Sinus tachycardia
B) Supraventricular tachycardia
C) Ventricular tachycardia
D) Atrial flutter

Question 566:   Which of the following fetal heart rate patterns is commonly associated with decreased blood flow?
A) Sinusoidal pattern
B) Accelerations
C) Early decelerations

D) Variable decelerations

Question 567:   A 30-year-old pregnant woman, Mrs. Johnson, at 38 weeks gestation presents for a nonstress test. The fetal heart rate baseline is 140 bpm, with moderate variability. Occasional accelerations are noted, but no contractions are observed during the 20-minute test. What is the interpretation of this nonstress test?
A) Reactive
B) Nonreactive
C) Equivocal
D) Abnormal

Question 568:   A 24-year-old primigravida at term presents to the labor and delivery unit with severe vaginal bleeding. The fetal heart rate (FHR) tracing reveals a baseline of 160 bpm, minimal variability, and late decelerations with contractions. What is the most appropriate immediate action?
A) Perform a sterile vaginal exam
B) Administer oxygen via face mask
C) Change maternal position
D) Prepare for immediate cesarean delivery

Question 569:   Mrs. Smith, 32 years old, is in her 36th week of gestation and is admitted to the labor and delivery unit for an electively scheduled repeat cesarean delivery. During continuous electronic fetal monitoring, the nurse notices ectopic beats on the fetal monitor strip. What action is most appropriate for the nurse to take?
A) Document the finding and continue monitoring the fetal heart rate.
B) Notify the obstetrician immediately.
C) Administer oxygen to the mother.
D) Prepare for an emergency cesarean delivery.

Question 570:   Lisa, a 32-year-old pregnant woman at 37 weeks of gestation, is undergoing electronic fetal monitoring. The fetal heart rate has a baseline variability of more than 25 bpm. What does this finding indicate?
A) It suggests fetal distress and the need for immediate intervention.
B) It is within the normal range for baseline variability.
C) It indicates normal fetal oxygenation and well-being.
D) It is an abnormal finding requiring further evaluation.

Question 571:   Ms. Ramirez, a 33-year-old pregnant woman at 34 weeks gestation with a history of previous myomectomy, presents to the labor and delivery unit with abdominal pain and vaginal bleeding. On examination, there is a tender, firm, and palpable mass in the lower uterine segment. The fetal heart rate tracing shows late decelerations. What is the most likely diagnosis?
A) Uterine rupture
B) Placental abruption
C) Placenta previa
D) Fibroid degeneration

Question 572:   Ms. Rodriguez, a 25-year-old primigravida at 28 weeks gestation, visits the clinic for a routine prenatal check-up. During auscultation of the fetal heart, you note an irregular fetal heart rate (FHR) with frequent pauses. What is the most likely cause of this finding?
A) Umbilical cord compression
B) Maternal fever
C) Fetal tachycardia

D) Fetal arrhythmia

Question 573: Olivia, a 28-year-old pregnant woman at 32 weeks gestation, presents to the clinic reporting decreased fetal movements. On examination, the fetal heart rate is within normal limits. The healthcare provider suspects decreased fetal movement due to maternal positioning. What is the appropriate advice for the healthcare provider to give Olivia?
A) Encourage Olivia to lie on her left side and monitor fetal movements.
B) Instruct Olivia to drink a sugary beverage and monitor fetal movements.
C) Advise Olivia to take a warm bath and monitor fetal movements.
D) Recommend Olivia to perform abdominal exercises and monitor fetal movements.

Question 574: Mrs. Anderson, a 28-year-old pregnant woman, is scheduled for an elective cesarean section under spinal anesthesia. During the procedure, she experiences a sudden decrease in blood pressure. Which of the following physiological changes associated with spinal anesthesia is most likely responsible for this hypotensive episode?
A) Decreased sympathetic outflow
B) Increased cardiac output
C) Decreased systemic vascular resistance
D) Increased plasma volume

Question 575: Which maternal condition can negatively impact fetal oxygenation by reducing the availability of oxygen for transfer?
A) Maternal hypertension
B) Maternal anemia
C) Maternal hyperthyroidism
D) Maternal obesity

Question 576: What is the recommended intervention for a sinusoidal pattern in electronic fetal monitoring?
A) No intervention is necessary as it is a benign finding.
B) Administer tocolytic medications to suppress uterine contractions.
C) Perform a complete maternal-fetal assessment and consider prompt delivery.
D) Increase the maternal fluid intake to improve fetal oxygenation.

Question 577: Which of the following is an example of an appropriate fetal movement assessment method?
A) External cephalic version
B) Doppler ultrasound
C) Contraction stress test
D) Biophysical profile

Question 578: Which of the following is NOT considered a potential cause of fetal demise?
A) Maternal hypertension
B) Maternal hyperthyroidism
C) Maternal diabetes
D) Maternal hypotension

Question 579: Mrs. Anderson, a 32-year-old pregnant woman at 38 weeks gestation, presents to the maternity unit in active labor. Upon auscultation of the fetal heart rate (FHR), the nurse notices a sudden drop in the FHR immediately after a uterine contraction. This observation is concerning for:
A) Fetal distress
B) Fetal tachycardia

C) Fetal bradycardia
D) Fetal heart block

Question 580: Mrs. Johnson, a pregnant patient, comes to the clinic for her prenatal visit. During her examination, you notice that she has gained excessive weight and her blood pressure is significantly elevated. You suspect that Mrs. Johnson may have developed gestational hypertension. What is your ethical obligation in this situation?
A) Inform the patient of your concerns and recommend further evaluation and monitoring.
B) Ignore the findings and continue with the regular prenatal care.
C) Discuss the findings with a colleague and seek their opinion.
D) Withhold the information from Mrs. Johnson to prevent unnecessary anxiety.

Question 581: Mrs. Johnson, a 38-year-old pregnant woman, is admitted to the antepartum unit for fetal monitoring. The fetal heart rate tracing appears abnormal with a sudden increase in baseline rate from 130 bpm to 180 bpm. On closer examination, you notice sharp and uniform spikes that are unrelated to maternal movement. What could be the possible artifact causing this abnormal tracing?
A) Maternal movement
B) Fetal scalp electrode
C) Radiofrequency interference
D) Uterine activity monitoring

Question 582: Which of the following statements about uteroplacental circulation is true?
A) It is maintained entirely by fetal cardiovascular mechanisms,
B) Maternal and fetal circulations are completely separate,
C) It is primarily regulated by maternal factors,
D) Placenta acts as a barrier preventing exchange between maternal and fetal blood

Question 583: During a quality improvement committee meeting, the team discusses the importance of effective communication in healthcare. Which of the following statements accurately reflects the role of communication in promoting quality improvement?
A) Effective communication is only necessary between healthcare providers.
B) Communication is not essential in quality improvement initiatives.
C) Proper communication enhances patient safety, reduces errors, and improves overall healthcare outcomes.
D) Communication within the healthcare team is not significant in quality improvement projects.

Question 584: Which of the following is not a management option for hypoxemia in the fetus?
A) Maternal repositioning
B) Fluid administration
C) Fetal blood sampling
D) Immediate delivery

Question 585: Ms. Garcia is a 28-year-old multiparous woman who is currently 40 weeks pregnant. She visits her obstetrician for a routine antenatal check-up. The obstetrician assesses the patient's uterine activity by performing an external tocodynamometry. Which of the following patterns would be considered normal during this assessment?
A) Regular contractions lasting 90 seconds

B) Uterine activity occurring every two minutes
C) Multiple episodes of strong contractions with a frequency of six minutes
D) Contractions lasting for 30 seconds or less

Question 586: Which of the following devices is commonly used for external uterine monitoring?
A) Colposcope
B) Laparoscope
C) Ultrasound transducer
D) Fetal blood sampling catheter

Question 587: Which hormone is responsible for maintaining the uterine lining during pregnancy?
A) Estrogen
B) Progesterone
C) Testosterone
D) Prolactin

Question 588: Emma, a 36-week gestation pregnant woman, is in active labor. The fetal heart rate (FHR) monitoring reveals a pattern of consistent smooth waves with a uniform frequency of 2-3 cycles per minute. The FHR ranges between 110-130 beats per minute, and there are no accelerations or decelerations. What is the most appropriate nursing intervention?
A) Administer Oxytocin to augment labor
B) Prepare for an emergency cesarean section
C) Administer oxygen to the mother via face mask
D) Perform a scalp electrode insertion to assess fetal well-being

Question 589: Which of the following can cause interference with electronic fetal monitoring equipment?
A) Mobile phones
B) Fluorescent lights
C) Wi-Fi routers
D) All of the above

Question 590: Which of the following is a contraindication for nonstress testing (NST)?
A) Maternal hypertension
B) Gestational diabetes
C) Twin gestation
D) Previous cesarean delivery

Question 591: What is the most common clinical manifestation of placental abruption?
A) Painful vaginal bleeding
B) Painless vaginal bleeding
C) Abdominal cramping
D) Loss of fetal movements

Question 592: Which fetal condition can impair fetal oxygenation due to decreased oxygen exchange in the placenta?
A) Fetal tachycardia
B) Fetal macrosomia
C) Fetal growth restriction
D) Fetal bradycardia

Question 593: When encountering a prolonged deceleration pattern on the fetal heart rate tracing, what should be the immediate action of the healthcare provider?
A) Document the pattern and continue monitoring.
B) Administer oxygen to the mother.
C) Change the mother's position.
D) Perform a vaginal examination.

Question 594: Which of the following interventions is recommended for a fetus diagnosed with congenital heart block?
A) Fetal heart rate monitoring every 12 hours
B) Maternal administration of corticosteroids
C) Intrauterine blood transfusion
D) Immediate delivery via cesarean section

Question 595: Ms. Rodriguez, a 29-year-old G1P0 at 39 weeks gestation, presents to the labor and delivery unit with sudden onset dyspnea and chest pain. On examination, she is tachypneic and presents with low oxygen saturation. The electronic fetal monitoring (EFM) shows variable decelerations. Which intervention is a priority in managing this maternal complication?
A) Administer oxygen via nasal cannula
B) Obtain a chest x-ray to rule out pulmonary embolism
C) Administer intravenous furosemide
D) Prepare the patient for immediate cesarean delivery

Question 596: Sarah, a 35-year-old pregnant woman, is admitted to the labor and delivery unit for fetal monitoring. She is receiving epidural anesthesia for pain management. Which of the following statements is true regarding the use of electronic monitoring equipment in this scenario?
A) Electronic monitoring equipment is not suitable for monitoring the fetus in women receiving epidural anesthesia.
B) External monitoring devices are more accurate than internal monitoring devices for assessing the fetal heart rate in this scenario.
C) Internal monitoring devices are preferred for accurate fetal assessment in women receiving epidural anesthesia.
D) Electronic monitoring equipment should only be used during the second stage of labor in this scenario.

Question 597: What is the definition of postdates pregnancy?
A) Pregnancy that extends beyond 42 weeks
B) Pregnancy between 35 and 40 weeks
C) Pregnancy that occurs after the woman's due date
D) Pregnancy before 37 weeks

Question 598: Mrs. Johnson, a 32-year-old pregnant woman at 38 weeks gestation, presents to the antenatal clinic for a routine check-up. During the fetal monitoring, you notice short-term variability with fetal heart rate accelerations. Which of the following statements regarding fetal heart rate accelerations is true?
A) Fetal heart rate accelerations are a sign of fetal distress.
B) Fetal heart rate accelerations are typically seen during contractions.
C) Fetal heart rate accelerations are an indicator of fetal well-being.
D) Fetal heart rate accelerations are only observed during the active phase of labor.

Question 599: Dr. Thompson, an obstetrician, is responsible for interpreting fetal heart rate tracings during labor and delivery. According to legal considerations, which of the following actions should Dr. Thompson undertake?
A) Clearly document the interpretation and any concerns in the medical record.
B) Inform the nursing staff promptly about the interpretation findings.
C) Ensure appropriate actions are taken based on the interpretation, involving the expectant mother in decision-making.

D) All of the above actions should be undertaken by Dr. Thompson.

Question 600: Which of the following is a possible complication of chronic hypertension in pregnancy?
A) Preterm birth
B) Oligohydramnios
C) Hyperglycemia
D) Fetal macrosomia

Question 601: A pregnant patient has been diagnosed with preeclampsia. Which maternal factor is primarily influenced by this condition and can impact fetal oxygenation?
A) Renal function
B) Hematocrit levels
C) Blood pressure
D) Uterine contractions

Question 602: Which of the following laboratory findings is associated with preeclampsia-eclampsia?
A) Increased platelet count
B) Normal liver function tests
C) Elevated serum creatinine levels
D) Decreased levels of uric acid

Question 603: When should internal fetal heart rate monitoring be discontinued?
A) When the mother requests to switch to external monitoring.
B) When the baby's heart rate pattern becomes abnormal.
C) When there is a need to assess the mother's blood pressure.
D) When the cervix is fully dilated and delivery is imminent.

Question 604: Sarah, a 32-year-old primigravida at 36 weeks gestation, has been diagnosed with chronic essential hypertension. During an antenatal visit, her blood pressure is measured as 150/95 mmHg. Which intervention is most appropriate for managing her hypertension during pregnancy?
A) Initiation of antihypertensive medication
B) Dietary modification and increased physical activity
C) Serum creatinine and uric acid level monitoring
D) Close monitoring of fetal well-being

Question 605: Julia, a 28-year-old primigravida at 39 weeks gestation, presents to the antenatal clinic complaining of reduced fetal movements. On examination, the fetal heart rate is normal, but a fundal height measurement reveals less growth compared to the previous visit. What is the most appropriate next step?
A) Immediate induction of labor
B) Fetal kick count for 2 hours
C) Ultrasonography for fetal biophysical profile (BPP)
D) Doppler velocimetry of umbilical artery

Question 606: Mrs. Smith, a 31-year-old multiparous woman at 40 weeks of gestation, presents to the emergency department with severe abdominal pain, vaginal bleeding, and uterine tenderness. Hemodynamic instability is noted on initial assessment. Which of the following uteroplacental complications is the most likely cause of her presentation?
A) Placental abruption
B) Uterine rupture
C) Placenta previa
D) Placenta accreta

Question 607: Mrs. Brown, a 34-year-old multiparous woman at 39 weeks of gestation, presents to the labor and delivery unit with rupture of membranes and contractions every 2 minutes. Electronic fetal monitoring shows late decelerations in fetal heart rate associated with a reduced baseline variability. The cervical examination reveals a fully dilated cervix. What is the most appropriate next step in managing this situation?
A) Perform a biophysical profile
B) Administer intravenous fluids
C) Administer terbutaline
D) Prepare for immediate instrumental delivery

Question 608: During labor, a pregnant woman experiences repetitive and severe variable decelerations on the electronic fetal monitoring (EFM) tracing. What intervention should the nurse prioritize?
A) Administering intravenous fluids
B) Applying oxygen via a face mask
C) Changing the mother's position
D) Preparing for immediate cesarean delivery

Question 609: Emma, a 28-year-old pregnant woman at 38 weeks gestation, presents to the emergency department with complaints of dizziness and decreased fetal movement. On examination, the fetal heart rate is noted to be consistently below 100 beats per minute. The maternal heart rate is normal. Which of the following is the most likely diagnosis for this fetal heart rate pattern?
A) Fetal bradyarrhythmia
B) Sinus tachycardia
C) Ventricular tachycardia
D) Supraventricular tachycardia

Question 610: During a labor and delivery shift, Nurse Roberts notices a prolonged deceleration on the fetal monitor tracing of Mrs. Brown, a 30-year-old pregnant woman. The nurse promptly notifies the obstetrician who orders an emergency cesarean section. However, another nurse interrupts Nurse Roberts before she can pass on the information about the deceleration. What should Nurse Roberts do to ensure legal compliance?
A) Document the deceleration and nursing actions in Mrs. Brown's medical record.
B) Immediately inform the obstetrician again about the prolonged deceleration.
C) Seek guidance from the hospital's legal department regarding the situation.
D) Both A and B

Answers

with

Detailed

Explanation

Question 1:
Correct Answer: C) Placenta previa
Rationale: Placenta previa is a condition in which the placenta implants in the lower uterine segment, partially or completely covering the cervix. The classic presentation includes painless vaginal bleeding, typically occurring after 28 weeks of gestation. Placental abruption and uterine rupture may cause painful bleeding, while placenta accreta involves abnormal placental attachment to the uterine wall and is not usually associated with painless bleeding.

Question 2:
Correct Answer: B) Ectopic pregnancy
Rationale: Ectopic pregnancy, where implantation occurs outside the uterus, can lead to maternal hemorrhage if untreated. Hyperemesis gravidarum is severe vomiting but does not typically result in hemorrhage. Amniotic fluid embolism is a rare, life-threatening condition characterized by the entry of amniotic fluid into the maternal circulation. Gestational diabetes, a metabolic disorder, does not directly cause hemorrhage.

Question 3:
Correct Answer: D) Prepare for an emergency cesarean section
Rationale: Recurrent late decelerations coupled with decreased beat-to-beat variability indicate severe fetal compromise. This requires prompt delivery as the fetal condition could worsen rapidly. Preparing for an emergency cesarean section is the most appropriate action to ensure a timely delivery and optimize fetal well-being. Administering oxygen, beginning continuous fetal monitoring, and starting intravenous fluids may be important interventions in other scenarios but are not the most appropriate actions based on the given information.

Question 4:
Correct Answer: C) Fetal hypoxia
Rationale: Ectopic beats in a fetus may occur due to various factors, including fetal hypoxia. When the fetus experiences inadequate oxygen supply, it can lead to irregular heartbeats, known as ectopic beats. Other potential causes of ectopic beats include maternal anxiety, umbilical cord compression, and certain fetal sleep patterns. However, fetal hypoxia is a significant contributing factor as it affects the normal electrical conduction system of the heart, resulting in irregular beats. Therefore, careful monitoring and timely intervention are crucial to prevent further hypoxia and promote fetal well-being.

Question 5:
Correct Answer: C) Maternal hypoglycemia
Rationale: Maternal hypoglycemia is not a potential cause of tachycardia in fetal monitoring. Tachycardia can be caused by factors such as maternal fever, fetal hypoxia, and fetal anemia. It is important to identify and address the underlying cause of tachycardia to ensure appropriate management and intervention.

Question 6:
Correct Answer: B) Assisting with intrauterine resuscitation.
Rationale: In cases of tachysystole, the priority nursing action is to assist with intrauterine resuscitation to improve fetal oxygenation and reduce the risk of fetal acidemia. This includes repositioning the patient, discontinuing oxytocin (if in use), administering oxygen, and administering intravenous fluids. Decreasing the maternal pushing efforts may be indicated if the mother is pushing during a contraction, which can further stress the fetus. Meperidine administration is not the priority in this case. Immediate delivery by vacuum extraction is not indicated solely based on tachysystole.

Question 7:
Correct Answer: B) Deceleration that begins before the contraction peak and returns to baseline after the contraction ends
Rationale: Early decelerations are benign and mirror image of uterine contractions. They start before the contraction peak and return to baseline after the contraction ends. They are usually a result of head compression during contractions and are not associated with fetal distress.

Question 8:
Correct Answer: C) Reassure the mother and continue with regular prenatal care
Rationale: In the absence of symptoms or concerns from the mother, isolated tachycardia without other signs of distress is not an immediate cause for alarm. It is important to continue with regular prenatal care and monitor the fetal heart rate during subsequent visits. If the tachycardia persists or is accompanied by other worrisome findings, further evaluation may be warranted. However, immediate hospitalization or informing the obstetrician is not necessary at this time.

Question 9:
Correct Answer: A) Fetal heart rate
Rationale: External fetal monitoring involves measuring the fetal heart rate using a Doppler or ultrasound device placed on the mother's abdomen. This allows healthcare providers to assess the well-being of the fetus by monitoring changes in the fetal heart rate pattern. Maternal blood pressure, uterine contractions, and fetal breathing movements are not measured during external fetal monitoring.

Question 10:
Correct Answer: B) Offer her empathy and actively listen to her concerns.
Rationale: Patient-centered care is a fundamental ethical principle in healthcare. When a patient expresses feeling neglected or unheard, it is crucial to offer empathy and actively listen to their concerns. Validating the patient's feelings and providing support can help build trust and improve the patient's experience of care. Ignoring or dismissing the patient's concerns may lead to dissatisfaction, poor outcomes, and a breakdown in the patient-provider relationship. Active listening promotes patient empowerment, satisfaction, and better healthcare outcomes.

Question 11:
Correct Answer: A) Fetal bradycardia
Rationale: Fetal bradycardia is a fetal complication that is characterized by a decrease in variability, repetitive late decelerations, and absence of accelerations. It refers to a persistently low heart rate below the normal range. Fetal bradycardia can be a sign of fetal distress and may indicate inadequate oxygenation and perfusion to the fetus. Prompt recognition and intervention are necessary to minimize potential adverse outcomes for the fetus.

Question 12:
Correct Answer: C) Fetal distress
Rationale: Fetal distress is a fetal complication that is characterized by persistent late decelerations, decreased variability, and repetitive variable decelerations. It refers to a state in which the fetus is experiencing compromised oxygenation and perfusion. Fetal distress can be caused by various factors, such as placental insufficiency, umbilical

cord compression, or maternal hypotension. Timely recognition and intervention are critical to prevent further fetal compromise and minimize potential adverse outcomes.

Question 13:
Correct Answer: B) Arterioarterial anastomosis
Rationale: In monochorionic-diamniotic twin pregnancies, where the twins share one placenta and two amniotic sacs, the most common type of placental vascular anastomosis is arterioarterial (AA) anastomosis. AA anastomosis refers to direct connections between the arterial circulation of the two twins. These anastomoses can lead to imbalances in blood flow between the twins and contribute to complications such as twin-to-twin transfusion syndrome (TTTS) or selective intrauterine growth restriction (sIUGR). Arteriovenous anastomosis, venovenous anastomosis, and venous-arterial anastomosis are less commonly observed in monochorionic-diamniotic twin pregnancies. Understanding the type of placental vascular anastomosis is crucial for managing the pregnancy and monitoring for potential complications.

Question 14:
Correct Answer: D) Administer oxygen to the pregnant woman
Rationale: Sudden loss of fetal heart rate variability with repetitive decelerations suggests fetal compromise. Administering oxygen to the pregnant woman helps improve fetal oxygenation and can potentially improve fetal well-being. Other interventions may be necessary depending on the specific circumstances but ensuring adequate oxygen supply is crucial.

Question 15:
Correct Answer: B) Category III
Rationale: In Category III, the baseline rate is bradycardic (<110 bpm) or tachycardic (>160 bpm) with absent variability, recurrent late decelerations, recurrent variable decelerations, or bradycardia. The provided EFM tracing shows a baseline rate of 170 bpm, increased variability of 30 bpm, and recurrent variable decelerations lasting 30 seconds. This corresponds to Category III, indicating an abnormal and non-reassuring fetal status.

Question 16:
Correct Answer: D) Relaxin
Rationale: Relaxin is a hormone secreted by the corpus luteum and placenta during pregnancy. One of its important functions is to induce uteroplacental vasodilation. This vasodilation enhances blood flow to the placenta, ensuring adequate oxygen and nutrient supply to the developing fetus. Progesterone and estrogen also play crucial roles during pregnancy but do not directly induce uteroplacental vasodilation. Oxytocin is involved in uterine contractions during labor and does not have a direct effect on uteroplacental blood flow. Therefore, the correct answer is Relaxin.

Question 17:
Correct Answer: B) Uterine contractions
Rationale: While monitoring the fetal heart rate during induction of labor in a patient with gestational diabetes, the nurse should be particularly vigilant about uterine contractions. Uterine contractions can have an impact on placental blood flow and may lead to fetal distress, especially in patients with diabetes. Monitoring the frequency, duration, and intensity of contractions is essential to detect any signs of compromised fetal well-being. Fetal movement patterns should also be monitored, but contraction patterns are of higher priority in this situation. Blood glucose levels and maternal blood pressure should be closely monitored as per

routine care but are not directly related to assessing fetal well-being during labor induction.

Question 18:
Correct Answer: A) Late decelerations
Rationale: Late decelerations are characterized by visually apparent, gradual decreases in the FHR that occur after the onset of a contraction and return to the baseline after the contraction ends. Late decelerations are usually associated with uteroplacental insufficiency and require immediate intervention. In this scenario, the regular, symmetrical FHR decelerations beginning at the onset of the contractions and persisting beyond their end suggest late decelerations, indicating a compromised fetal well-being that requires prompt evaluation and intervention.

Question 19:
Correct Answer: C) Fetal blood sampling
Rationale: The correct option is C. Fetal blood sampling (also known as cordocentesis or fetal blood sampling) is a fetal assessment method that involves sampling and analysis of the fetal blood obtained from the umbilical cord. This invasive procedure is performed under ultrasound guidance and allows for direct assessment of the fetal blood gases, acid-base status, and other important parameters. It is commonly used in situations where there is a need for more specific information about the fetal condition, such as in cases of suspected fetal hypoxia or acidemia.

Question 20:
Correct Answer: A) Reposition the mother
Rationale: A sudden decrease in the amplitude of uterine contractions may indicate a change in fetal and maternal position, which can impede the transmission of pressure to the IUPC. Repositioning the mother, such as turning her side-to-side or changing her position, can help improve uterine contraction amplitude. Administering an IV fluid bolus, providing oxygen, or calling the obstetrician may be necessary depending on the assessment findings, but repositioning is the initial action to try to resolve the issue.

Question 21:
Correct Answer: C) Maternal hyperglycemia
Rationale: Maternal hyperglycemia is not a common cause of fetal bradycardia. Fetal bradycardia can be caused by various factors, including maternal hypotension, fetal anemia, and umbilical cord compression. Maternal hypotension reduces blood flow to the placenta, leading to decreased oxygen supply to the fetus. Fetal anemia reduces the oxygen-carrying capacity of the blood, resulting in bradycardia. Umbilical cord compression can also lead to bradycardia by restricting blood flow to the fetus.

Question 22:
Correct Answer: D) All of the above
Rationale: Several methods can be employed to minimize artifact in EFM. Using adhesive electrodes can improve the quality of electrical contact and reduce artifact caused by loose electrodes. Ensuring tight electrode application can also help maintain proper contact and prevent signal interference. Additionally, providing clear instructions to the patient regarding movements and positions during monitoring can minimize artifacts caused by patient-related factors. By combining these measures, healthcare providers can improve the accuracy and reliability of EFM tracings.

Question 23:
Correct Answer: B) Variability increases with increasing gestational age

Rationale: Fetal heart rate variability is influenced by gestational age. As the pregnancy progresses, the fetal autonomic nervous system matures, leading to an increase in variability. This increase is attributed to the developing regulation of the sympathetic and parasympathetic systems, allowing for more fluctuations in the heart rate. Variability is minimal in preterm fetuses and gradually increases in term pregnancies. Therefore, it is important to consider gestational age when interpreting the variability pattern and assessing fetal well-being.

Question 24:
Correct Answer: A) Deceleration that occurs after a contraction
Rationale: Late decelerations are pathological and occur after the peak of a contraction. They represent inadequate oxygenation to the fetus and are often indicative of uteroplacental insufficiency or fetal hypoxia. Immediate intervention and evaluation are required when late decelerations are present.

Question 25:
Correct Answer: A) Decreased maternal blood pressure
Rationale: During anesthesia, decreased maternal blood pressure can significantly impact fetal oxygenation. Maternal hypotension can lead to decreased uteroplacental blood flow, compromising oxygen delivery to the fetus. It can result in fetal hypoxia and acidemia. Therefore, it is crucial to monitor maternal blood pressure closely and ensure adequate perfusion to maintain optimal fetal oxygenation.

Question 26:
Correct Answer: B) 6/10
Rationale: The biophysical profile assigns a score based on the assessment of five parameters: fetal breathing movements, fetal tone, gross body movements, reactive fetal heart rate, and amniotic fluid volume. A score of 8/10 or 10/10 is considered normal, indicating a healthy fetus. A score of 6/10 suggests the need for further evaluation due to potential compromise and the possibility of fetal well-being deteriorating. It is important to identify such cases promptly and take appropriate actions to prevent adverse outcomes. Scores below 6/10 are often indicative of fetal distress and may require immediate intervention.

Question 27:
Correct Answer: C) If there is persistent fetal hypoxia
Rationale: An obstetrician should be consulted for hypertonus during labor if there is persistent fetal hypoxia. Persistent fetal hypoxia indicates an ongoing compromise in fetal well-being and requires immediate medical attention. Elevated maternal blood pressure, cervical dilation less than 4 cm, and irregular contractions are important considerations but do not warrant an immediate consultation with an obstetrician like persistent fetal hypoxia does.

Question 28:
Correct Answer: A) Type 1 diabetes
Rationale: Type 1 diabetes is an autoimmune disease in which the body's immune system attacks and destroys the insulin-producing cells in the pancreas. This leads to a lack of insulin production, resulting in high blood sugar levels. Type 1 diabetes is usually diagnosed in childhood or early adulthood and requires lifelong insulin therapy. It is not related to lifestyle or obesity, unlike type 2 diabetes. Type 1 diabetes accounts for approximately 5-10% of all diabetes cases.

Question 29:

Correct Answer: A) When the mother is unable to tolerate external monitoring.
Rationale: Internal fetal heart rate monitoring may be necessary when the mother's condition or the position of the baby makes it difficult to obtain an accurate reading using external monitoring methods. For example, if the mother is obese or has excessive abdominal fat, the external monitor may not provide clear signals. In such cases, internal monitoring allows for a direct and reliable measurement of the fetal heart rate.

Question 30:
Correct Answer: B) Fetal hypoxemia
Rationale: Late decelerations are typically associated with fetal hypoxemia. Uterine hyperstimulation may lead to variable or prolonged decelerations. Maternal hypoglycemia would present with variable decelerations. Fetal tachycardia would have an increased baseline FHR, not late decelerations.

Question 31:
Correct Answer: A) To assess fetal heart rate reactivity
Rationale: Fetal acoustic stimulation is included in the biophysical profile (BPP) to assess fetal heart rate reactivity. This test involves the use of sound to stimulate the fetus and evaluate its response by monitoring the fetal heart rate. Fetal heart rate reactivity is an important indicator of fetal well-being. The BPP also evaluates other parameters such as amniotic fluid volume, fetal movements, fetal tone, and fetal breathing movements. Fetal acoustic stimulation, along with these parameters, provides a comprehensive assessment of fetal well-being.

Question 32:
Correct Answer: D) Uterine activity has no impact on fetal heart rate.
Rationale: Uterine contractions help with cervical effacement and dilation, allowing for the progression of labor. The frequency of contractions is measured from the beginning of one contraction to the beginning of the next. Intensity of contractions refers to the strength of the contraction, which can be measured using palpation or an electronic fetal monitoring device. Uterine activity does have an impact on fetal heart rate, as contractions can temporarily decrease blood flow to the placenta, affecting fetal oxygenation.

Question 33:
Correct Answer: C) Uterine fibroids
Rationale: Uterine contraction intensity can be affected by various factors, including uterine fibroids. Uterine fibroids are noncancerous growths in the uterus that can alter the normal anatomy and function of the uterus. Depending on their size and location, they can interfere with the strength and coordination of uterine contractions, impacting the intensity. Other factors, such as maternal age, fetal position, and amniotic fluid volume, may have indirect effects on labor progress but do not directly influence contraction intensity.

Question 34:
Correct Answer: C) Variable decelerations
Rationale: The described pattern is indicative of variable decelerations. Variable decelerations represent abrupt, temporary decreases in the FHR that vary in onset, depth, and duration. They are associated with cord compression and can occur in response to changes in fetal position or umbilical cord compression during contractions. The pattern observed does not fit the characteristics of early decelerations, variability, or a sinusoidal pattern. Close

monitoring and appropriate management are necessary to ensure fetal well-being.

Question 35:
Correct Answer: A) Duration refers to the time from the beginning to the end of a contraction.
Rationale: Duration refers to the time from the beginning of a contraction to the end of that contraction. It is an essential parameter to assess the progress of labor and ensure adequate uterine activity. Consistency in the duration of contractions is important, as variability can be an indication of abnormal labor patterns. Contractions should typically last between 45 to 80 seconds during the active phase of labor.

Question 36:
Correct Answer: D) Acceleration in the fetal heart rate
Rationale: Sinusoidal pattern in electronic fetal monitoring can be caused by various factors, including fetal anemia, maternal administration of opioids, and maternal hypotension. However, an acceleration in the fetal heart rate is not a cause of sinusoidal pattern. An acceleration is a normal finding that indicates fetal well-being and adequate oxygenation.

Question 37:
Correct Answer: C) Category I
Rationale: In Category I, the baseline rate is 110-160 bpm, variability is moderate (6-25 bpm), with no late or variable decelerations, and early decelerations or accelerations may be present. This is considered a reassuring pattern, indicating fetal well-being. The provided EFM tracing shows a baseline rate of 140 bpm, variability of 7 bpm, and no decelerations, which corresponds to Category I.

Question 38:
Correct Answer: C) Fetal movement monitoring provides an indirect measure of fetal well-being.
Rationale: Fetal movement monitoring involves monitoring the baby's movements, commonly known as kicks or counts, as a way to assess fetal well-being. It provides an indirect measure of fetal health and can help identify potential issues, such as decreased fetal movement, which may be a sign of fetal distress or compromise. Fetal heart rate can be assessed through electronic fetal monitoring (EFM), fetal movements do not predict the due date, and fetal movement monitoring is important throughout the third trimester to ensure the baby's well-being.

Question 39:
Correct Answer: D) To monitor uterine contractions
Rationale: The primary purpose of using an Intrauterine Pressure Catheter (IUPC) during labor is to monitor uterine contractions. It provides essential information about the frequency, duration, and intensity of contractions, allowing healthcare providers to assess the progress of labor and make informed decisions regarding the well-being of both the mother and the fetus. Options A, B, and C are incorrect as they do not accurately describe the purpose of using an IUPC.

Question 40:
Correct Answer: C) Preeclampsia
Rationale: Preeclampsia, a condition characterized by high blood pressure and organ damage in pregnant women, is associated with an increased risk of abnormal fetal heart rate patterns. The placental dysfunction in preeclampsia can lead to fetal hypoxia, resulting in abnormal heart rate patterns.

Question 41:
Correct Answer: C) Toco transducer

Rationale: The toco transducer is a noninvasive method used to monitor uterine contractions. It is placed on the maternal abdomen and measures uterine activity by sensing changes in pressure. The toco transducer is used to measure the frequency and duration of contractions, allowing healthcare professionals to assess the progress of labor and identify any abnormal patterns or uterine hyperactivity. External monitoring refers to the use of sensors placed on the maternal abdomen to monitor fetal heart rate and contractions. Internal monitoring involves the placement of a fetal scalp electrode and an intrauterine pressure catheter for more accurate and direct measurement.

Question 42:
Correct Answer: A) Uteroplacental circulation actively transports drugs from the maternal circulation to the fetal circulation.
Rationale: Uteroplacental circulation plays a significant role in drug transfer to the fetus. It actively transports drugs from the maternal circulation to the fetal circulation, allowing drugs to reach the developing fetus. The placenta acts as a filter, allowing certain substances to pass through while restricting others. Drug transfer primarily occurs through the umbilical vein, not the umbilical artery. Therefore, the correct answer is A) Uteroplacental circulation actively transports drugs from the maternal circulation to the fetal circulation.

Question 43:
Correct Answer: B) Change the maternal position
Rationale: Persistent variable decelerations on EFM suggest umbilical cord compression and potential hypoxemia. The initial intervention should be to change the maternal position to relieve cord compression. This can be done by turning the patient to a lateral position or performing a knee-chest position. Administering oxygen is important but is not the most appropriate initial intervention in this scenario. Inserting an IUPC or increasing the rate of oxytocin infusion may exacerbate the cord compression and should be avoided until the cause of the decelerations is addressed.

Question 44:
Correct Answer: A) Ensuring the equipment is properly calibrated
Rationale: Proper calibration of the equipment used in electronic fetal monitoring is crucial to ensure accurate and reliable results. Inaccurate readings can lead to misinterpretation of the fetal condition and potentially harm the patient. Educating the patient about the procedure and any potential risks is also important for informed consent and shared decision-making but not directly related to minimizing the risk of harm. Monitoring the maternal blood pressure is important but not specific to electronic fetal monitoring. Taking frequent breaks during the monitoring process may cause interruptions and compromise the continuous monitoring required.

Question 45:
Correct Answer: A) Oxygen tension
Rationale: The primary mechanism regulating blood flow to the placenta is oxygen tension. Decreased oxygen levels in the placenta stimulate the release of vasodilatory substances, such as nitric oxide and prostaglandins, which in turn increase blood flow. Conversely, high oxygen tension leads to vasoconstriction, reducing blood flow. This mechanism ensures an adequate oxygen supply to the developing fetus and helps maintain a balance between oxygen delivery and demand.

Question 46:
Correct Answer: B) 6-10 mmHg

Rationale: The optimal resting tone of the uterus between contractions during labor is approximately 6-10 mmHg. This range indicates a state of uterine relaxation necessary for adequate placental perfusion, allowing for optimal fetal oxygenation and nutrient exchange. Resting tone below 6 mmHg may suggest uterine atony, while resting tone above 10 mmHg may indicate excessive uterine activity which can compromise oxygen supply to the fetus.

Question 47:
Correct Answer: C) Avoiding unnecessary discussions about the patient in the presence of others
Rationale: Maintaining patient privacy is crucial during electronic fetal monitoring to ensure confidentiality and protect the patient's dignity. Healthcare providers should avoid unnecessary discussions about the patient's personal information and medical history in the presence of others who are not involved in the care. Using curtains or screens to create privacy and minimizing the number of healthcare providers present in the room can also help maintain privacy. Allowing visitors to stay during the monitoring process may compromise privacy and confidentiality.

Question 48:
Correct Answer: A) Uterine hyperstimulation
Rationale: A sudden increase in the duration of uterine contractions may indicate uterine hyperstimulation, which is characterized by contractions lasting longer than 90 seconds. This can lead to inadequate fetal oxygenation and potential fetal distress. The nurse should assess for other signs of uterine hyperstimulation, such as frequent contractions (more than five in ten minutes) or hypertonic contractions. Fetal distress, maternal fatigue, or IUPC dislodgment may have different presenting signs and symptoms.

Question 49:
Correct Answer: C) Inaccuracy in assessing fetal heart rate
Rationale: One potential limitation of external fetal monitoring is inaccuracy in assessing the fetal heart rate. Factors such as maternal obesity, fetal position, and maternal movement can affect the quality of the signal obtained by the external monitor, leading to difficulties in accurately detecting the fetal heart rate. External monitoring allows the mother to maintain mobility during labor, unlike invasive methods such as internal fetal monitoring. The risk of infection to the fetus is not directly associated with external monitoring. Monitoring uterine contractions can be achieved through external monitoring using a tocometer.

Question 50:
Correct Answer: D) Sinusoidal pattern
Rationale: A sinusoidal pattern is characterized by a consistent smooth, wavelike motion with a uniform frequency of 3-5 cycles per minute. It is typically unrelated to uterine contractions and persists for at least 20 minutes. The FHR ranges between 120-160 beats per minute, but there are no periodic changes. It is a concerning pattern as it is often associated with severe fetal anemia or hypoxia, intrauterine infection, or fetal bleeding. Immediate evaluation and intervention are necessary to determine the cause and provide appropriate management.

Question 51:
Correct Answer: C) Performing a fetal scalp blood sampling
Rationale: In the scenario described, the management of prolonged decelerations should involve further assessment of the fetal acid-base status. Performing a fetal scalp blood sampling involves obtaining a blood sample from the baby's scalp for analysis of pH and oxygenation. This provides valuable information on fetal well-being. Administering magnesium sulfate is not indicated for prolonged decelerations. Immediate delivery via cesarean section is not warranted solely based on the presence of prolonged decelerations. Applying gentle fundal pressure is contraindicated as it may further compromise fetal oxygenation.

Question 52:
Correct Answer: C) Preconception counseling helps to optimize glycemic control before pregnancy.
Rationale: Preconception counseling is crucial for women with diabetes, especially type 1 diabetes. It plays a significant role in optimizing glycemic control before pregnancy, reducing the risk of adverse pregnancy outcomes. Through preconception counseling, women can receive education regarding the importance of tight glycemic control, adjusting medications, managing potential complications, and ensuring adequate folic acid supplementation. It helps to establish a solid foundation for a healthy pregnancy and increases the chances of a successful outcome. Glycemic control during pregnancy significantly impacts fetal outcomes, and preconception counseling plays a vital role in achieving and maintaining optimal glycemic control.

Question 53:
Correct Answer: A) Early deceleration
Rationale: Early decelerations are benign, mirror-image decelerations that are related to head compression during contractions. They are considered a normal physiological response and are not associated with fetal compromise. The deceleration begins at the onset of the contraction and returns to baseline by the end of the contraction.

Question 54:
Correct Answer: D) Mechanical transducer malfunction
Rationale: Mechanical transducer malfunction can cause irregular oscillations on the paper printout of the fetal heart rate tracing but may not be apparent on the monitor screen. This artifact can be caused by issues with the recording mechanism or the paper feed system. It is important to troubleshoot and resolve the mechanical malfunction to obtain an accurate representation of the fetal heart rate and effectively monitor the well-being of the fetus during labor.

Question 55:
Correct Answer: A) Insulin resistance
Rationale: Obesity is associated with insulin resistance, which can affect fetal oxygenation. Insulin resistance in pregnant women with obesity disrupts glucose metabolism, leading to gestational diabetes. This condition increases the risk of fetal hypoxia due to elevated maternal blood glucose levels and impaired placental function. Gestational diabetes can affect fetal oxygenation and result in macrosomia (large fetus), which can further compromise oxygenation during labor and delivery. Regular monitoring and management of glucose levels are crucial in pregnant patients with obesity to optimize fetal oxygenation.

Question 56:
Correct Answer: D) All of the above
Rationale: Maternal conditions such as diabetes, hypertension, and obesity can impact fetal oxygenation during labor. Diabetes can lead to increased fetal size and decreased placental function, causing hypoxia. Hypertension can reduce uteroplacental blood flow, resulting in fetal hypoxia. Obesity increases the risk of complications,

including umbilical cord compression and reduced blood flow to the fetus, leading to oxygen deprivation. These maternal factors should be carefully monitored during labor to ensure optimal fetal oxygenation and reduce the risk of birth complications.

Question 57:
Correct Answer: D) Detect uterine contractions
Rationale: Uterine monitoring during pregnancy is primarily used to detect and monitor uterine contractions. It helps in assessing the frequency, duration, and intensity of contractions and identifying any abnormal patterns. Uterine contractions play a crucial role in the progression of labor, and monitoring them is essential in ensuring a safe delivery. Assessing uterine blood flow, evaluating cervix dilation, and monitoring fetal growth are important aspects of prenatal care but are not the primary purpose of uterine monitoring specifically.

Question 58:
Correct Answer: A) Vertex presentation
Rationale: In multiple gestations, the most common fetal presentation is vertex, which means the baby's head is positioned to come out first during birth. This is the preferred presentation for a vaginal delivery as it allows for a smoother and more efficient delivery process. Breech presentation, where the baby's buttocks or feet come out first, is less common in multiple gestations. Transverse presentation, where the baby is positioned horizontally across the uterus, and compound presentation, where two or more body parts present together, are even less common. It is important to know the fetal presentation in multiple gestations to determine the mode of delivery and plan appropriate interventions if needed.

Question 59:
Correct Answer: B) Uteroplacental circulation is responsible for transporting oxygen and nutrients from the placenta to the fetus.
Rationale: Uteroplacental circulation refers to the blood flow between the uterus and the placenta. It is responsible for the exchange of oxygen, nutrients, and waste products between the maternal blood and the fetal blood. Oxygen and nutrients are transported from the placenta to the fetus through the placental circulation, while waste products and carbon dioxide are transported from the fetal blood to the maternal blood for elimination. Uteroplacental circulation is primarily regulated by the maternal uterine arteries, which dilate to increase blood flow to the placenta during pregnancy.

Question 60:
Correct Answer: A) Administer oxygen to the mother
Rationale: Late decelerations are associated with uteroplacental insufficiency and can indicate fetal hypoxemia. The first action in addressing this situation is to administer oxygen to the mother to improve oxygenation and perfusion. Repositioning the mother may also be done to relieve any potential pressure on the uterus, but administering oxygen takes priority. Increasing the intravenous fluid rate may be considered to improve maternal blood volume, but it is not the first action to be taken. Performing a vaginal examination is not necessary at this time and does not address the immediate concern of fetal hypoxemia.

Question 61:
Correct Answer: A) Uteroplacental insufficiency
Rationale: Prolonged decelerations on the FHR tracing can be caused by uteroplacental insufficiency. The intense uterine contractions lasting longer than 90 seconds can lead

to decreased blood flow to the placenta, resulting in fetal hypoxemia and prolonged decelerations. Maternal hypotension, fetal head compression, and nuchal cord are associated with different patterns of decelerations on the FHR tracing.

Question 62:
Correct Answer: B) Biophysical profile (BPP)
Rationale: The correct option is B. The biophysical profile (BPP) is a fetal assessment method that provides continuous monitoring of fetal heart rate, uterine activity, and fetal movement. It is a noninvasive test that combines ultrasound evaluation with a nonstress test (NST) to assess the overall well-being of the fetus. A BPP score of 8 or 10 is considered reassuring, while a score of 6 or less may indicate fetal compromise and the need for further intervention.

Question 63:
Correct Answer: A) Administer tocolytic medications
Rationale: High-frequency contractions, defined as more than 5 contractions in 10 minutes, may indicate tachysystole, which can be harmful to the fetus and the progress of labor. In such cases, the management approach involves administering tocolytic medications to inhibit uterine activity and reduce the frequency of contractions. This helps to ensure adequate fetal oxygenation and prevent uterine hyperstimulation. Monitoring the fetal heart rate closely is important; however, in cases of high-frequency contractions, immediate intervention with tocolytic medications is necessary. Encouraging maternal rest and hydration may be beneficial but alone may not be sufficient to resolve the issue. Performing a vaginal examination does not directly address the high frequency of contractions.

Question 64:
Correct Answer: A) Nonstress test (NST)
Rationale: The correct option is A. The nonstress test (NST) is a fetal assessment method that involves the measurement of the fetal heart rate in response to fetal movement. It is a noninvasive test performed during pregnancy to assess fetal well-being. The NST monitors the fetal heart rate patterns at rest (non-stressful conditions) and evaluates accelerations (increases in the heart rate) in response to fetal movement. The presence of accelerations is a reassuring sign and indicates a healthy fetus.

Question 65:
Correct Answer: A) Measurement of fetal heart rate variability
Rationale: A non-stress test (NST) is a common fetal assessment method used to evaluate fetal well-being. It involves the measurement of fetal heart rate variability, which refers to the changes in the fetal heart rate in response to fetal movements. The non-stress test helps assess the baby's oxygenation and neurological status. Visualization of the placental position is typically done through ultrasound, assessment of fetal movements is part of kick counting or fetal movement monitoring, and evaluation of amniotic fluid volume is performed using techniques like the amniotic fluid index (AFI) or pocket measurements.

Question 66:
Correct Answer: A) Macrosomia
Rationale: Poorly controlled diabetes during pregnancy can lead to macrosomia in the neonate. Macrosomia refers to a larger-than-average birth weight, usually over 8 pounds, 13 ounces (4,000 grams). It increases the risk of birth injuries and cesarean delivery. Premature rupture of membranes, ectopic pregnancy, and gestational hypertension are not

directly associated with poorly controlled diabetes during pregnancy.

Question 67:
Correct Answer: C) Placental abruption
Rationale: Placental abruption occurs when the placenta separates prematurely from the uterine wall, leading to significant bleeding and compromising the oxygen supply to the fetus. This condition can result in fetal hypoxia and distress. Maternal hypertension, umbilical cord compression, and placenta previa are all potential factors that may impact fetal oxygenation but are not directly related to placental abruption.

Question 68:
Correct Answer: A) Fetal heart rate variability
Rationale: Fetal heart rate variability is the fluctuation in the interval between consecutive fetal heartbeats. It is an essential characteristic of a normal, healthy fetus. Fetal distress refers to a condition in which the fetus is not receiving enough oxygen or nutrients. Fetal bradycardia is a slow heart rate, usually less than 110 beats per minute. Fetal tachycardia is an abnormally fast heart rate, usually above 160 beats per minute.

Question 69:
Correct Answer: D) Order a biophysical profile score
Rationale: In this scenario, the patient presents with decreased fetal movements and a non-reassuring FHR tracing characterized by minimal variability and infrequent accelerations. The next appropriate step in management would be to order a biophysical profile (BPP) score. The BPP combines a non-stress test (NST) for assessing FHR reactivity with four additional ultrasound components to assess fetal well-being. This comprehensive evaluation helps determine the fetal risk and guides appropriate interventions.

Question 70:
Correct Answer: A) Human Chorionic Gonadotropin (hCG)
Rationale: Human Chorionic Gonadotropin (hCG) is a hormone produced by the placenta during early pregnancy. It is responsible for maintaining the corpus luteum, which, in turn, secretes progesterone. Progesterone is necessary to support the thickening and maintenance of the uterine lining, ensuring a favorable environment for the developing embryo. The presence of hCG is detected in pregnancy tests, and its levels gradually decrease as the pregnancy progresses.

Question 71:
Correct Answer: C) Maternal age over 35
Rationale: Uterine rupture/scar dehiscence is a serious complication that can occur during labor, particularly in women with a history of previous cesarean section. The risk is further increased by the use of oxytocin for labor induction or augmentation and pregnancy with multiple gestations. However, maternal age over 35 is not directly associated with an increased risk of uterine rupture/scar dehiscence.

Question 72:
Correct Answer: A) Perform a biophysical profile (BPP) immediately
Rationale: Given the persistent loss of beat-to-beat variability of the fetal heart rate below 5 bpm for more than 10 minutes, an immediate BPP is necessary. BPP combines NST (non-stress test) and ultrasound evaluation including fetal breathing, movement, tone, and amniotic fluid volume. BPP will provide valuable information about the well-being of the fetus and help determine if further intervention is required.

Question 73:
Correct Answer: A) Increased risk of preterm delivery
Rationale: Monoamniotic-monochorionic twins share both the same amniotic sac and placenta. This type of twin pregnancy carries a higher risk of complications, especially preterm delivery. The risk of cord entanglement and compression is also higher in monoamniotic-monochorionic twins. Close monitoring and early intervention may be necessary to minimize the risk of adverse outcomes.

Question 74:
Correct Answer: A) Proper hand hygiene before and after the procedure
Rationale: Maintaining proper hand hygiene is crucial to prevent infection during electronic fetal monitoring. This includes washing hands with soap and water or using alcohol-based hand sanitizers before and after the procedure. Using sterile gloves during the procedure can further reduce the risk of infection. Administering antibiotics prophylactically is not a standard practice for electronic fetal monitoring. Lubricating jelly is often used during the procedure to ensure a comfortable insertion of the fetal monitor and does not increase the risk of infection.

Question 75:
Correct Answer: C) Syphilis
Rationale: Syphilis is a sexually transmitted infection that can be transmitted from mother to fetus through the placenta. This can lead to congenital syphilis, which may cause severe complications such as stillbirth, prematurity, and neurological abnormalities. Early detection and treatment of syphilis in pregnancy are essential to prevent these adverse outcomes.

Question 76:
Correct Answer: B) Normal pH
Rationale: A normal fetal scalp pH range is considered to be between 7.25 and 7.35. In this scenario, the fetal scalp pH is 7.24, which falls within the normal range. Therefore, the interpretation of the fetal scalp pH in this situation would be a normal pH.

Question 77:
Correct Answer: B) Fetal tachycardia
Rationale: Fetal tachycardia is a fetal complication that is characterized by a sudden, transient increase in the fetal heart rate. It refers to a persistently high heart rate above the normal range. Fetal tachycardia can be caused by various factors, including maternal fever, fetal infection, maternal or fetal medications, and fetal hypoxia. Close monitoring and intervention are necessary to determine the cause of fetal tachycardia and prevent potential complications.

Question 78:
Correct Answer: D) 24-hour urine protein collection
Rationale: In the management of chronic essential hypertension during pregnancy, the assessment of proteinuria is important. A 24-hour urine protein collection is the gold standard for evaluating protein excretion. This helps in identifying early signs of preeclampsia, a complication often associated with chronic hypertension. While assessing fasting blood glucose levels may be important in the management of gestational diabetes, it is not specific to chronic hypertension. A CBC and renal ultrasound are not routinely indicated in the evaluation of chronic essential hypertension unless there are specific concerns.

Question 79:
Correct Answer: A) Placental abruption
Rationale: The symptoms of lower abdominal pain, feeling of "something tearing," closed cervix, prolonged fetal bradycardia, and ultrasound findings of a retroplacental hematoma are suggestive of placental abruption. This is a serious obstetric emergency and prompt delivery may be necessary depending on the severity of the abruption and fetal status. Uterine rupture typically presents with a different clinical picture, including a tense and tender uterus and variable decelerations.

Question 80:
Correct Answer: B) Variable deceleration
Rationale: Variable decelerations are visually apparent, abrupt decelerations that vary in duration, timing, and depth. They are associated with cord compression and can occur at any time in the labor cycle, not just during contractions. Immediate interventions, such as repositioning the mother, may be required.

Question 81:
Correct Answer: C) Fetal heart murmur
Rationale: The continuous, high-pitched, musical sound heard during auscultation of the fetal heart rate (FHR) is suggestive of a fetal heart murmur. Fetal heart murmurs are relatively common and can occur due to various factors, such as blood flow abnormalities or structural abnormalities in the heart. It is important to further evaluate the murmur to determine its cause and potential impact on the fetus.

Question 82:
Correct Answer: D) Notify the obstetrician for further evaluation
Rationale: A sinusoidal fetal heart rate pattern is an abnormal finding and may indicate fetal distress. The obstetrician should be notified for further evaluation and management. Prompt intervention is crucial to ensure the well-being of the fetus.

Question 83:
Correct Answer: B) Preeclampsia
Rationale: Preeclampsia is a maternal complication commonly associated with postdates pregnancy. Preeclampsia is characterized by high blood pressure and damage to organs, most commonly the liver and kidneys. It usually develops after 20 weeks of gestation and can lead to serious complications for both the mother and the baby, including placental abruption, fetal growth restriction, and preterm birth. It is essential to closely monitor blood pressure and other signs of preeclampsia in postdates pregnancies to ensure early detection and appropriate management, which may include close observation, blood pressure control, and potential delivery if symptoms worsen.

Question 84:
Correct Answer: A) Progesterone supplementation
Rationale: Progesterone supplementation has been shown to be the most effective intervention in preventing preterm labor in women with a history of preterm birth. It helps to reduce the risk of preterm birth by providing hormonal support to the uterine lining and preventing early contractions. Progesterone supplementation can be administered through various routes, including intramuscular injections, vaginal suppositories, or oral tablets. Bed rest, induction of labor, and increased fluid intake are not proven interventions for preventing preterm labor and may not have significant benefits or evidence-based support in this context.

Question 85:

Correct Answer: B) The foramen ovale connects the right and left atria of the fetal heart.
Rationale: The foramen ovale is an opening between the right and left atria of the fetal heart. It allows the majority of blood to bypass the fetal lungs, as they are not functional in utero. This allows oxygenated blood to flow directly from the right atrium to the left atrium and then into the systemic circulation. Options A, C, and D are incorrect statements. Oxygenated blood is carried from the placenta to the fetus through the umbilical vein, the ductus arteriosus connects the pulmonary artery and the aorta, and the umbilical artery carries deoxygenated blood from the fetus to the placenta.

Question 86:
Correct Answer: C) Both the nurse and physician share the responsibility for the fetal monitoring process.
Rationale: In the scenario described, both the nurse and the physician have legal responsibilities in the fetal monitoring process. The nurse's role includes promptly notifying the physician of any concerning findings, whereas the physician is accountable for taking appropriate actions based on the nurse's notification. Collaboration between the nurse and physician ensures optimal care for the pregnant woman and her fetus, with shared responsibility for the monitoring process.

Question 87:
Correct Answer: A) Maternal diabetes
Rationale: Maternal diabetes is a known risk factor for decreased fetal heart rate variability. This can be due to placental insufficiency and impaired oxygen and nutrient delivery to the fetus. Fetal sleep cycles typically lead to increased variability. Maternal smoking can also affect fetal heart rate variability but is not as significant as diabetes. Fetal anemia can lead to decreased variability due to compromised oxygen-carrying capacity, but this would usually be associated with other characteristics on the monitor strip.

Question 88:
Correct Answer: B) Poor electrode connection
Rationale: Poor electrode connection can lead to signal ambiguity, resulting in an unstable baseline fetal heart rate tracing and frequent signal dropouts. In this scenario, the nurse should ensure that the electrodes are properly attached and securely connected to the mother's abdomen. This will help establish a reliable signal and prevent further signal ambiguities while monitoring the fetal heart rate.

Question 89:
Correct Answer: C) Electronic fetal monitor
Rationale: Continuous external fetal monitoring during labor is achieved using an electronic fetal monitor. This device combines the measurement of the fetal heart rate, uterine contractions, and maternal vital signs into a single monitoring system. Fetal heart rate monitors and Doppler ultrasounds are used for intermittent external monitoring, while a tocodynamometer is used to measure uterine contractions.

Question 90:
Correct Answer: D) Preeclampsia
Rationale: Maternal obesity is a known risk factor for several complications during pregnancy. Preeclampsia, a condition characterized by high blood pressure and organ damage, is one of the complications commonly observed in obese pregnant women. Other complications associated with maternal obesity include gestational diabetes, preterm birth, and shoulder dystocia. However, preeclampsia has been particularly linked to maternal obesity due to the underlying inflammation and metabolic dysregulation associated with

obesity. This knowledge is crucial for healthcare providers involved in the management of obese pregnant women to ensure appropriate monitoring and timely intervention to prevent adverse outcomes.

Question 91:
Correct Answer: A) Absent variability
Rationale: Fetal demise is characterized by the absence of fetal heart rate variability, meaning the absence of fluctuations in the baseline heart rate. This finding is a sign of fetal compromise and is often associated with a non-reassuring fetal heart rate tracing. Accelerations, early decelerations, and fetal tachycardia are not typically observed in cases of fetal demise.

Question 92:
Correct Answer: B) It provides more accurate measurement of uterine contractions compared to an external tocodynamometer
Rationale: An internal uterine pressure catheter provides a more accurate measurement of uterine contractions compared to an external tocodynamometer. It is an invasive method that involves the insertion of a catheter into the uterine cavity. It provides continuous and direct measurement of intrauterine pressure. Rupture of the membranes is necessary for the insertion of an internal uterine pressure catheter. It is contraindicated in cases of placenta previa due to the risk of injury or hemorrhage.

Question 93:
Correct Answer: A) Inform the patient that this is a normal finding.
Rationale: A baseline variability of 4-6 bpm is within the normal range. It indicates a slightly decreased but still acceptable variability. It is not suggestive of fetal distress or the need for immediate intervention. Informing the patient that this finding is normal reassures them about the fetal well-being.

Question 94:
Correct Answer: C) 8-10 contractions in 10 minutes
Rationale: During the active phase of labor, the typical frequency range for uterine contractions is 8-10 contractions in 10 minutes. This frequency pattern indicates regular and effective uterine activity necessary for progressive cervical dilation and descent of the fetus. Contractions occurring less frequently may be insufficient to promote cervical dilation, whereas contractions occurring more frequently may lead to inadequate uterine relaxation which can compromise fetal oxygenation.

Question 95:
Correct Answer: B) Absence of accelerations in the fetal heart rate
Rationale: The absence of accelerations in the fetal heart rate is considered a non-reassuring finding on an external fetal monitoring test. Accelerations are temporary increases in fetal heart rate that indicate fetal well-being. A fetal heart rate of 150 bpm is within the normal range. A reactive non-stress test, which shows appropriate accelerations with fetal movement, is a reassuring finding. The duration of uterine contractions does not directly indicate fetal well-being in the context of external fetal monitoring.

Question 96:
Correct Answer: A) Increased risk of infection.
Rationale: One of the main risks associated with internal fetal heart rate monitoring is an increased risk of infection. Since the procedure involves the insertion of an electrode into the baby's scalp, there is a small risk of introducing infection into the birth canal. However, healthcare providers take precautions to minimize this risk by following strict sterile techniques during insertion. The benefits of continuous and accurate monitoring often outweigh the potential risk of infection, especially in high-risk situations where close monitoring is necessary for the well-being of the baby.

Question 97:
Correct Answer: D) Fetal weight
Rationale: Ultrasound is a commonly used fetal assessment method that utilizes sound waves to create images of the fetus. It provides valuable information about the fetus, including its size, anatomical structures, and growth. Fetal weight estimation is often done during ultrasound examinations to assess the baby's growth and evaluate its well-being. Fetal heart rate can be assessed using electronic fetal monitoring (EFM), fetal movements are subjective observations by the mother, and placental position is typically determined through ultrasound or clinical examination.

Question 98:
Correct Answer: B) Emergency cesarean section
Rationale: The recommended management for uterine rupture/scar dehiscence is an emergency cesarean section. This is necessary to ensure the safety of both the mother and the baby. Immediate vaginal delivery is contraindicated due to the risk of further uterine rupture and fetal compromise. Tocolytic agents are not effective in the management of uterine rupture/scar dehiscence. Observation without intervention would not address the potentially life-threatening situation.

Question 99:
Correct Answer: B) 1 contraction every 150 seconds
Rationale: The frequency of contractions is determined by the time interval between the start of one contraction and the start of the next contraction. In this scenario, since each contraction lasts for 75 seconds, there is a 150-second interval between contractions, resulting in a frequency of 1 contraction every 150 seconds.

Question 100:
Correct Answer: C) Administer oxygen to the mother
Rationale: Repetitive late decelerations in the FHR tracing are suggestive of uteroplacental insufficiency and fetal hypoxia. Administering oxygen to the mother helps improve oxygenation and blood flow to the fetus, reducing the risk of fetal injury. Administering intravenous fluids, changing the mother's position, or performing an episiotomy are not the primary interventions indicated in this scenario.

Question 101:
Correct Answer: C) Normal uterine activity
Rationale: A resting uterine tone of 10 mmHg indicates normal uterine activity. Normal resting tone ranges between 5-20 mmHg. In this scenario, there are no signs of excessive or inadequate uterine activity, which suggests a normal uterine tone.

Question 102:
Correct Answer: B) Uterine contractions
Rationale: Decreased fetal heart rate variability can be caused by uterine contractions. During contractions, the fetal heart rate may become momentarily suppressed, leading to reduced variability.

Question 103:
Correct Answer: D) Prepare for immediate delivery

Rationale: In this scenario, the fetal heart rate of 100 bpm, absence of fetal movement, and the presence of variable decelerations indicate fetal distress. Immediate delivery is necessary to prevent further compromise and ensure optimal outcomes for both the mother and the baby.

Question 104:
Correct Answer: D) Multiple gestation
Rationale: Multiple gestation (e.g., twins, triplets) is not a risk factor for gestational hypertension. However, obesity, teenage pregnancy, and a history of preeclampsia in previous pregnancies are known risk factors for the development of gestational hypertension. It is essential for healthcare providers to identify these risk factors early on to closely monitor pregnant individuals and provide appropriate intervention and management to reduce complications associated with gestational hypertension.

Question 105:
Correct Answer: A) Dizygotic
Rationale: Dizygotic (fraternal) twins are more common than monozygotic (identical) twins. Dizygotic twins result from the fertilization of two separate eggs by two separate sperm, resulting in two genetically distinct embryos. On the other hand, monozygotic twins occur when a single fertilized egg splits into two embryos. Understanding the zygosity of twins is essential for appropriate management and counseling of multiple gestations.

Question 106:
Correct Answer: B) Regular physical exercise
Rationale: Regular physical exercise is recommended as an intervention for pregnant women with diabetes to reduce the risk of fetal complications. Exercise helps control blood sugar levels, improves insulin sensitivity, and promotes a healthy pregnancy. Increased caffeine intake, smoking, and heavy alcohol consumption are not advisable during pregnancy and can have detrimental effects on both the mother and the fetus.

Question 107:
Correct Answer: B) Promoting equality in the distribution of healthcare resources
Rationale: The principle of justice in medical ethics focuses on promoting fairness and equality in the distribution of healthcare resources, ensuring that all individuals have equal access to appropriate medical care and treatment. This principle emphasizes the equitable allocation of resources, such as medical facilities, personnel, and technology, to avoid any form of discrimination or bias based on socio-economic status, ethnicity, or other factors.

Question 108:
Correct Answer: B) Hypertension
Rationale: Hypertension, particularly conditions such as preeclampsia or chronic hypertension, is associated with an increased risk of preterm labor. These hypertensive disorders can lead to complications such as placental insufficiency, poor fetal growth, and uteroplacental vascular abnormalities, which can ultimately result in preterm birth. Regular blood pressure monitoring and appropriate management of hypertension during pregnancy are essential to reduce the risk of preterm labor and improve maternal and fetal outcomes. Gestational diabetes, ovarian cysts, and thyroid disorders are not directly linked to an increased risk of preterm labor.

Question 109:
Correct Answer: A) Initiate antiviral treatment with oseltamivir within 48 hours of symptom onset

Rationale: Pregnant women with suspected or confirmed influenza should receive antiviral treatment with oseltamivir within 48 hours of symptom onset to reduce the severity and duration of illness. Antibiotics targeting atypical pathogens are unnecessary in this case as the diagnosis is H1N1 influenza. Admission to the intensive care unit is not indicated unless the patient develops severe respiratory distress or complications. Bed rest and symptomatic treatment alone may not be sufficient to manage influenza in pregnancy.

Question 110:
Correct Answer: A) Contractions in the active phase of labor are usually irregular.
Rationale: Contractions in the active phase of labor are usually irregular, with a frequency of three to five contractions in ten minutes. As labor progresses, contractions become more regular, intense, and frequent. The latent phase of labor, on the other hand, is characterized by irregular, mild contractions with longer intervals. Contractions in the active phase of labor are also generally longer in duration when compared to the latent phase. Pain during contractions progressively increases as labor advances.

Question 111:
Correct Answer: C) Oxytocin
Rationale: Oxytocin is a hormone released by the pituitary gland that plays a significant role in initiating and regulating labor contractions. During labor, oxytocin is released in increasing amounts, stimulating the uterus to contract. These contractions help to facilitate cervical dilation, effacement, and ultimately the delivery of the baby. Oxytocin also plays a crucial role in the bonding between the mother and the newborn and in promoting the release of breast milk during breastfeeding.

Question 112:
Correct Answer: D) Montvield Units (MU)
Rationale: The intensity of uterine contractions is measured in Montvield Units (MU). This unit helps in assessing the strength or power of the contraction. It is measured using an intrauterine pressure catheter (IUPC) or external tocodynamometer. The normal range of intensity is typically between 40-100 MU, with higher values indicating stronger contractions. Monitoring the intensity of contractions is essential in evaluating the progress of labor, determining the effectiveness of interventions, and ensuring the well-being of the fetus.

Question 113:
Correct Answer: B) Cocaine
Rationale: Cocaine is a potent vasoconstrictor that can reduce blood flow to the uterus, leading to decreased oxygen supply to the fetus. This drug can also increase the risk of placental abruption, further compromising fetal oxygenation and potentially resulting in fetal distress or death.

Question 114:
Correct Answer: C) Report the incident to a supervisor or the appropriate authority.
Rationale: Patient safety should always be a priority in healthcare settings. Mishandling of fetal monitoring equipment can lead to inaccurate readings, potentially compromising the well-being of the mother and the baby. It is your ethical responsibility to report such incidents to a supervisor or appropriate authority to ensure that corrective measures are taken. This helps maintain the highest standards of patient care and promotes a culture of safety within the healthcare facility.

Question 115:
Correct Answer: C) Umbilical cord prolapse
Rationale: Umbilical cord prolapse refers to the displacement of the umbilical cord into the birth canal before the fetal presenting part. This condition can cause compression of the cord, leading to fetal distress. It is considered one of the most common causes of cord compression during labor. Maternal positioning, uterine contractions, and fetal movement may contribute to cord compression, but they are not the primary cause.

Question 116:
Correct Answer: A) Perform a fetal scalp pH sampling
Rationale: The presence of meconium-stained amniotic fluid and repetitive variable decelerations suggests possible fetal compromise. In this situation, it would be most appropriate to perform a fetal scalp pH sampling to assess the fetal acid-base status. Administering oxygen to the mother can be considered, but fetal assessment should take priority. Immediate cesarean section may be indicated if there are signs of severe fetal distress or worsening decelerations. Continuing monitoring while awaiting the second stage of labor is not the most proactive approach in this situation.

Question 117:
Correct Answer: A) Verify the accuracy of the tocodynamometer placement
Rationale: A high frequency of uterine activity on the EFM tracing can occur if the tocodynamometer is not accurately placed on the mother's abdomen. Verifying the placement of the tocodynamometer is the first step in troubleshooting this issue. Stopping the oxytocin infusion, changing the mother's position, and assessing for signs of uterine hyperstimulation should be done after verifying the tocodynamometer placement.

Question 118:
Correct Answer: C) Review the patient's laboratory results, specifically renal function.
Rationale: Levofloxacin is primarily excreted through the kidneys, and patients with impaired renal function may require dosage adjustments. Therefore, it is essential for the nurse to review the patient's laboratory results, specifically renal function, to ensure safe administration of the medication and prevent adverse reactions.

Question 119:
Correct Answer: B) Fetal anemia
Rationale: A sinusoidal fetal heart rate pattern, accompanied by decreased fetal movements, is highly suggestive of fetal anemia. Fetal anemia can occur due to conditions such as isoimmunization (Rh incompatibility) or severe fetal hemorrhage. Gestational diabetes, preeclampsia, or fetal tachycardia would not typically present with a sinusoidal fetal heart rate pattern and decreased fetal movements.

Question 120:
Correct Answer: C) Expectant management with no specific interventions.
Rationale: First-degree AV block in a fetus is generally considered a benign finding, and expectant management with no specific interventions is typically recommended. Immediate medical termination of the pregnancy is not warranted for a first-degree AV block. Serial fetal echocardiography is not necessary as there is no evidence to suggest progression to a higher-degree block. Initiation of transplacental therapy with corticosteroids is not indicated in the management of first-degree AV block.

Question 121:
Correct Answer: B) Tachysystole is defined as more than two contractions in ten minutes.
Rationale: Tachysystole is defined as more than five contractions in ten minutes. It is an abnormal pattern in fetal heart rate and contraction frequency. Tachysystole can lead to decreased fetal heart rate variability and potential fetal compromise. It is important to monitor closely and intervene appropriately when tachysystole is identified to prevent adverse outcomes.

Question 122:
Correct Answer: B) Facilitate a change in maternal position.
Rationale: In the scenario presented, the nurse observes a FHR pattern suggestive of tachysystole, as the contractions occur more frequently than every 2 minutes. Tachysystole is often associated with decreased fetal oxygenation. The first intervention should be to facilitate a change in maternal position, such as moving the patient to the side or using a knee-chest position, to improve fetal oxygenation and alleviate the repetitive late decelerations. Tocolytic medications are not indicated unless other interventions have failed. Oxygen administration is not the priority in this case. An emergency cesarean delivery may be considered if nonreassuring fetal status persists despite implementing corrective measures.

Question 123:
Correct Answer: B) A deceleration lasting 30 seconds or longer.
Rationale: A prolonged deceleration pattern in fetal heart rate monitoring refers to a deceleration lasting 30 seconds or longer. This pattern may indicate possible fetal compromise and should be carefully evaluated by healthcare providers. It is important to differentiate prolonged decelerations from shorter decelerations that may not carry the same clinical significance. Close monitoring and appropriate interventions are necessary to ensure the well-being of the fetus.

Question 124:
Correct Answer: D) Maternal hyperoxygenation
Rationale: Maternal hyperoxygenation is a technique used to improve oxygen delivery to the fetus during labor. It involves the administration of high concentrations of oxygen to the mother. Maternal hyperoxygenation can improve oxygen transfer across the placenta and alleviate fetal hypoxemia. Therefore, it is not a cause of hypoxemia in the fetus but a potential intervention to address it.

Question 125:
Correct Answer: A) Autonomy
Rationale: The primary principle of medical ethics is autonomy, which refers to the respect for the patient's right to make decisions and choices about their own healthcare. Autonomy ensures that patients have the freedom to give informed consent or refuse treatment based on their values, beliefs, and preferences. This principle promotes patient empowerment and reinforces the importance of respecting their autonomy while considering medical interventions.

Question 126:
Correct Answer: D) All of the above
Rationale: Artifact in EFM can be caused by various factors such as maternal movement, fetal movement, and loose electrodes. Maternal movement, such as repositioning or walking, can result in signal interference on the monitor.

Fetal movement, including kicking or rolling, can also cause temporary disruption in the EFM tracings. Additionally, loose electrodes can lead to poor electrical contact, resulting in artifact. It is important to minimize these factors and ensure proper electrode placement to obtain accurate fetal monitoring tracings.

Question 127:
Correct Answer: A) Variable decelerations are caused by umbilical cord compression.
Rationale: Variable decelerations in the fetal heart rate are caused by umbilical cord compression. These decelerations are characterized by an abrupt decrease in FHR that varies in shape, duration, and depth. Unlike early decelerations, variable decelerations are not related to contractions. They can occur at any time during labor and are often associated with cord prolapse or cord compression. Immediate intervention, such as changing the mother's position or relieving cord compression, is necessary to ensure adequate oxygenation to the fetus.

Question 128:
Correct Answer: A) Maternal anemia
Rationale: Maternal anemia, characterized by low levels of red blood cells or hemoglobin, can result in decreased fetal oxygenation due to reduced blood volume. Anemia decreases the oxygen-carrying capacity of maternal blood, leading to fetal hypoxia. Conditions such as gestational diabetes and hypothyroidism do not directly contribute to reduced blood volume and, therefore, do not impair fetal oxygenation in the same manner as maternal anemia.

Question 129:
Correct Answer: C) Hypotonic uterine dysfunction
Rationale: Hypotonic uterine dysfunction is characterized by weak and prolonged uterine contractions. This can lead to ineffective cervical dilation and prolonged labor. Uterine tachysystole refers to excessive uterine contractions. Uterine hyperstimulation syndrome occurs when uterine contractions are too frequent or too strong. Hypertonic uterine dysfunction is characterized by increased resting tone between contractions.

Question 130:
Correct Answer: B) Placenta previa
Rationale: Placenta previa refers to the implantation of the placenta over or near the internal os of the cervix. It can cause painless, bright red vaginal bleeding. In cases of placenta previa, minimal variability may be seen in the fetal heart rate tracing due to the relative lack of oxygen perfusion from the compromised placenta. Placental abruption typically presents with painful bleeding. Uterine rupture would have more severe fetal heart rate changes. Placental insufficiency may cause variable decelerations rather than minimal variability.

Question 131:
Correct Answer: A) Non-stress test (NST)
Rationale: The non-stress test (NST) is the recommended fetal surveillance test for postdates pregnancy. It involves monitoring the baby's heart rate in response to its own movements. The NST is a non-invasive and reliable test that helps assess fetal well-being by evaluating the baby's heart rate patterns. A reactive NST, characterized by the presence of at least two accelerations in a 20-minute period, indicates a healthy, oxygenated fetus. In cases of non-reactive NST or abnormalities in the heart rate patterns, further tests such as a biophysical profile or Doppler velocimetry may be required.

Question 132:

Correct Answer: A) Supine position
Rationale: The supine position should be avoided to prevent cord compression. In this position, the weight of the gravid uterus can compress the inferior vena cava, reducing venous return and potentially compromising blood flow to the fetus. This can increase the risk of cord compression and fetal distress. Lateral position, semi-Fowler's position, and Trendelenburg position are commonly used to alleviate cord compression and improve blood flow to the fetus.

Question 133:
Correct Answer: C) Placenta previa
Rationale: Placenta previa, a condition in which the placenta implants in the lower uterine segment, is commonly associated with small-for-gestational-age fetuses. The abnormal placental implantation may lead to inadequate blood flow and nutrient exchange, resulting in fetal growth restriction. Placental abruption, uterine rupture, and placenta accreta may cause other complications but are not specifically associated with small-for-gestational-age fetuses.

Question 134:
Correct Answer: A) Decreased fetal heart rate variability
Rationale: Inhalation anesthetics can easily cross the placenta and affect the central nervous system of the fetus. The most common effect observed is a decrease in fetal heart rate variability. This decrease signifies fetal distress and is an important indicator of fetal well-being. Increased fetal movement, elevated fetal arterial oxygen saturation, and increased uterine blood flow are not expected effects of inhalation anesthetics.

Question 135:
Correct Answer: B) 50-60mmHg
Rationale: Normal uterine contractions usually have a peak intensity between 50-60mmHg. Contractions with a peak intensity of less than 25mmHg are classified as weak, while contractions with a peak intensity between 25-50mmHg are classified as moderate. Intensity greater than 150mmHg would be considered hyperstimulation.

Question 136:
Correct Answer: A) Prostaglandin E2 gel
Rationale: Prostaglandin E2 gel is the most appropriate method for cervical ripening in a postdates pregnancy. It is administered intracervically or intra-vaginally to soften and ripen the cervix before induction of labor. Cervical Foley catheter can also be used for cervical ripening by mechanical dilation. Oxytocin infusion is used for induction of labor once the cervix is favorable. Amniotomy is the artificial rupture of membranes and is not the most appropriate method for cervical ripening.

Question 137:
Correct Answer: C) Moderate variability
Rationale: Moderate variability in the baseline heart rate is considered normal in electronic fetal monitoring. It indicates a healthy autonomic nervous system and adequate oxygenation to the fetus. Absence or minimal variability may suggest fetal compromise, while marked variability may indicate fetal distress or umbilical cord compression.

Question 138:
Correct Answer: A) Uterine rupture
Rationale: The sudden increased pain, fetal distress, loss of contraction pattern, palpable fetal head above the symphysis pubis, and abdominal wall bulging are indicative of uterine rupture. In this scenario, the patient's previous low transverse cesarean scar likely dehisced leading to rupture

of the uterus. Immediate delivery via emergency cesarean section is necessary to prevent further complications.

Question 139:
Correct Answer: B) Prodromal labor
Rationale: Prodromal labor refers to a pattern of irregular contractions that may occur during the antepartum period. These contractions are typically not associated with cervical dilation and are often considered preparatory in nature. They are not considered true labor contractions and are commonly referred to as false labor or Braxton Hicks contractions. Contractions of labor are regular and progressive contractions that lead to cervical dilation and fetal descent. Hypertonic contractions are excessive, uncoordinated contractions that can impede cervical dilation, while hypotonic contractions are weak and ineffective contractions.

Question 140:
Correct Answer: D) Ensuring proper contact and alignment with the fetal heart
Rationale: To obtain accurate and reliable results during external fetal heart rate monitoring, it is essential to ensure proper contact and alignment between the transducer and the fetal heart. The transducer should be positioned on the mother's abdomen over the area where the fetal heart sounds are best heard. It is important to avoid placing the transducer over the umbilical cord, as this may interfere with the detection of the fetal heart rate. Additionally, excessive pressure should be avoided to prevent discomfort to the mother and potential interference with the transducer's functionality.

Question 141:
Correct Answer: C) Placental abruption
Rationale: Placental abruption is a potential cause of decreased blood flow to the fetus. It occurs when the placenta partially or completely separates from the uterine wall, interrupting the delivery of oxygen and nutrients to the fetus. Maternal hypertension and hyperglycemia may have separate effects on the fetus, but they do not directly impact blood flow. Fetal tachycardia is an increased heart rate but does not necessarily imply decreased blood flow.

Question 142:
Correct Answer: D) Rubella
Rationale: Rubella infection during pregnancy can cause serious congenital disabilities known as congenital rubella syndrome, which includes deafness, visual impairments, and heart abnormalities. It is crucial for women to be vaccinated against rubella before becoming pregnant to prevent these complications.

Question 143:
Correct Answer: A) Placenta previa
Rationale: Placenta previa is a condition in which the placenta partially or completely covers the opening of the cervix, leading to potential uteroplacental complications such as bleeding during pregnancy and increased risk of preterm birth. It is important to recognize placenta previa early in pregnancy to monitor and manage potential complications.

Question 144:
Correct Answer: C) Reposition the client
Rationale: In this scenario, the nurse identifies variable decelerations in the FHR tracing. Variable decelerations are often associated with cord compression. The most appropriate initial action for managing variable decelerations is to reposition the client. Changing the client's position can alleviate cord compression and subsequently resolve the variable decelerations. Reassessing the client's blood

pressure, administering oxygen via face mask, and preparing for a rapid delivery are not the first interventions for variable decelerations.

Question 145:
Correct Answer: C) 8 to 10 contractions in 10 minutes
Rationale: During active labor, the normal frequency of contractions should be between 8 to 10 contractions in a 10-minute period. This frequency indicates effective uterine activity to promote cervical dilation and fetal descent. Contractions that occur more frequently or less frequently may indicate abnormal uterine activity and should be assessed further. Monitoring the frequency of contractions helps identify patterns and enables appropriate interventions if necessary. It is important to monitor this aspect closely to ensure the progress of labor and the well-being of both the mother and the fetus.

Question 146:
Correct Answer: C) Internal monitoring devices are preferred for accurate assessment of uterine contractions in women with a history of previous cesarean delivery.
Rationale: Women with a history of previous cesarean delivery may require accurate assessment of uterine contractions during labor. Internal monitoring devices are preferred in this scenario as they provide more accurate measurement of uterine contractions. External monitoring devices may be influenced by the presence of scar tissue from the previous surgery, resulting in less accurate assessment. Internal monitoring allows for direct measurement of uterine contractions using a catheter inserted into the uterus, ensuring accurate assessment and appropriate management.

Question 147:
Correct Answer: C) Initiate continuous fetal monitoring
Rationale: Variable decelerations can be caused by umbilical cord compression. In this scenario, the appropriate intervention is to initiate continuous fetal monitoring to closely observe the fetal heart rate pattern for any further changes. Administering oxygen to the mother is indicated in cases of late decelerations, not variable decelerations. Performing a fetal scalp blood sample may be considered if further assessment of fetal well-being is needed. Performing an amniotomy is not indicated in this situation as it does not address the underlying cause of variable decelerations.

Question 148:
Correct Answer: C) Analgesics
Rationale: Analgesics, such as opioids, are commonly used for pain relief during labor. However, they can cross the placenta and cause respiratory depression in the fetus. This can lead to decreased oxygenation of the fetal tissues, posing a risk to the well-being of the baby.

Question 149:
Correct Answer: D) Absent Variability
Rationale: Absent variability is characterized by a flat line with no discernible variability and is a concerning finding. It indicates fetal hypoxia or acidemia and requires immediate intervention. Moderate variability is considered to be a reassuring pattern and is associated with a normal fetal acid-base balance. Marked variability is characterized by a sinusoidal pattern with a frequency of 2-5 cycles per minute, indicating a well-oxygenated and healthy fetus. Minimal variability suggests fetal compromise and should be further evaluated.

Question 150:

Correct Answer: B) Provide additional training and support to the healthcare providers who are struggling.
Rationale: When a quality issue arises due to healthcare providers struggling to use a new system, the most appropriate action is to provide additional training and support. It is essential to recognize that not all individuals adapt to change at the same pace. By offering further training, guidance, and support, healthcare providers can develop the necessary skills to effectively use the new EFM system. Punishment does not address the underlying issue and may discourage healthcare providers from seeking assistance or reporting difficulties. Reverting to the old paper-based monitoring method would negate the potential benefits of the new system and hinder progress in quality improvement.

Question 151:
Correct Answer: B) Systolic ? 140 mm Hg or diastolic ? 90 mm Hg
Rationale: The diagnostic threshold for gestational hypertension is a systolic blood pressure of ? 140 mm Hg or a diastolic blood pressure of ? 90 mm Hg on two or more occasions, at least 4 hours apart, after 20 weeks of gestation in a previously normotensive individual. It is crucial to diagnose gestational hypertension accurately to initiate appropriate management and monitor the health of both the mother and the fetus.

Question 152:
Correct Answer: C) 120 bpm
Rationale: Tachycardia in fetal monitoring is defined as a baseline heart rate greater than 120 bpm. A fetal heart rate below 110 bpm is considered bradycardia, while a baseline heart rate between 110-120 bpm is within the normal range. Tachycardia may indicate fetal distress or underlying medical conditions and requires further evaluation and intervention.

Question 153:
Correct Answer: B) 5 to 10 movements
Rationale: A normal range of fetal movements during a 60-minute period is typically considered to be between 5 to 10 movements. This indicates normal fetal activity and well-being. Fewer than 5 movements may indicate fetal distress, while more than 10 movements can also be normal. However, an excessive number of movements may warrant further evaluation to rule out potential issues. It is important for pregnant women to keep track of fetal movements as a decrease or change in movement pattern may indicate potential problems and should be reported to their healthcare provider.

Question 154:
Correct Answer: B) Oxytocin augmentation
Rationale: Oxytocin augmentation is recommended for a fetus with bradycardia that persists despite maternal repositioning. Oxytocin can stimulate uterine contractions, thereby improving fetal oxygenation. Amnioinfusion involves the infusion of sterile fluid into the amniotic cavity and is indicated for variable decelerations caused by cord compression. Fetal scalp stimulation can be performed to elicit a response from the fetus if the bradycardia is suspected to be due to fetal sleep or sedation. Epidural administration is not a specific intervention for managing bradycardia.

Question 155:
Correct Answer: C) 1 contraction every 90 seconds
Rationale: The frequency of contractions is determined by the time interval between the start of one contraction and the start of the next contraction. In this scenario, since each contraction lasts for 45 seconds, there is a 90-second interval between contractions, resulting in a frequency of 1 contraction every 90 seconds.

Question 156:
Correct Answer: C) Normal variation
Rationale: A fetal baseline heart rate above 160 bpm may indicate normal variation in fetal heart rate. This can occur during fetal movement or maternal activity. However, it is important to assess the overall pattern and consider other factors to ensure the well-being of the fetus.

Question 157:
Correct Answer: D) Cord compression
Rationale: Irregular baseline fluctuations on the monitor that are not related to uterine contractions may indicate cord compression. Cord compression can lead to transient changes in fetal heart rate due to impaired blood flow. The nurse should assess for other signs of cord compression, such as variable decelerations, and promptly intervene by repositioning the mother or relieving pressure on the cord. Fetal tachycardia, uterine rupture, or chorioamnionitis may have different characteristics on the fetal heart rate monitor.

Question 158:
Correct Answer: C) Variable decelerations
Rationale: Variable decelerations are a characteristic pattern associated with tachycardia in fetal monitoring. Variable decelerations are abrupt and visually apparent decreases in fetal heart rate below the baseline. They are typically caused by umbilical cord compression and can be associated with tachycardia. Monitoring and intervention are necessary to improve fetal well-being.

Question 159:
Correct Answer: B) Cardiac output
Rationale: Maternal smoking significantly affects cardiac output, leading to impaired oxygen delivery to the fetus. Smoking causes vasoconstriction and reduces blood flow to the placenta, resulting in decreased oxygen availability for fetal oxygenation. Nicotine and carbon monoxide from cigarette smoke contribute to increased heart rate and decreased stroke volume, leading to reduced cardiac output. It is crucial for healthcare providers to educate pregnant patients about the harms of smoking and encourage smoking cessation to optimize fetal oxygenation.

Question 160:
Correct Answer: B) Placental Abruption
Rationale: Placental abruption refers to the premature separation of the placenta from the uterine wall before delivery. It can present with sudden, painful vaginal bleeding, uterine tenderness, and signs of fetal distress. Risk factors include maternal hypertension, trauma, advanced maternal age, smoking, and cocaine use. Ultrasound may be used for diagnosis, but the clinical presentation is often sufficient. Management depends on the severity of the abruption and the gestational age of the fetus, ranging from observation to immediate delivery.

Question 161:
Correct Answer: B) Prepare the patient for immediate delivery via cesarean section
Rationale: In cases where preterm labor, ruptured membranes, and late decelerations are present, immediate delivery via cesarean section is the intervention of choice. This would improve fetal oxygenation and reduce the risk of fetal distress. Corticosteroids for fetal lung maturation should have been administered prior to this scenario. Magnesium sulfate for fetal neuroprotection is typically indicated in cases

of imminent preterm birth, but the presence of late decelerations warrants immediate delivery. Vaginal delivery with continuous fetal monitoring would not be appropriate in this situation due to the increased risk for fetal compromise.

Question 162:
Correct Answer: B) Formation of adhesions
Rationale: Previous cesarean sections can result in the formation of adhesions, which can make surgery and anesthesia more challenging. Adhesions may obscure the surgical field and increase the risk of injury to surrounding structures. Increased uterine blood flow, decreased risk of uterine rupture, and enhanced tolerance to anesthetic agents are not associated with previous cesarean sections and do not increase the risk of complications during anesthesia.

Question 163:
Correct Answer: B) False
Rationale: Fetal heart rate accelerations are not a reliable indicator of fetal acidemia. They are considered a reassuring sign of fetal well-being but cannot accurately assess fetal acid-base status. Other indicators, such as decelerations or the presence of a prolonged deceleration, may suggest acidemia. Fetal blood sampling or other diagnostic tests would be required to confirm the presence of acidemia.

Question 164:
Correct Answer: D) Abnormal
Rationale: An abnormal nonstress test is characterized by absent or minimal variability in the fetal heart rate, indicating poor oxygenation or fetal distress. In this scenario, Mrs. Wilson's test shows a fetal heart rate baseline of 120 bpm with absent variability, and no accelerations or decelerations are observed. These findings suggest an abnormal test result, requiring further evaluation.

Question 165:
Correct Answer: A) Obesity
Rationale: Obesity is a known risk factor for the development of gestational hypertension. It increases the risk of developing hypertension during pregnancy due to its association with insulin resistance, endothelial dysfunction, and inflammation. Nulliparity, young maternal age, and multiparity are not directly associated with an increased risk of gestational hypertension. However, it is important to consider these factors along with obesity and other medical conditions when assessing a patient's risk for hypertensive disorders in pregnancy.

Question 166:
Correct Answer: A) Immediate delivery
Rationale: The patient is presenting with symptoms of HELLP syndrome, including right upper quadrant pain, malaise, and elevated liver enzymes. Though her platelet count is normal, immediate delivery is the most appropriate management for this patient as HELLP syndrome can rapidly progress to life-threatening complications. Delivery is the definitive treatment and should be undertaken promptly, even if the fetus is premature.

Question 167:
Correct Answer: A) Magnesium sulfate
Rationale: Magnesium sulfate is not contraindicated but can be used to manage severe hypertension associated with preeclampsia. It acts as a central nervous system depressant and prevents seizures in women with severe preeclampsia or eclampsia. The other options mentioned, hydralazine, labetalol, and nifedipine, are also commonly used in the management of hypertension in pregnant women.

Question 168:
Correct Answer: D) Perform a Cesarean section
Rationale: Prolonged decelerations indicate a significant interruption in fetal oxygenation and may require immediate intervention. In this scenario, the appropriate action is to perform a Cesarean section to expedite the delivery and relieve the potential hypoxemia in the fetus. Administering oxygen to the mother may be considered, but it does not address the underlying cause of the prolonged decelerations. Performing a fetal scalp blood sample may provide additional information about fetal well-being, but immediate delivery is necessary if prolonged decelerations persist. Applying pressure to the fetal head is not indicated and may cause harm to the fetus.

Question 169:
Correct Answer: B) Perform a scalp stimulation test
Rationale: In the scenario described, the presence of prolonged decelerations on the EFM indicates potential fetal compromise. Prioritizing the assessment of the fetal well-being is crucial. Performing a scalp stimulation test involves applying pressure to the fetal scalp to elicit a reactive acceleration in the heart rate, confirming fetal well-being. Administering oxygen is generally reserved for nonreassuring patterns such as severe variable or late decelerations. Placing the patient in the Trendelenburg position is not indicated for prolonged decelerations. Initiating an IV infusion of oxytocin is contraindicated in the presence of nonreassuring fetal status and decelerations, as it may further compromise fetal oxygenation.

Question 170:
Correct Answer: C) Severe headaches
Rationale: Severe headaches are a common symptom of preeclampsia-eclampsia. Headaches may be persistent and not relieved by usual treatments. It is important to monitor for this symptom as it can be an early warning sign of worsening preeclampsia and impending eclampsia. Other symptoms may include high blood pressure, proteinuria, edema, blurred vision, and upper abdominal pain. Early recognition and management of preeclampsia are crucial to prevent complications for both the mother and the baby.

Question 171:
Correct Answer: A) Decreased cardiac output
Rationale: Spinal anesthesia can cause sympathetic blockade, leading to a decrease in systemic vascular resistance and venous return, ultimately resulting in decreased cardiac output. The effects on uterine blood flow, blood pressure, and respiratory rate are not significant with the administration of spinal anesthesia.

Question 172:
Correct Answer: C) Fetal growth rate
Rationale: Close monitoring of the fetal growth rate is crucial in cases of chronic (essential) hypertension during pregnancy. Hypertensive disorders can negatively affect the placenta and restrict the baby's growth. Regular ultrasound scans and measurements are used to assess fetal growth and ensure adequate nutrition and oxygen supply to the fetus. Fetal heart rate variability, fetal movement count, and fetal limb movements are important parameters but not specifically related to chronic hypertension monitoring.

Question 173:
Correct Answer: A) Administer a prophylactic dose of hepatitis B immune globulin (HBIG) and initiate hepatitis B vaccination to the newborn

Rationale: Pregnant women who test positive for HBsAg should be managed to prevent perinatal transmission of hepatitis B. Administration of both a prophylactic dose of HBIG and hepatitis B vaccination to the newborn significantly reduces the risk of transmission. Hepatitis B vaccination alone is not sufficient to prevent perinatal transmission. Delaying HBIG administration until after delivery increases the risk of transmission. Intervention is necessary for HBsAg-positive mothers to prevent transmission to the newborn.

Question 174:
Correct Answer: A) Fetal heart rate accelerations of 10 bpm for at least 10 seconds, occurring twice in a 20-minute period
Rationale: A reactive nonstress test (NST) is characterized by the presence of fetal heart rate accelerations of at least 10 bpm for at least 10 seconds, occurring twice in a 20-minute period. This indicates normal fetal well-being and is reassuring. Fetal heart rate decelerations, absence of accelerations, or a baseline variability less than 10 bpm are considered abnormal findings on NST and may require further evaluation.

Question 175:
Correct Answer: C) Insulin therapy initiation
Rationale: The management of gestational diabetes involves multiple interventions, including dietary modification, exercise, self-monitoring of blood glucose levels, and insulin therapy initiation when glycemic control is inadequate. Insulin therapy allows for better control of blood glucose levels and reduces the risks associated with uncontrolled gestational diabetes. Avoiding exercise, strict dietary restriction, and frequent fasting during the day are not recommended interventions for managing glucose levels during pregnancy.

Question 176:
Correct Answer: C) Late decelerations are often associated with umbilical cord compression and prolonged fetal hypoxia.
Rationale: Late decelerations occur as a result of impaired placental perfusion due to uteroplacental insufficiency. This can occur during periods of maternal hypotension, uterine hyperstimulation, or any condition that compromises blood flow to the placenta. Late decelerations are frequently observed with umbilical cord compression, leading to fetal hypoxia. Prompt intervention is necessary to prevent further fetal compromise and initiate appropriate management.

Question 177:
Correct Answer: A) Maternal movement
Rationale: Maternal movement, such as coughing or sneezing, can cause sudden, brief accelerations in the fetal heart rate tracing. These movements create temporary pressure changes within the abdomen, resulting in transient changes in fetal circulation. It is important to differentiate such artifacts from true fetal accelerations to avoid misleading interpretations and ensure accurate assessment of fetal well-being during electronic fetal monitoring.

Question 178:
Correct Answer: D) Uterine perforation
Rationale: Uterine perforation is the most common complication associated with the use of an Intrauterine Pressure Catheter (IUPC). It occurs when the catheter punctures or perforates the uterine wall. This complication can lead to uterine bleeding, infection, or damage to surrounding organs. Options A, B, and C are incorrect as they represent other complications that are not directly associated with the use of an IUPC.

Question 179:
Correct Answer: B) Fetal heart rate
Rationale: Fetal tachycardia, characterized by a persistent baseline heart rate above 160 bpm, increases the cardiac workload and oxygen demand of the fetus. This increased demand puts pressure on the umbilical blood flow, potentially compromising fetal oxygenation and nutrient supply. Therefore, an increased fetal heart rate places an additional burden on the umbilical blood flow, making it an important factor to consider in assessing fetal well-being.

Question 180:
Correct Answer: B) Interuterine pressure catheter
Rationale: IUPC stands for Intrauterine Pressure Catheter. It is a device used for monitoring the strength and frequency of uterine contractions during labor. It is inserted through the cervix into the uterus and measures the pressure changes within the uterine cavity. By accurately measuring uterine contractions, IUPC helps in assessing the progress of labor and determining the appropriate management strategies for the well-being of both the mother and the fetus. Options A, C, and D are incorrect as they do not correctly represent the abbreviation of IUPC.

Question 181:
Correct Answer: B) Late deceleration
Rationale: Late decelerations are defined as an abrupt and sustained decrease in fetal heart rate that occurs after the peak of the contraction. This pattern is often indicative of uteroplacental insufficiency, where there is inadequate oxygenation and perfusion to the fetus during contractions. Early decelerations are characterized by a gradual decrease and return to baseline, and they mirror the contractions. Variable decelerations are characterized by a sharp drop, variable in duration and depth, often associated with cord compression. Accelerations are transient increases in fetal heart rate.

Question 182:
Correct Answer: B) Chronic hypertension
Rationale: Chronic hypertension is commonly associated with late decelerations due to compromised uteroplacental perfusion. The elevated blood pressure can impair placental blood flow, resulting in fetal hypoxia and subsequent late decelerations on the fetal heart rate tracing. Gestational diabetes, placenta previa, and oligohydramnios may have other fetal heart rate patterns but are not directly linked to late decelerations.

Question 183:
Correct Answer: C) Placental insufficiency
Rationale: Chronic hypertension can lead to reduced blood flow through the uterine arteries, resulting in placental insufficiency. This condition impairs the placenta's ability to deliver adequate oxygen and nutrients to the fetus, potentially leading to fetal growth restriction, preterm birth, or stillbirth. Close monitoring of fetal well-being and timely intervention are crucial in managing pregnancies complicated by chronic hypertension.

Question 184:
Correct Answer: B) Fetal tone
Rationale: The biophysical profile assesses five parameters to evaluate fetal well-being. Fetal tone is one of these parameters and represents the presence or absence of limb or body movements. It is assessed by observing the flexion or extension of the fetal limbs on ultrasound. Fetal breathing movements, amniotic fluid volume, and the nonstress test are the other parameters considered in the biophysical

profile, but they do not directly measure fetal body movements. Fetal tone reflects the integrity of the central nervous system and is an essential component in assessing fetal health.

Question 185:
Correct Answer: B) Induction of labor
Rationale: The recommended management approach in cases of fetal demise is the induction of labor. This allows for the timely delivery of the fetus and the placenta, reducing the risk of maternal complications and enabling the parents to have closure. Immediate cesarean delivery may be considered in certain situations, such as a non-reassuring maternal condition or logistical limitations. Expectant management is not recommended in cases of fetal demise as the risks of infection and other complications increase with time. External cephalic version is a procedure performed to turn a breech fetus and is not relevant to the management of fetal demise.

Question 186:
Correct Answer: C) Accelerations
Rationale: Accelerations are transient increases in the FHR above the baseline, usually lasting less than 2 minutes. They are a reassuring sign and often indicate fetal well-being. In this scenario, the consistent accelerations of at least 15 beats per minute above the baseline FHR suggest a good fetal response and a normal pattern.

Question 187:
Correct Answer: C) Document the findings and continue to monitor the patient closely.
Rationale: The patient's EFM tracing shows a baseline fetal heart rate within a normal range, moderate variability, no accelerations, and no decelerations, indicating a reassuring fetal status. Therefore, it is important to document these findings and continue to closely monitor the patient, as there is no indication for immediate intervention or delivery.

Question 188:
Correct Answer: D) It is less convenient compared to internal uterine monitoring.
Rationale: While external uterine monitoring is a non-invasive technique, it is considered less convenient compared to internal uterine monitoring. External monitoring may not provide accurate information about the strength of contractions as it relies on external sensors placed on the maternal abdomen. Internal uterine monitoring, such as the intrauterine pressure catheter (IUPC), provides more precise measurements by directly measuring the pressure within the uterus. Fetal heart rate monitoring is typically performed separately using a fetal scalp electrode (FSE) or ultrasound.

Question 189:
Correct Answer: D) HELLP syndrome
Rationale: The patient is presenting with epigastric pain, nausea, vomiting, elevated blood pressure, and low platelet count. These symptoms are consistent with the diagnosis of HELLP syndrome. Although laboratory results indicate normal liver enzymes, it is essential to consider HELLP syndrome as a potential diagnosis due to its clinical presentation and associated complications.

Question 190:
Correct Answer: D) Multidisciplinary approach
Rationale: Managing maternal obesity during pregnancy requires a comprehensive and multidisciplinary approach. This includes combining various interventions such as nutritional counseling, exercise guidance, and behavioral therapy. A low-calorie diet alone or high-intensity aerobic

exercises may not be appropriate during pregnancy as they can pose risks to the developing fetus. Similarly, weight loss medications are generally contraindicated during pregnancy due to their potential adverse effects. A multidisciplinary approach involving healthcare providers such as obstetricians, dietitians, psychologists, and physical therapists ensures holistic care and improves maternal and fetal outcomes. This approach helps address the complex issues associated with obesity and provides tailored interventions and support throughout pregnancy.

Question 191:
Correct Answer: C) Report the incident to the nurse manager or supervisor
Rationale: Patient-centered care and maintaining professional conduct are vital in healthcare settings. Witnessing a colleague's unprofessional behavior should not be tolerated. The nurse should report the incident to the nurse manager or supervisor, providing accurate details of the situation. This action helps ensure proper follow-up, appropriate intervention, and corrective measures, which are necessary for maintaining a safe and professional environment for both patients and healthcare providers. By reporting the incident, the nurse contributes to upholding professional standards and maintaining patient trust.

Question 192:
Correct Answer: C) They usually last for at least 30 seconds.
Rationale: Fetal heart rate accelerations are brief increases in the fetal heart rate above the baseline and are considered a reassuring sign of fetal well-being. They are typically induced by fetal movement and can last for as short as 15 seconds. The duration of accelerations is usually not specified, but they do not necessarily need to last for at least 30 seconds.

Question 193:
Correct Answer: A) Cord compression
Rationale: The sudden deceleration in the fetal heart rate associated with the onset of maternal contractions, as well as the symmetric pattern with an onset to nadir time of 20 seconds and a recovery time of 30 seconds, is consistent with cord compression. Cord compression occurs when there is a mechanical obstruction or squeezing of the umbilical cord, leading to a temporary decrease in blood flow and oxygenation to the fetus. This can result in fetal heart rate decelerations. Other signs of cord compression may include a rapid onset of deceleration, a prolonged deceleration phase, and a rapid recovery phase. Fetal tachycardia, late decelerations, and variable decelerations are less likely in this scenario based on the given information.

Question 194:
Correct Answer: A) The baseline fetal heart rate is 120 bpm.
Rationale: A reassuring result in nonstress testing (NST) is obtained when the baseline fetal heart rate is within normal limits, typically between 110 and 160 bpm. A baseline variability of <5 bpm, absence of accelerations, or presence of decelerations would be considered abnormal findings.

Question 195:
Correct Answer: A) Fetal growth restriction
Rationale: Reduced placental perfusion can lead to inadequate nutrient and oxygen supply to the fetus, resulting in fetal growth restriction. This condition is characterized by a fetus that is smaller than expected for the gestational age. Close monitoring of fetal growth and interventions to

optimize placental perfusion are essential in managing this uteroplacental complication.

Question 196:
Correct Answer: A) Doppler ultrasound
Rationale: Doppler ultrasound is a commonly used imaging technique to assess blood flow to the fetus. It allows healthcare providers to evaluate the speed and direction of blood flow in various fetal vessels, providing important information about the adequacy of blood supply. Fetal blood sampling is performed to assess pH and oxygen levels and is not directly related to blood flow assessment. Fetal scalp stimulation test and electronic fetal heart rate monitoring are techniques used to evaluate fetal well-being but do not specifically assess blood flow.

Question 197:
Correct Answer: C) Equivocal
Rationale: An equivocal nonstress test is characterized by insufficient data to confirm a reactive or nonreactive result. In this scenario, Mrs. Davis's test shows a fetal heart rate baseline of 150 bpm with increased variability, indicating a good fetal oxygenation. However, the absence of accelerations or decelerations makes the interpretation equivocal, as further assessment may be needed.

Question 198:
Correct Answer: D) Change the patient's position
Rationale: In the scenario described, the presence of prolonged decelerations during labor warrants immediate intervention to improve fetal well-being. Changing the patient's position, such as turning from the supine to a lateral position, can help relieve compression on the umbilical cord and improve fetal oxygenation. Administering tocolytic medications is not indicated for prolonged decelerations. Performing an amnioinfusion involves infusing sterile fluid into the amniotic cavity to alleviate variable decelerations, not prolonged decelerations. Increasing the rate of IV fluids may be appropriate for certain situations but is not the primary intervention for prolonged decelerations.

Question 199:
Correct Answer: A) Administer intravenous ampicillin and continue prophylactic antibiotics until delivery
Rationale: In the setting of PPROM and GBS colonization, the most appropriate management is to administer intravenous ampicillin and continue prophylactic antibiotics until delivery. This is done to prevent neonatal early-onset GBS infection. Vancomycin is not typically used for prophylaxis but can be considered for patients allergic to beta-lactam antibiotics. Cefazolin is not recommended for GBS prophylaxis. Delaying prophylactic antibiotics until the onset of labor increases the risk of neonatal infection.

Question 200:
Correct Answer: A) Cephalohematoma
Rationale: Cephalohematoma is the injury characterized by the presence of scalp swelling due to the accumulation of blood beneath the periosteum. It occurs as a result of trauma during delivery, causing rupture of blood vessels in the scalp. Cephalohematoma is usually confined to a specific cranial bone and does not cross suture lines. Although it does not pose an immediate threat to the infant's well-being, close monitoring for potential complications such as jaundice is essential.

Question 201:
Correct Answer: D) All of the above
Rationale: When differentiating between true FHR patterns and artifacts, several factors can be considered. Increased baseline variability is a desirable characteristic of a valid FHR pattern and can help distinguish it from artifact-induced fluctuations. Consistent accelerations are often observed in response to fetal movement and can also indicate the presence of a true FHR pattern. Furthermore, the absence of uterine contractions during the period of irregularities can further support the presence of artifact rather than a true FHR pattern.

Question 202:
Correct Answer: A) Immediate induction of labor
Rationale: Severe preeclampsia is a serious condition that poses risks to both the mother and fetus. Delivery is the definitive management for severe preeclampsia at or beyond 34 weeks of gestation. Immediate induction of labor is the most appropriate option in this scenario. Administering corticosteroids for fetal lung maturity can be considered if the gestational age is less than 34 weeks. Close monitoring of blood pressure and fetal well-being should be done during the management, but delivery is necessary. Performing an emergency cesarean delivery is not indicated in this case.

Question 203:
Correct Answer: A) Group B Streptococcus
Rationale: Group B Streptococcus (GBS) is the leading cause of neonatal sepsis. It can be transmitted to the fetus during delivery and can cause serious infections, including pneumonia, meningitis, and sepsis. Pregnant women are typically screened for GBS colonization in the third trimester, and if positive, they receive intrapartum antibiotic prophylaxis to reduce the risk of transmission.

Question 204:
Correct Answer: B) Document and communicate your concerns to the appropriate supervisor or authority.
Rationale: In this situation, it is crucial to advocate for the safety and well-being of the patient and her baby. If the obstetrician dismisses your concerns and decides not to intervene, it is important to take appropriate action by documenting the concerns and communicating them to the appropriate supervisor or authority. This ensures that the patient's case is reviewed by someone with the authority to intervene and make decisions based on the best interest of the patient and her baby.

Question 205:
Correct Answer: D) None of the above
Rationale: Gestational diabetes is associated with pregnancy, while type 1 and type 2 diabetes can occur at any age. Type 1 diabetes is usually diagnosed in childhood or early adulthood and is an autoimmune disease. Type 2 diabetes, on the other hand, is often associated with lifestyle factors and usually develops in adulthood. It is important to differentiate between the types of diabetes as each requires different management strategies and monitoring.

Question 206:
Correct Answer: B) Change the mother's position.
Rationale: Early decelerations are considered benign and do not require any specific intervention. However, changing the mother's position, such as turning her to her side or elevating her legs, can help alleviate any potential compression on the fetal head and improve blood flow to the fetus. This simple intervention can often resolve the early decelerations and ensure adequate fetal oxygenation. Administering oxygen or performing a fetal scalp stimulation is not necessary for managing early decelerations as they do not indicate fetal distress.

Question 207:

Correct Answer: D) Hyperbilirubinemia
Rationale: Selective serotonin reuptake inhibitors (SSRIs) are commonly used to treat depressive disorders during pregnancy. These medications have been associated with an increased risk of neonatal complications, including jitteriness, irritability, and poor neonatal adaptation. One of the common complications is hyperbilirubinemia or an increase in the levels of bilirubin in the newborn's blood. This can occur due to delayed clearance of bilirubin from the liver, leading to jaundice.

Question 208:
Correct Answer: D) Intensity is a measure of the strength or power of contractions.
Rationale: Intensity is a measure of the strength or power of uterine contractions. It refers to how strong the contractions are and is typically measured in Montvield Units (MU). Intensity is assessed using an intrauterine pressure catheter (IUPC) or external tocodynamometer. It is independent of the frequency, duration, or distance between contractions. Monitoring the intensity is crucial in managing labor, as it helps in determining the progress of contractions, evaluating the effectiveness of interventions, and ensuring optimal fetal well-being.

Question 209:
Correct Answer: D) Both A and B
Rationale: The Society for Maternal-Fetal Medicine (SMFM) and the Association of Women's Health, Obstetric and Neonatal Nurses (AWHONN) are professional organizations that provide resources and guidelines for continuing education in EFM. They offer conferences, workshops, online courses, and publications to help healthcare providers stay updated with the latest evidence-based practices in fetal monitoring. The National Association of Neonatal Nurses (NANN) and the American Academy of Pediatrics (AAP) focus more on neonatal care rather than EFM education.

Question 210:
Correct Answer: B) It provides continuous fetal heart rate monitoring.
Rationale: One advantage of external uterine monitoring is that it is often used in combination with continuous fetal heart rate monitoring. This allows for the simultaneous monitoring of both uterine contractions and fetal heart rate without the need for invasive procedures. However, external monitoring may be affected by maternal movement and may not provide direct measurement of intrauterine pressure, which is possible with internal monitoring using an intrauterine pressure catheter (IUPC).

Question 211:
Correct Answer: A) Sinusoidal pattern is characterized by a regular, smooth, and continuous waveform with a baseline resembling a sine wave.
Rationale: Sinusoidal pattern is characterized by a regular, smooth, and continuous waveform with a baseline resembling a sine wave. It is an abnormal fetal heart rate pattern that is associated with fetal distress and requires immediate intervention. The pattern often indicates severe fetal anemia or other conditions that impair oxygen delivery to the fetus. It is important to recognize the sinusoidal pattern and take appropriate actions, such as performing a complete maternal-fetal evaluation and considering prompt delivery if necessary.

Question 212:
Correct Answer: C) It bypasses the liver sinusoids, allowing oxygenated blood to enter the fetal systemic circulation.

Rationale: The ductus venosus bypasses the liver sinusoids, allowing oxygenated blood from the umbilical vein to enter the fetal systemic circulation. It connects the umbilical vein with the inferior vena cava, ensuring that well-oxygenated blood flows directly to the fetal heart and brain. This bypass is essential as the fetal liver's metabolic functions are relatively immature, and it avoids any potential interference with oxygen delivery to vital organs.

Question 213:
Correct Answer: A) Expectant management
Rationale: With a closed, firm, and posterior cervix at term, expectant management is the most appropriate initial approach. Many women with postdates pregnancies will go into spontaneous labor if given time. Prostaglandin cervical ripening and oxytocin induction of labor are interventions used when expectant management fails. A membrane sweep is a procedure that can be performed as part of expectant management to stimulate labor, but it is not the most appropriate initial management option in this scenario.

Question 214:
Correct Answer: A) Administering oxygen to the mother
Rationale: In the presence of tachycardia in fetal monitoring, administering oxygen to the mother is an appropriate intervention. Oxygen therapy helps improve oxygenation to the fetus and may alleviate the underlying cause of tachycardia, such as fetal hypoxia. Other interventions such as performing a scalp stimulation test, increasing intravenous fluids, or applying a fetal scalp electrode may be considered based on the specific clinical situation and healthcare provider's assessment.

Question 215:
Correct Answer: B) Placenta
Rationale: During pregnancy, the placenta acts as the primary source of oxygen supply to the fetus. The placenta is a specialized organ that develops in the uterus during pregnancy and facilitates the exchange of oxygen, nutrients, and waste products between the mother and the fetus. The umbilical cord connects the fetus to the placenta, providing a pathway for the exchange of these substances. The lungs of the fetus do not play a significant role in oxygenation until birth, as they are filled with amniotic fluid during intrauterine life. The liver is involved in various metabolic processes but is not the primary source of oxygen supply to the fetus.

Question 216:
Correct Answer: C) Lack of standardized medication labeling and packaging.
Rationale: One of the primary factors contributing to medication errors related to wrong dosage administration is the lack of standardized medication labeling and packaging. Inconsistent or confusing labeling can lead to misunderstanding, resulting in incorrect dosages being administered. Implementing clear and standardized labeling and packaging systems is crucial in reducing medication errors. Adequate staffing and workload distribution, implementation of double-check systems, and efficient medication reconciliation processes are important strategies to improve patient safety and quality of care but may not directly address the specific issue of wrong dosage administration caused by labeling and packaging inconsistencies.

Question 217:
Correct Answer: C) A drop in heart rate lasting more than 2 minutes

Rationale: A prolonged deceleration in fetal heart rate is defined as a drop in heart rate lasting more than 2 minutes but less than 10 minutes. It is an abnormal finding that may indicate fetal hypoxia or asphyxia. The duration of a prolonged deceleration sets it apart from other types of decelerations. A drop in heart rate lasting less than 30 seconds would be classified as an early deceleration.

Question 218:
Correct Answer: A) Prepare the patient for immediate cesarean delivery
Rationale: The clinical presentation of Mrs. Thompson with vaginal bleeding, abdominal pain, uterine tenderness, and abnormal EFM tracing (absent variability and late decelerations) suggests placental abruption. Placental abruption is a severe maternal complication that requires immediate intervention to prevent further harm to both the mother and the fetus. Immediate cesarean delivery is the most appropriate action to ensure the best outcome for both patients.

Question 219:
Correct Answer: D) Maintaining continuous fetal monitoring for further assessment
Rationale: In a situation where uterine activity is minimal and there are concerns about fetal well-being, maintaining continuous fetal monitoring for further assessment is the most appropriate intervention. Administering oxytocin to stimulate uterine contractions may not be necessary if the fetal heart rate is reassuring. Placing the patient in the lithotomy position or encouraging ambulation does not directly address the concern of decreased uterine activity. Continuous fetal monitoring allows for ongoing evaluation of the fetal heart rate and uterine activity, ensuring timely intervention if needed.

Question 220:
Correct Answer: D) Late decelerations during contractions
Rationale: During an NST, the presence of late decelerations during contractions is considered abnormal and indicative of fetal compromise. Late decelerations suggest decreased uteroplacental circulation, which can be concerning in the setting of gestational diabetes. Absence of fetal movements is also abnormal and requires further evaluation. Two accelerations in 20 minutes and a baseline heart rate of 150 bpm are within normal limits for a non-stress test.

Question 221:
Correct Answer: A) Non-stress test
Rationale: The non-stress test is the most appropriate method to assess fetal well-being in a postdates pregnancy. It involves monitoring fetal heart rate in response to fetal movement. This test is non-invasive and has a high sensitivity and specificity for identifying fetal compromise. Biophysical profile is another option for assessing fetal well-being and includes additional parameters such as fetal breathing, fetal movement, fetal tone, amniotic fluid volume, and reactive non-stress test. However, in this case, the non-stress test is the most appropriate initial monitoring technique.

Question 222:
Correct Answer: B) Variable deceleration
Rationale: Variable decelerations are abrupt and transient decreases in the fetal heart rate from the baseline. They can be caused by umbilical cord compression, which may occur during contractions or spontaneously, leading to an irregular pattern.

Question 223:
Correct Answer: D) All of the above
Rationale: Quality improvement in healthcare involves identifying problems and errors, assessing current processes and outcomes, and implementing evidence-based practices to enhance patient care and outcomes. By identifying problems and errors, healthcare professionals can address areas for improvement and prevent future occurrences. Assessing current processes and outcomes allows for the identification of areas that require enhancement or modification. Implementing evidence-based practices ensures that healthcare interventions are based on research and best practices, resulting in improved patient outcomes. Therefore, all of the options mentioned are essential components of quality improvement in healthcare.

Question 224:
Correct Answer: A) Twin-to-twin transfusion syndrome
Rationale: The triangle sign, or the ? sign, is a characteristic finding in twin-to-twin transfusion syndrome (TTTS). TTTS is a serious condition that can occur in monochorionic twin pregnancies, where there is an imbalance in blood flow between the twins through the shared placenta. The ? sign represents the intertwin membrane separating the amniotic sacs and is an important indicator for the diagnosis of TTTS. Early detection and appropriate management are crucial to improve outcomes in TTTS cases.

Question 225:
Correct Answer: B) Absence of P waves on the electrocardiogram (ECG)
Rationale: Supraventricular tachycardia (SVT) in a fetus is characterized by the absence of P waves on the electrocardiogram (ECG). This is due to the fast, abnormal electrical activity originating above the ventricles, resulting in a rapid heart rate. The absence of P waves suggests that the electrical signals bypass the normal conduction pathway. Other features may include irregular or poorly defined QRS complexes on the ECG, a heart rate usually over 200 bpm, and occurrence during both fetal sleep and awake periods.

Question 226:
Correct Answer: C) Serial fetal echocardiography to assess for further progression of the AV block.
Rationale: In cases of fetal congenital heart block, serial fetal echocardiography is essential to assess for further progression of the AV block and any associated structural abnormalities. Termination of pregnancy is not recommended for all cases of congenital heart block, especially if the block is not complete or severe. Initiating dexamethasone is not indicated in the management of congenital heart block. Expectant management with close monitoring is appropriate, but serial fetal echocardiography is necessary to detect any changes in the fetal heart rate and cardiac function.

Question 227:
Correct Answer: D) All of the above
Rationale: Maternal factors such as a previous cesarean section, multiple gestation (e.g., twins or triplets), and intrauterine growth restriction (IUGR) can increase the risk of uterine rupture during labor. A previous cesarean section scar weakens the uterine wall, making it more prone to rupture. Multiple gestation pregnancies stretch the uterus excessively, increasing the risk of rupture. In cases of IUGR, the weakened uterine wall may not be able to handle the stress of labor, leading to uterine rupture. Identification of these risk factors is crucial in determining the appropriate

management and delivery plan for ensuring both maternal and fetal well-being.

Question 228:
Correct Answer: A) Non-stress test (NST) twice weekly
Rationale: After 32 weeks gestation, close monitoring of twin pregnancies is necessary to assess fetal well-being. One recommended intervention is the non-stress test (NST) performed twice weekly. NST involves monitoring the fetal heart rate and uterine contractions to evaluate the baby's response to movement. This test helps to ensure that both babies are receiving enough oxygen and nutrients and that there are no signs of distress. Biophysical profile (BPP) is another form of fetal assessment but is typically done once weekly. Ultrasound examination every 4 weeks can provide important information on fetal growth and amniotic fluid levels but may not be sufficient for precise fetal monitoring. Fetal fibronectin (fFN) testing every 2 weeks is more commonly used for predicting the likelihood of preterm labor rather than monitoring fetal well-being.

Question 229:
Correct Answer: B) Intrauterine growth restriction (IUGR)
Rationale: Intrauterine growth restriction is a condition in which the fetus fails to reach its growth potential, resulting in a smaller size and reduced placental blood flow. This can have a direct impact on fetal oxygen supply, potentially leading to hypoxia and fetal distress. Gestational diabetes, preterm labor, and polyhydramnios can all have implications for fetal oxygenation but do not directly impair placental blood flow.

Question 230:
Correct Answer: D) Prepare for an emergency cesarean delivery
Rationale: Prolonged decelerations lasting more than two minutes are indicative of severe fetal compromise and hypoxia. Immediate intervention is necessary to prevent fetal harm. Preparing for an emergency cesarean delivery is the priority action in this situation, as it provides a quick delivery method to improve fetal outcomes. The other interventions may be implemented in conjunction with this action but are not the priority.

Question 231:
Correct Answer: A) Severe abdominal pain
Rationale: The most common symptom of uterine rupture/scar dehiscence is severe abdominal pain. This pain is often described as sudden and sharp and may be accompanied by a tearing sensation. Other signs and symptoms may include vaginal bleeding, fetal distress, and maternal hypotension, but severe abdominal pain is the hallmark symptom.

Question 232:
Correct Answer: C) Administer oxygen via a face mask
Rationale: Late decelerations are a sign of uteroplacental insufficiency and decreased fetal blood flow. Administering oxygen via a face mask can help improve oxygenation and increase blood flow to the uterus, thereby reducing the occurrence of late decelerations. This intervention can help improve fetal well-being and prevent further compromise during labor.

Question 233:
Correct Answer: C) Fetal hydrops
Rationale: Fetal hydrops is a possible complication of supraventricular tachycardia (SVT) in a fetus. SVT can cause severe and sustained rapid heart rates, leading to increased cardiac workload and compromised cardiac function. This can result in fluid accumulation in various fetal tissues, leading to edema and hydrops. Other complications of SVT may include fetal distress, decreased fetal movement, and abnormal fetal growth. Ventricular septal defect, hypoglycemia, and umbilical cord prolapse are not directly associated with SVT.

Question 234:
Correct Answer: C) It is an abnormal finding requiring further evaluation.
Rationale: A baseline variability of less than 5 bpm is considered absent or minimal. This can indicate fetal hypoxemia or acidemia. It is an abnormal finding that requires further evaluation and intervention, as it suggests compromised fetal well-being.

Question 235:
Correct Answer: A) Preeclampsia
Rationale: Chronic (essential) hypertension during pregnancy can increase the risk of developing preeclampsia, a condition characterized by high blood pressure and damage to organs such as the liver and kidneys. Preeclampsia can have serious complications for both the mother and the baby. Gestational diabetes, ectopic pregnancy, and preterm labor are not directly associated with chronic hypertension during pregnancy.

Question 236:
Correct Answer: B) Provides continuous and accurate measurement
Rationale: Internal uterine monitoring, which involves the use of an intrauterine pressure catheter, provides more accurate and continuous measurement of uterine contractions compared to external monitoring methods. The intrauterine pressure catheter is placed inside the uterus and directly measures the pressure changes during contractions. This allows healthcare professionals to have a more precise assessment of uterine activity and better identify any abnormal patterns. Although external monitoring, such as the toco transducer, is noninvasive and allows mobility during labor, it may not provide the same level of accuracy and consistency as internal monitoring.

Question 237:
Correct Answer: A) Anti-Ro (SSA) antibodies
Rationale: Anti-Ro (SSA) antibodies are strongly associated with congenital heart block in infants of mothers with SLE. These antibodies can cross the placenta and cause inflammation and fibrosis of the conducting system in the developing fetus. Anti-La (SSB) antibodies are also associated with certain cardiac manifestations in infants of mothers with SLE but are less strongly associated with heart block. Anti-double-stranded DNA antibodies and Anti-Smith antibodies are not specifically associated with congenital heart block in infants of mothers with SLE.

Question 238:
Correct Answer: B) Placenta previa
Rationale: Placenta previa occurs when the placenta implants low in the uterus, partially or completely covering the cervix. This abnormal implantation can lead to bleeding during pregnancy and delivery, increasing the risk of fetal hypoxia. Placental abruption refers to premature separation of the placenta, while placental calcification and insufficiency are related to the functional capacity of the placenta but not its implantation site.

Question 239:
Correct Answer: B) Pulmonary hypertension

Rationale: Pulmonary hypertension is a potential long-term complication of congenital heart block. The altered fetal circulatory patterns associated with the condition can lead to increased vascular resistance in the pulmonary artery, resulting in pulmonary hypertension. Neonatal jaundice, gastroschisis, and anencephaly are not directly related to congenital heart block.

Question 240:
Correct Answer: D) Improving fetal oxygenation
Rationale: The primary goal of managing hypertonus during labor is to improve fetal oxygenation. Hypertonus can restrict blood flow to the placenta, leading to fetal hypoxia and distress. By managing hypertonus and reducing uterine contractions, fetal oxygenation can be improved. Restoring normal fetal heart rate patterns is important, but it is not the primary goal of managing hypertonus. Reducing the risk of postpartum hemorrhage and promoting active labor progression are not direct goals of managing hypertonus.

Question 241:
Correct Answer: C) 2 contractions every 60 seconds
Rationale: The frequency of contractions is determined by the time interval between the start of one contraction and the start of the next contraction. In this scenario, since each contraction lasts for 60 seconds and there are two contractions within that time frame, the frequency is 2 contractions every 60 seconds.

Question 242:
Correct Answer: C) Contractions lasting 40-60 seconds with a frequency of 2-3 every 10 minutes.
Rationale: The normal uterine contraction pattern during labor involves contractions lasting 40-60 seconds with a frequency of 2-3 every 10 minutes. Contractions should have a regular pattern and increase in intensity as labor progresses. Contractions lasting less than 20 seconds and with a frequency of 1 every 5 minutes are too infrequent to be considered normal. Contractions lasting more than 60 seconds and with a frequency of 4 every 20 minutes are too long in duration and too infrequent. Contractions lasting more than 80 seconds and with a frequency of 1 every 15 minutes are also abnormal.

Question 243:
Correct Answer: B) Hypotonic uterus
Rationale: A resting uterine tone of 0 mmHg indicates a hypotonic uterus, which suggests inadequate uterine activity. Normal resting tone ranges between 5-20 mmHg. In this scenario, the absence of any uterine tone implies reduced uterine contractions, which may necessitate further evaluation and intervention.

Question 244:
Correct Answer: D) Fetal acidemia
Rationale: Fetal acidemia is a fetal complication that is characterized by an abnormal pH value in the fetal blood. It indicates an imbalance in acid-base status, with a pH below the normal range. Fetal acidemia can be associated with conditions such as fetal hypoxia, asphyxia, or metabolic disturbances. Close surveillance and appropriate intervention are necessary to identify and address the underlying cause of fetal acidemia, as it can have significant implications for the fetal well-being and long-term outcomes.

Question 245:
Correct Answer: D) Inadequate gel application
Rationale: Inadequate gel application between the transducer and the skin can lead to signal ambiguity, resulting in intermittent signal loss on both the tocodynamometer and the fetal heart rate tracing. It is essential for the nurse to ensure sufficient gel is applied to provide good conductivity and optimize the signal transmission between the transducer and the skin. This will help minimize signal ambiguities and maintain an accurate fetal monitoring.

Question 246:
Correct Answer: A) It refers to the frequency, duration, and intensity of contractions.
Rationale: Uterine activity refers to the frequency, duration, and intensity of contractions. It is an important factor that affects fetal oxygenation and determines the progress of labor. The frequency of contractions is the time between the beginning of one contraction and the beginning of the next. The duration is the length of time a contraction lasts, and the intensity is the strength of the contraction. Monitoring uterine activity helps assess the adequacy of fetal oxygenation and progression of labor. Maternal heart rate does not directly influence uterine activity, and it plays a significant role in cervical dilation.

Question 247:
Correct Answer: D) Maternal body mass index (BMI)
Rationale: Maternal factors such as body mass index (BMI) can influence fetal movement perception. Women with a higher BMI may have a harder time perceiving fetal movements due to the additional layers of adipose tissue. This can make it difficult to distinguish between fetal movements and other sensations. Maternal age, previous pregnancies, and gestational age do not directly impact the perception of fetal movement.

Question 248:
Correct Answer: B) Perform a biophysical profile evaluation
Rationale: In the scenario described, the presence of prolonged decelerations during induction of labor warrants further assessment of the fetal well-being. Performing a biophysical profile evaluation involves assessing multiple parameters, including fetal heart rate, fetal breathing movements, gross body movements, fetal tone, and amniotic fluid volume. This evaluation provides a comprehensive assessment of fetal well-being. Administering terbutaline is not indicated for prolonged decelerations. Preparing the patient for an emergency cesarean section would be premature without further assessment. Placing the patient in a knee-to-chest position is unlikely to resolve the prolonged decelerations.

Question 249:
Correct Answer: D) Category IV
Rationale: In Category IV, there is absent baseline variability with any of the following: recurrent late decelerations, recurrent variable decelerations, or bradycardia. The provided EFM tracing shows a baseline rate of 135 bpm, normal variability of 10 bpm, and recurrent late decelerations. This corresponds to Category IV, indicating an abnormal tracing associated with fetal hypoxemia.

Question 250:
Correct Answer: A) Twin-to-twin transfusion syndrome
Rationale: Monochorionic twin pregnancies have a higher risk of developing complications compared to dichorionic twin pregnancies. One of the most common complications seen in monochorionic twins is twin-to-twin transfusion syndrome (TTTS), where blood flow between the twins is imbalanced, leading to one twin receiving too much blood and the other receiving too little. This can result in various

complications for both twins, such as growth abnormalities, heart failure, and even death. Twin reversed arterial perfusion sequence (TRAP), preterm premature rupture of membranes (PPROM), and gestational hypertension are complications that can occur in both monochorionic and dichorionic twin pregnancies, but their frequency may vary.

Question 251:
Correct Answer: A) Headache
Rationale: Headache is a common clinical manifestation of hypertensive disorders in pregnancy. It is often described as persistent and severe, and it may be accompanied by visual disturbances. Vaginal bleeding, excessive fetal movement, and palpitations are not typically associated with hypertensive disorders in pregnancy. It is important to recognize and monitor the symptoms of hypertension in order to provide appropriate management and prevent complications.

Question 252:
Correct Answer: B) Perform an emergency cesarean section
Rationale: In the case of fetal hypoxemia and acidemia during suspected preterm labor, the most appropriate intervention to improve fetal oxygenation is to perform an emergency cesarean section. This allows for prompt delivery, reducing the duration of compromised oxygenation. Tocolytic medication may temporarily halt contractions, but it does not address the underlying cause of fetal distress. Administering corticosteroids for fetal lung maturity is essential in preterm labor but does not directly address the fetal hypoxemia. Oxygen administration to the mother can benefit fetal oxygenation to some extent but is not the most appropriate immediate intervention in this scenario.

Question 253:
Correct Answer: A) The frequency and intensity increase gradually over time.
Rationale: In a normal labor pattern, uterine contractions generally progress by increasing in frequency and intensity over time. This progression helps with cervical effacement and dilation, promoting the progress of labor. The duration of contractions may remain relatively stable or slightly increase toward the end of labor. The intensity of contractions may also remain constant or increase as labor advances. The pattern of contractions plays a crucial role in achieving effective uterine activity during labor and ensuring optimal fetal oxygenation.

Question 254:
Correct Answer: A) Flowchart
Rationale: A flowchart is a visual representation of a process, allowing healthcare professionals to understand the sequence of steps and identify potential areas for improvement. It helps in analyzing existing processes by visually mapping out the steps, decision points, and interactions involved. By using a flowchart, healthcare providers can identify bottlenecks, redundancies, and inefficiencies in the process, leading to potential improvements. Flowcharts are commonly used in quality improvement initiatives to enhance process understanding and streamline healthcare delivery.

Question 255:
Correct Answer: B) Maternal tachycardia
Rationale: Selective beta-2 agonists stimulate beta-2 receptors, resulting in bronchodilation. However, these medications can cross the placenta and affect the maternal cardiovascular system. Maternal tachycardia is a common side effect, which may decrease uterine blood flow and compromise fetal oxygenation. The increase in heart rate can lead to decreased perfusion and efficiency of oxygen delivery to the fetus, negatively impacting fetal heart rate variability.

Question 256:
Correct Answer: C) Terbutaline
Rationale: Tachysystole is defined as more than 5 contractions in a 10-minute period, averaged over a 30-minute window. When conservative measures fail to correct tachysystole, a tocolytic agent can be administered to decrease uterine activity. Among the options provided, terbutaline is commonly used for this purpose. Oxytocin is a uterotonic medication used to induce or augment labor and is not appropriate for managing tachysystole. Nifedipine is a calcium channel blocker used as a tocolytic, but its use for tachysystole is not as common. Methylergonovine is used to prevent or treat postpartum hemorrhage.

Question 257:
Correct Answer: A) Bed rest
Rationale: Bed rest is no longer recommended as an intervention for the management of gestational hypertension. Instead, regular monitoring of blood pressure, administration of antihypertensive medications if necessary, and induction of labor at term or earlier if indicated are the preferred approaches. Bed rest has not been shown to improve outcomes and may lead to other complications such as deep vein thrombosis and muscle atrophy. It is important for healthcare providers to stay up-to-date with the current guidelines to provide optimal care to individuals with gestational hypertension.

Question 258:
Correct Answer: C) Spinal cord injury
Rationale: Spinal cord injury is associated with damage to the spinal cord, resulting in motor and sensory deficits. This type of injury can occur during a difficult delivery, particularly when excessive force is applied to the fetal neck or back. Spinal cord injury can lead to long-term neurological impairments and may require specialized medical and rehabilitative interventions.

Question 259:
Correct Answer: B) The chorionic villi are responsible for oxygen and carbon dioxide exchange in the placenta.
Rationale: The chorionic villi are finger-like projections present in the placenta. They contain fetal blood vessels and are responsible for oxygen and carbon dioxide exchange between the maternal and fetal circulations. Oxygenated blood flows from the placenta to the fetus through the umbilical vein, not vice versa. The uterine artery carries oxygenated blood to the placenta, and the intervillous space contains oxygenated maternal blood. Therefore, the correct answer is B) The chorionic villi are responsible for oxygen and carbon dioxide exchange in the placenta.

Question 260:
Correct Answer: A) Obtain a fetal heart rate tracing
Rationale: Contractions that are lasting for 90 seconds and occurring every 2 minutes indicate a hyperstimulation of contractions. This may compromise fetal well-being, and thus, obtaining a fetal heart rate tracing will help assess the fetal response to these contractions. Administering tocolytic medications is not necessary in this situation. Preparing for a cesarean section or encouraging pushing would be premature actions without knowing the fetal well-being.

Question 261:
Correct Answer: D) Late decelerations during labor

Rationale: Late decelerations during labor are considered a non-reassuring fetal heart rate pattern. They indicate inadequate placental perfusion and fetal hypoxia. Immediate action should be taken to address the underlying cause and improve fetal oxygenation. Variability of 1-5 beats per minute is within the normal range, accelerations are a reassuring sign, and early decelerations are benign and mirror the contractions.

Question 262:
Correct Answer: B) Order a biophysical profile (BPP) to assess fetal well-being.
Rationale: Decreased fetal movements in the later stages of pregnancy can be a cause for concern. While the fetal heart rate is within normal limits, the healthcare provider should further assess fetal well-being to ensure the baby is not in distress. A biophysical profile (BPP) is a comprehensive assessment that includes fetal heart rate monitoring, fetal movement assessment, amniotic fluid volume assessment, and fetal breathing movements. By ordering a BPP, the healthcare provider can gather more information about the overall well-being of the fetus and make appropriate decisions regarding further management.

Question 263:
Correct Answer: D) Uterine contractions
Rationale: Repetitive late decelerations on fetal heart rate monitoring indicate compromised umbilical blood flow and potential placental insufficiency. Uterine contractions that occur close together or are too frequent may reduce the time for intervillous space reperfusion and compromise placental blood flow. This impairs the exchange of oxygen and nutrients between the mother and fetus, leading to persistent hypoxemia and late decelerations. Hence, uterine contractions play a crucial role in determining the adequacy of umbilical blood flow.

Question 264:
Correct Answer: D) All of the above.
Rationale: When documenting electronic fetal monitoring (EFM) findings, it is essential to ensure the accuracy of the recorded data. Accurate documentation provides a comprehensive record of the fetal heart rate patterns and associated events during labor. Including the interpretation of the EFM tracings is crucial as it demonstrates the healthcare professional's assessment and decision-making process. Timely notification of abnormal findings to the healthcare team allows for prompt interventions if necessary. Therefore, all the options mentioned in the Question are essential when documenting EFM findings in a legal context.

Question 265:
Correct Answer: C) Maternal infection
Rationale: Maternal infections, such as chorioamnionitis, can cause an increase in the fetal heart rate due to the release of inflammatory mediators. The fever in the mother is indicative of an infection, which can be transmitted to the fetus. Fetal distress may cause tachycardia, but it would typically be associated with other signs such as decelerations. Maternal dehydration and uteroplacental insufficiency are less likely to cause a sustained increase in the fetal heart rate.

Question 266:
Correct Answer: A) Administer oxygen to the mother
Rationale: In this scenario, the fetal heart rate of 80 bpm indicates severe bradycardia. Administering oxygen to the mother can increase oxygenation to the fetus, thereby potentially improving the fetal heart rate. Close monitoring should continue, and further interventions may be necessary based on the response to oxygen administration.

Question 267:
Correct Answer: B) Perform an amnioinfusion
Rationale: The severe variable decelerations lasting more than 60 seconds, associated with a slow return to baseline and unresponsive to maternal oxygenation, are suggestive of umbilical cord compression. In this situation, performing an amnioinfusion would be the most appropriate next step as it can help relieve cord compression by increasing the volume of amniotic fluid. Administering terbutaline, preparing for immediate operative vaginal delivery, or preparing for immediate cesarean delivery would not address the underlying cause of the decelerations.

Question 268:
Correct Answer: C) Placement of a transducer on the mother's abdomen
Rationale: External fetal heart rate monitoring is a non-invasive technique that involves placing a transducer on the mother's abdomen to detect and record the fetal heart rate. This method allows for continuous monitoring of the fetal heart rate during labor and delivery without requiring any invasive procedures or electrode insertion. The transducer is usually held in place with an elastic belt to ensure proper contact and accurate monitoring. This technique is commonly used in clinical practice due to its effectiveness and ease of use.

Question 269:
Correct Answer: A) Ultrasound
Rationale: Ultrasound is commonly used as a diagnostic tool to confirm uterine rupture/scar dehiscence. It can help visualize the presence of free fluid in the abdominal cavity or the extension of the uterine rupture. Fetal heart rate monitoring is important for assessing fetal well-being but may not directly confirm uterine rupture. Magnetic resonance imaging (MRI) and maternal blood tests are not typically used for the diagnosis of uterine rupture/scar dehiscence.

Question 270:
Correct Answer: C) Standard of care
Rationale: The legal principle that governs the use of electronic fetal monitoring (EFM) in healthcare is the standard of care. The standard of care refers to the level of care and skill that a healthcare professional should provide, based on the accepted practices and guidelines within their particular field. In the case of EFM, healthcare professionals are expected to provide care that adheres to the established standards of fetal monitoring during labor and childbirth. Deviating from the standard of care may result in legal implications, such as allegations of medical negligence or malpractice.

Question 271:
Correct Answer: C) Document the finding and continue monitoring the fetal heart rate.
Rationale: The priority nursing intervention when ectopic beats are noted on the fetal heart rate strip during labor is to document the finding and continue monitoring the fetal heart rate. Ectopic beats are usually benign and self-resolving. Administering oxygen or increasing fluid administration is not indicated in this situation.

Question 272:
Correct Answer: B) Propofol
Rationale: Among the given options, propofol is considered the safest anesthesia agent during pregnancy. It has a short duration of action and rapid recovery time, minimizing the

risk to the fetus. Sevoflurane and nitrous oxide should be used with caution due to potential negative effects on fetal oxygenation. Ketamine may cause uterine hypertonicity and should be used judiciously, especially during labor.

Question 273:
Correct Answer: B) Placental infarction
Rationale: Placental infarction refers to the ischemic necrosis of an area of the placenta caused by insufficient blood flow. This can compromise the oxygenation of the fetus and lead to prolonged decelerations in the fetal heart rate tracing. Decreased intervillous space is not associated with prolonged decelerations. Placental previa and placental abruption can result in acute fetal heart rate changes but are not typically associated with prolonged decelerations.

Question 274:
Correct Answer: A) Decreased oxygen content in the blood
Rationale: Hypoxemia is a condition characterized by a decreased level of oxygen in the blood. It can occur due to various reasons such as impaired oxygen delivery, decreased oxygen availability, or increased oxygen demand. Hypoxemia can lead to fetal hypoxia, which is associated with fetal distress and potential long-term complications. Monitoring oxygen levels in the blood is crucial in assessing fetal well-being and determining appropriate interventions to optimize oxygen delivery.

Question 275:
Correct Answer: A) Clear goals and objectives
Rationale: Successful quality improvement initiatives require clear goals and objectives to guide the improvement process. Clear goals provide a direction for the initiative and help in measuring progress and success. Inadequate data collection hinders the ability to track improvement and make informed decisions. Stakeholder involvement is crucial for a successful quality improvement initiative as it ensures diverse perspectives and engages all key players. A reactive approach to problem-solving may lead to temporary fixes instead of sustainable improvements. Therefore, clear goals and objectives are an essential characteristic of a successful quality improvement initiative.

Question 276:
Correct Answer: B) Uterine contractions intensity
Rationale: External fetal monitoring allows the assessment of uterine contractions intensity by measuring the pressure changes on the maternal abdomen. It provides information about the frequency, duration, and strength of contractions. Fetal heart rate variability is an assessment of the variation between fetal heartbeats and is typically evaluated using internal fetal monitoring methods. Fetal scalp pH is obtained through an invasive procedure and is used to assess fetal well-being during labor. Fetal oxygen saturation is not directly measured using external fetal monitoring.

Question 277:
Correct Answer: D) All of the above
Rationale: The fetal baseline heart rate can be influenced by various factors. Maternal age, fetal position, and maternal emotions can all impact the baseline heart rate. It is important to consider these factors when interpreting fetal heart rate patterns and making clinical decisions during labor.

Question 278:
Correct Answer: B) 120-160 bpm
Rationale: The normal range for fetal baseline heart rate is 120-160 beats per minute (bpm). This range indicates a healthy and stable heart rate for the fetus. It is important to monitor the baseline heart rate throughout labor to assess the well-being of the fetus.

Question 279:
Correct Answer: A) Normal uterine activity
Rationale: A contraction duration of 45-50 seconds during labor indicates normal uterine activity. This duration falls within the typical range for contractions during the active phase of labor. Inadequate contractions may have shorter durations, while tachysystole refers to excessively frequent contractions.

Question 280:
Correct Answer: B) 30 seconds to 2 minutes.
Rationale: Early decelerations usually have a duration ranging from 30 seconds to 2 minutes. These decelerations generally coincide with the contraction and recover before or shortly after its peak. The transient nature and short duration of early decelerations indicate that they are related to the fetal head compression rather than a prolonged period of compromised fetal oxygenation. It is essential to differentiate the duration of early decelerations from other deceleration patterns as it helps in determining the appropriate management and intervention for fetal well-being.

Question 281:
Correct Answer: C) Administration of oxytocin.
Rationale: Various factors can affect uterine activity. Maternal hydration level is important for maintaining uteroplacental blood flow but does not directly influence uterine contractions. Fetal position can affect the progress of labor but does not directly influence uterine activity. Administration of oxytocin, a synthetic form of the hormone that stimulates uterine contractions, can significantly affect uterine activity. Maternal age does not directly impact uterine activity.

Question 282:
Correct Answer: A) Category II
Rationale: In Category II, the baseline rate is 110-160 bpm, variability may be decreased (<6 bpm) or normal (6-25 bpm), and either the presence of minimal or absent variability with no recurrent decelerations or tachycardia. The provided EFM tracing shows a baseline rate of 135 bpm, decreased variability of 2 bpm, and the presence of early decelerations. This corresponds to Category II.

Question 283:
Correct Answer: C) Fetal atrial flutter
Rationale: The fetal heart rate pattern described in this scenario is consistent with fetal atrial flutter. Fetal atrial flutter is characterized by a rapid and regular heart rate with sudden accelerations and decelerations. The baseline fetal heart rate is often normal. It is important to assess other fetal parameters and consider further evaluation and management to ensure the well-being of the fetus.

Question 284:
Correct Answer: B) Calcium channel blockers
Rationale: Calcium channel blockers are commonly used for the management of chronic (essential) hypertension during pregnancy. They help relax the blood vessels and lower blood pressure. Angiotensin-converting enzyme (ACE) inhibitors and nonsteroidal anti-inflammatory drugs (NSAIDs) are contraindicated during pregnancy as they can cause harm to the developing fetus. Diuretics may be used in certain cases, but calcium channel blockers are generally preferred.

Question 285:
Correct Answer: A) Administering oxygen to the mother
Rationale: Administering oxygen to the mother helps to improve oxygenation and perfusion to the fetus. This intervention can enhance oxygen transfer across the placenta, potentially alleviating fetal distress caused by late decelerations. Terbutaline is used to decrease uterine contractions, and its administration would not directly address the underlying cause of late decelerations. Performing a vaginal examination or applying fundal pressure during contractions may further compromise the fetal well-being and is contraindicated in the presence of late decelerations.

Question 286:
Correct Answer: C) Place the mother in a side-lying position
Rationale: Late decelerations are caused by uteroplacental insufficiency and can be improved by optimizing maternal blood flow to the placenta. Placing the mother in a side-lying position helps reduce pressure on the vena cava, improves blood flow, and promotes fetal oxygenation. Increasing the rate of oxytocin infusion may worsen the fetal hypoxemia. Administering a tocolytic medication is not indicated as it is used to delay preterm labor. Administering a fluid bolus is also not indicated in this situation.

Question 287:
Correct Answer: A) Maternal smoking
Rationale: Maternal smoking can contribute to reduced fetal oxygenation by impairing placental blood flow. Smoking leads to vasoconstriction of the maternal vessels, including those in the uteroplacental circulation. This vasoconstriction can decrease blood flow to the placenta, resulting in decreased oxygen supply to the fetus. Maternal diabetes, anxiety, and hypothyroidism can also affect fetal oxygenation, but they do not primarily impair placental blood flow.

Question 288:
Correct Answer: B) The foramen ovale connects the right and left ventricles of the fetal heart
Rationale: During fetal development, the foramen ovale is an opening between the right and left atria of the heart. This allows oxygenated blood from the placenta to bypass the developing lungs and enter the left atrium, which is then pumped to the rest of the fetal body. The ductus arteriosus, not the umbilical vein, connects the pulmonary artery to the aorta, allowing most of the blood from the right ventricle to bypass the lungs. The umbilical arteries carry deoxygenated blood from the fetus to the placenta.

Question 289:
Correct Answer: A) A baseline variability of 8-10 bpm is within the normal range.
Rationale: Baseline variability reflects the fluctuations in the fetal heart rate. A baseline variability of 8-10 bpm is considered normal. It indicates a healthy autonomic nervous system and normal oxygenation to the fetus. This variability is associated with a favorable fetal outcome and does not require immediate intervention.

Question 290:
Correct Answer: D) Normal fetal heart rate pattern
Rationale: An irregular pattern with frequent accelerations on the fetal heart rate tracing is considered a normal finding during external fetal monitoring. It indicates a healthy, responsive fetus with a normal autonomic nervous system.

Fetal distress, fetal tachycardia, and fetal arrhythmia would present with different patterns on the fetal heart rate tracing.

Question 291:
Correct Answer: B) Loose connection
Rationale: The most common cause of electronic fetal monitor failure in clinical settings is a loose connection. This can occur due to frequent movement and handling of the equipment, leading to disconnection of wires and sensors. It is important to ensure that all connections are secure to achieve accurate monitoring and prevent the loss of crucial fetal data. Regular inspection and proper handling of the equipment can minimize the occurrence of loose connections and optimize the reliability of electronic fetal monitoring systems.

Question 292:
Correct Answer: B) To assess fetal heart rate response to contractions
Rationale: Fetal acoustic stimulation is performed during a contraction stress test (CST) to assess the fetal heart rate response to contractions. This test is performed by applying a sound stimulus to the mother's abdomen, which triggers contractions. The response of the fetal heart rate to these contractions is monitored to evaluate fetal well-being. Fetal heart rate response to contractions provides valuable information about the fetal oxygenation and the presence of fetal distress. Other parameters evaluated during the CST include the presence of uterine contractions, amniotic fluid index, and fetal heart rate variability.

Question 293:
Correct Answer: B) It is not influenced by maternal factors.
Rationale: One of the advantages of auscultation as a fetal assessment method is that it is not influenced by maternal factors. Unlike certain technologies used for fetal monitoring, such as ultrasound or electronic fetal monitoring, auscultation relies solely on listening to fetal heart sounds with a stethoscope. This method allows healthcare providers to directly assess the baby's heart rate and rhythm without being affected by maternal factors such as obesity or excessive movement. The simplicity and accessibility of auscultation make it a valuable tool in fetal assessment, particularly in resource-limited settings.

Question 294:
Correct Answer: D) All of the above
Rationale: The resting tone during electronic fetal monitoring can be influenced by various factors. Fetal heart rate patterns, such as accelerations or decelerations, can affect the resting tone. Maternal position can also have an impact on uterine activity and resting tone. Certain positions, such as lateral tilt or supine position, can modify the resting tone. Additionally, the presence and intensity of uterine contractions can significantly alter the resting tone. Monitoring and assessing these factors are essential for understanding the uterine activity pattern and ensuring optimal fetal well-being.

Question 295:
Correct Answer: B) 120-160 beats per minute.
Rationale: During auscultation, the normal fetal heart rate range is 120-160 beats per minute. This range is considered normal and indicates a healthy fetal heart. Deviations from this range could be indicative of fetal distress or other complications. Healthcare providers carefully listen to the fetal heart sounds and observe any changes in heart rate patterns, which can provide valuable information about the baby's well-being. Regular auscultation of fetal heart sounds

is an essential component of antenatal care and helps monitor the baby's health throughout pregnancy.

Question 296:
Correct Answer: B) Perform a cord blood gas analysis
Rationale: Variable decelerations in the fetal heart rate can be a sign of cord compression and decreased blood flow to the fetus. Perform a cord blood gas analysis to assess fetal acid-base status and determine the need for further intervention. This test provides objective information about fetal well-being and can guide management decisions during labor.

Question 297:
Correct Answer: A) Two separate placentas and two amniotic sacs
Rationale: In a dichorionic-diamniotic twin pregnancy, each twin has its own placenta and amniotic sac. This is the most common type of twin pregnancy and is considered low-risk. It is important to differentiate between the different types of twin pregnancies as management and monitoring may vary based on the chorionicity and amnionicity of the pregnancy.

Question 298:
Correct Answer: D) HELLP syndrome
Rationale: Chronic essential hypertension during pregnancy is commonly associated with maternal complications such as HELLP syndrome. HELLP syndrome is characterized by hemolysis, elevated liver enzymes, and low platelet count and can lead to severe liver dysfunction and clotting abnormalities. Gestational diabetes is typically associated with maternal obesity and impaired glucose metabolism, not chronic hypertension. Preterm labor can occur in any pregnancy but is not specific to chronic hypertension. Placenta previa, a condition where the placenta covers the cervix, is not directly linked to chronic hypertension but can coexist in some cases.

Question 299:
Correct Answer: B) Report the incident to the unit manager or supervisor
Rationale: Privacy and confidentiality are crucial aspects of professional practice. Overhearing a conversation discussing a patient's medical condition without proper authorization violates the patient's privacy rights. The nurse should report the incident to the unit manager or supervisor, who can address the issue and reinforce the importance of maintaining patient confidentiality. Reporting such incidents helps maintain a culture of professionalism and patient privacy within the healthcare setting.

Question 300:
Correct Answer: A) Foramen ovale
Rationale: A congenital heart defect involving the atria would impact the foramen ovale. The foramen ovale is the opening between the right and left atria of the fetal heart that allows blood to bypass the non-functional fetal lungs. If there is an abnormality in the development or closure of the foramen ovale, it can lead to mixing of oxygenated and deoxygenated blood. Options B, C, and D are incorrect as they are not directly involved in the atrial defect.

Question 301:
Correct Answer: C) Prolonged decelerations
Rationale: Prolonged decelerations, characterized by a slow decline in the fetal heart rate lasting more than 2 minutes, are a common presenting sign of fetal demise during labor. Absence of fetal movements, meconium-stained amniotic fluid, and foul-smelling vaginal discharge may also occur in cases of fetal demise, but prolonged

decelerations are typically the most prominent and concerning finding.

Question 302:
Correct Answer: D) Hyperstimulation
Rationale: A resting uterine tone of 35 mmHg indicates hyperstimulation of the uterus. Normal resting tone ranges between 5-20 mmHg. In this scenario, the high resting tone value suggests excessive uterine contractions, which may lead to uteroplacental insufficiency and fetal distress if not appropriately managed.

Question 303:
Correct Answer: B) Electronic fetal monitoring using a handheld Doppler device
Rationale: The commonly used method for external fetal monitoring during a non-stress test is electronic fetal monitoring using a handheld Doppler device. This method allows the healthcare provider to assess the fetal heart rate by listening to the Doppler sound waves reflected from the fetal heart. It is a non-invasive and safe method that can be easily performed in the outpatient setting. Invasive monitoring with a fetal scalp electrode is usually reserved for high-risk situations or when external monitoring is inadequate. Real-time ultrasound monitoring is used for assessing fetal anatomy and growth, not specifically for monitoring fetal heart rate. Monitoring uterine contractions is done using a tocometer, which measures the frequency and intensity of contractions, but not the fetal heart rate.

Question 304:
Correct Answer: D) Reposition the patient onto her hands and knees
Rationale: Variable decelerations are often caused by umbilical cord compression. Repositioning the patient onto her hands and knees (all fours position) helps to relieve pressure on the umbilical cord and improve fetal oxygenation. This intervention should be implemented to alleviate the variable decelerations and prevent fetal compromise.

Question 305:
Correct Answer: D) Fetal head compression during labor
Rationale: Fetal head compression during labor can cause transient decelerations in the fetal heart rate but is unlikely to cause variability. Variability is primarily influenced by fetal well-being, oxygenation, and autonomic nervous system control.

Question 306:
Correct Answer: C) Sudden increase in heart rate
Rationale: Accelerations in fetal heart rate are characterized by a sudden increase in heart rate, usually reaching a peak of at least 15 beats per minute above the baseline. They are considered a reassuring sign and are often associated with fetal movement. Accelerations have a sudden onset and offset, differ from decelerations, and are not related to uterine contractions or variable durations.

Question 307:
Correct Answer: B) Reattach the FHR transducer to the mother's abdomen
Rationale: The first step in troubleshooting a flat line on the FHR tracing is to ensure that the transducer is properly attached to the mother's abdomen. A loose or detached transducer can lead to loss of signal and a flat line on the tracing. Checking the maternal vital signs and position, determining the correct mode, and assessing the mother for

distress are important steps but should be done after ensuring proper attachment of the transducer.

Question 308:
Correct Answer: A) Preeclampsia
Rationale: Mrs. Johnson's elevated blood pressure, along with the presence of headaches and swelling, are indicative of preeclampsia. Preeclampsia is a pregnancy-specific syndrome characterized by hypertension, proteinuria, and edema. It typically develops after 20 weeks gestation in previously normotensive women. In contrast, gestational hypertension refers to new-onset hypertension without proteinuria after 20 weeks gestation. Chronic hypertension refers to pre-existing hypertension before pregnancy or diagnosed before 20 weeks gestation. Essential hypertension is a term used for primary hypertension unrelated to pregnancy.

Question 309:
Correct Answer: A) Moderate Variability
Rationale: Moderate variability is characterized by a variance of 5-25 beats per minute and is considered a reassuring finding. It indicates a normal fetal acid-base balance and is associated with a well-oxygenated fetus. Absent variability is a concerning finding and suggests fetal hypoxia or acidemia. Marked variability is characterized by a sinusoidal pattern with a frequency of 2-5 cycles per minute, indicating a well-oxygenated and healthy fetus. Minimal variability suggests fetal compromise and should be further evaluated.

Question 310:
Correct Answer: C) Accelerated fetal heart rate
Rationale: Accelerated fetal heart rate is not a typical characteristic of fetal dysrhythmias. Fetal dysrhythmias are characterized by irregular fetal heart rate patterns, prolonged decelerations, and absence of beat-to-beat variability. Accelerations, on the other hand, are transient increases in the fetal heart rate and are considered reassuring signs of fetal well-being. Therefore, option C is the correct answer.

Question 311:
Correct Answer: B) Order a non-stress test (NST) to assess fetal well-being.
Rationale: Decreased fetal movements can be a sign of fetal distress. While the fetal heart rate is within normal limits, further assessment is warranted to ensure fetal well-being. A non-stress test (NST) is a common method used to evaluate fetal well-being by assessing fetal heart rate patterns in response to fetal movement. It is a non-invasive test that can provide valuable information about the oxygenation and overall health of the fetus. By ordering an NST, the healthcare provider can gather more information and make a more informed decision regarding further management.

Question 312:
Correct Answer: D) Perform a nonstress test to assess fetal well-being.
Rationale: Ectopic beats in the fetus can be a transient finding and do not always indicate fetal distress. The appropriate nursing action in this situation would be to perform a nonstress test to assess fetal well-being. This test involves monitoring the fetal heart rate and maternal contractions over a designated period to evaluate the fetus's response to movement.

Question 313:
Correct Answer: A) Induction of labor
Rationale: An amniotic fluid index less than 5 cm is considered low and may indicate fetal compromise in postdates pregnancy. In this scenario, induction of labor is the most appropriate management option. Induction of labor helps to prevent further complications associated with postdates pregnancy. Repeat biophysical profile in 24 hours may further confirm the need for induction. Cesarean section is not indicated based on the amniotic fluid index alone. Observation with daily fetal movement counts is not sufficient management for a low amniotic fluid index in postdates pregnancy.

Question 314:
Correct Answer: A) Fetal scalp stimulation
Rationale: Fetal scalp stimulation is a commonly recommended intervention for persistent fetal dysrhythmias. It involves gently applying pressure to the fetal scalp during a vaginal examination to elicit a response from the fetus. This stimulation can help evaluate the fetal heart rate response and determine the need for further intervention or monitoring. The other options listed are not specifically indicated for the management of fetal dysrhythmias.

Question 315:
Correct Answer: C) Consult the user manual
Rationale: When facing issues with electronic fetal monitoring equipment, consulting the user manual is a recommended troubleshooting step. The user manual provides information on how to operate, maintain, and troubleshoot the equipment. It contains valuable guidelines specific to the monitor, enabling users to identify and resolve common problems. By referring to the user manual, healthcare professionals can determine if the issue can be resolved independently or if further assistance is required.

Question 316:
Correct Answer: C) Metabolic acidosis
Rationale: A pH of 7.1 indicates acidemia, which suggests an acid-base imbalance. In this scenario, the low pH is indicative of metabolic acidosis in the newborn. Metabolic acidosis may occur in the setting of decreased placental perfusion or other causes leading to hypoxia and lactic acidosis.

Question 317:
Correct Answer: D) Vasa previa
Rationale: This patient's painless vaginal bleeding, non-tender uterus, fundus at the xiphoid level, and reassuring fetal heart rate pattern are suggestive of vasa previa. Vasa previa is a rare condition in which fetal blood vessels, unsupported by Wharton's jelly or the umbilical cord, traverse the cervical os. It can lead to painless vaginal bleeding due to vessel rupture, especially when the membranes rupture or during labor. Fetal compromise is a major concern in vasa previa, as rapid fetal exsanguination can occur if vessels are disrupted. Immediate intervention is warranted, with a cesarean delivery considered the optimal management.

Question 318:
Correct Answer: C) Less than 100 beats per minute
Rationale: Bradycardia during labor is defined as a fetal heart rate below 100 beats per minute. This condition requires immediate intervention and assessment to ensure the well-being of the fetus. Fetal bradycardia can indicate fetal distress and may be caused by factors such as umbilical cord compression, placental insufficiency, or maternal hypotension. Prompt identification and appropriate management of bradycardia are crucial to prevent adverse outcomes for the fetus.

Question 319:
Correct Answer: B) Inability to detect contractions accurately
Rationale: One potential limitation of external fetal heart rate monitoring is the inability to accurately detect uterine contractions. While the transducer placed on the mother's abdomen can monitor the fetal heart rate effectively, it may not provide accurate information about the intensity and frequency of contractions. This limitation can be addressed by combining external fetal heart rate monitoring with other methods, such as palpation or internal monitoring, to accurately assess the strength and pattern of uterine contractions during labor.

Question 320:
Correct Answer: B) Fetal hypoxemia
Rationale: The absence of variability in the fetal heart rate is concerning and is most commonly associated with fetal hypoxemia. Fetal hypoxemia can occur due to various reasons, such as placental insufficiency or umbilical cord compression. In this scenario, the absence of variability indicates an abnormal fetal heart rate pattern and a potential compromise in fetal oxygenation.

Question 321:
Correct Answer: C) Marked Variability
Rationale: Marked variability is characterized by a sinusoidal pattern with a frequency of 2-5 cycles per minute, indicating a well-oxygenated and healthy fetus. It is considered a normal finding and is associated with fetal well-being. Moderate variability is considered to be a reassuring pattern and is associated with a normal fetal acid-base balance. Minimal variability suggests fetal compromise and should be further evaluated. Absent variability is a concerning finding and indicates fetal hypoxia or acidemia.

Question 322:
Correct Answer: C) Weak
Rationale: Intensity of uterine contractions is measured in mmHg using an intrauterine pressure catheter (IUPC). Mild contractions have a peak intensity of less than 25mmHg. This intensity is considered weak. Moderate contractions have a peak intensity between 25-50mmHg, while strong contractions have a peak intensity above 50mmHg. Hyperstimulation refers to excessive uterine contractions, usually induced by administration of oxytocin or prostaglandins.

Question 323:
Correct Answer: A) Hypertonic uterine dysfunction
Rationale: In hypertonic uterine dysfunction, the resting tone between contractions is elevated, resulting in inadequate relaxation of the uterine muscle. This can lead to decreased perfusion of the placenta and fetal distress. Hypotonic uterine dysfunction is characterized by weak and ineffective contractions. Uterine tachysystole refers to excessive uterine contractions. Uterine hyperstimulation syndrome occurs when uterine contractions are too frequent or too strong, often as a result of medication administration.

Question 324:
Correct Answer: B) Begin tocolytic therapy with indomethacin
Rationale: Tocolytic therapy, such as indomethacin, is initiated to suppress contractions and delay preterm labor. This allows time for corticosteroid administration (such as betamethasone) to enhance fetal lung maturity. Magnesium sulfate is used for neuroprotection in cases of imminent preterm birth. Immediate cesarean section is not indicated at

this time unless there are other obstetric or fetal complications present.

Question 325:
Correct Answer: A) Braxton Hicks contractions
Rationale: The irregular, non-progressive contractions with a closed cervix are consistent with Braxton Hicks contractions. Braxton Hicks contractions are considered "practice contractions" and do not lead to cervical changes or preterm labor. Preterm labor contractions would lead to cervical changes. Dehydration can contribute to the intensity of contractions but would not cause irregular and non-progressive contractions. False labor contractions may be regular but do not lead to cervical changes.

Question 326:
Correct Answer: D) Monitor closely and repeat blood pressure measurements
Rationale: In this scenario, Mrs. Rodriguez has a history of chronic hypertension and her blood pressure is only significantly elevated on two consecutive occasions. Since she is asymptomatic, the initial step would be to monitor her closely and repeat blood pressure measurements. A single elevated blood pressure reading does not warrant immediate induction of labor or changing the antihypertensive medication regime. Increasing the dose of her current antihypertensive medication is not indicated unless her blood pressure remains persistently elevated.

Question 327:
Correct Answer: D) Severe metabolic acidosis
Rationale: A base deficit of -8 mmol/L indicates metabolic acidosis in the newborn. A more negative base deficit value indicates a more severe metabolic acidosis. This value suggests significant tissue hypoperfusion and acidemia, which may be associated with poor fetal oxygenation and potential adverse outcomes.

Question 328:
Correct Answer: D) Supraventricular tachycardia
Rationale: Supraventricular tachycardia (SVT) is the most likely diagnosis in this case. SVT is characterized by a regular fetal heart rate between 180-220 beats per minute. The maternal heart rate is usually normal. SVT can be confirmed by careful evaluation of other fetal heart rate characteristics such as absence of beat-to-beat variability and lack of response to fetal stimulation. Further evaluation and management should be initiated to assess the severity and potential risks associated with SVT in the fetus.

Question 329:
Correct Answer: C) Human Chorionic Gonadotropin (hCG)
Rationale: Human Chorionic Gonadotropin (hCG) is secreted by the developing placenta and plays a crucial role in initiating uteroplacental circulation. It stimulates the production of estrogen and progesterone, which further sustain pregnancy. The increase in hCG levels promotes the development of the maternal spiral arteries and uterine blood flow, thereby promoting the establishment of an effective uteroplacental circulation to meet the metabolic demands of the growing fetus.

Question 330:
Correct Answer: B) Placental abruption
Rationale: Mrs. Johnson's sudden onset abdominal pain, dark vaginal bleeding, uterine tenderness, and rigid abdomen, along with fetal heart rate monitoring showing late decelerations, are suggestive of placental abruption. Placental abruption is the premature separation of the

placenta from the uterine wall, leading to bleeding between the placenta and the uterine wall. The presenting symptoms include sudden onset abdominal pain and dark vaginal bleeding, along with signs of uterine tenderness and rigidity. Fetal heart rate abnormalities, including late decelerations, are commonly observed due to fetal hypoxia resulting from compromised placental perfusion.

Question 331:
Correct Answer: A) Reposition the patient on her left side
Rationale: Late decelerations are signs of fetal compromise due to impaired placental perfusion. Repositioning the patient on her left side helps to alleviate compression of the vena cava, improving blood flow to the placenta and enhancing fetal oxygenation. This intervention should be initiated immediately to prevent further fetal hypoxia and acidosis.

Question 332:
Correct Answer: D) Continue labor management and reassess fetal heart rate periodically.
Rationale: The absence of fetal heart rate accelerations does not necessarily indicate fetal distress. It is important to assess the overall fetal heart rate pattern and consider other factors such as baseline heart rate, variability, and decelerations. In this scenario, it would be appropriate to continue labor management and reassess the fetal heart rate periodically, as long as other reassuring signs are present. Continuous monitoring and close observation of the fetal heart rate tracing will provide valuable information about fetal well-being. Immediate intervention or cesarean section is not warranted based solely on the absence of fetal heart rate accelerations.

Question 333:
Correct Answer: D) Distorted tracings caused by maternal/fetal movement or loose cables
Rationale: Cable movement artifact refers to distorted tracings in EFM caused by factors such as maternal or fetal movement as well as loose cables. These movements can disrupt the electrical signals between the uterus and the monitoring device, resulting in irregular or distorted tracings. It is important to secure the cables properly and ensure minimal movement during monitoring to reduce the occurrence of cable movement artifact.

Question 334:
Correct Answer: A) It refers to a situation where the fetal heart rate signal is unclear and cannot be properly interpreted.
Rationale: Signal ambiguity occurs when the fetal heart rate signal obtained from electronic fetal monitoring equipment is unclear or distorted, making it difficult for healthcare providers to accurately interpret the fetal heart rate pattern. This can happen due to various factors such as maternal movement, poor contact between the transducer and the mother's abdomen, or the presence of artifacts. Signal ambiguity can lead to misinterpretation of the fetal heart rate and may result in inappropriate interventions or delays in necessary interventions. It is important for healthcare providers to troubleshoot and resolve signal ambiguity to ensure accurate fetal monitoring and optimal care for the mother and baby.

Question 335:
Correct Answer: A) Increase in heart rate of at least 15 bpm above the baseline.
Rationale: To classify as a fetal heart rate acceleration, there must be an increase in the heart rate of at least 15

bpm above the baseline. The duration of accelerations is not specified and can vary. There is no requirement for the acceleration to last for at least 10 seconds or to coincide with fetal movement.

Question 336:
Correct Answer: C) Ordering a complete blood count and liver function tests
Rationale: Severe headache, blurred vision, and hypertension in a pregnant woman with preeclampsia raise concerns for the development of eclampsia or HELLP syndrome. Before initiating any specific treatment, it is important to obtain a complete blood count to assess for thrombocytopenia and liver function tests to evaluate for hepatic involvement. Administering antihypertensive medications, initiating magnesium sulfate infusion, and scheduling a cesarean delivery should be considered after evaluating the patient's laboratory results.

Question 337:
Correct Answer: B) Cross-talk interference
Rationale: Cross-talk interference occurs when signals from one channel of electronic monitoring equipment are picked up by another channel, causing distortion and frequent signal interference. In this scenario, the nurse should investigate the possibility of cross-talk interference between the monitoring devices. Ensuring proper grounding and separation of the monitoring equipment can help minimize signal ambiguities and provide accurate fetal heart rate tracing.

Question 338:
Correct Answer: B) Sinusoidal pattern
Rationale: A sinusoidal pattern is commonly seen in pregnant women with maternal obesity and gestational diabetes mellitus (GDM). It is characterized by a smooth, undulating pattern resembling a sine wave in the fetal heart rate tracing. The exact etiology is unknown, but it is believed to be associated with severe fetal anemia or hypoxia. Monitoring fetal well-being and considering further evaluation for fetal anemia or distress is necessary when a sinusoidal pattern is observed. Early decelerations, accelerations, and variable decelerations are not typically associated with maternal obesity and GDM.

Question 339:
Correct Answer: C) Prepare for immediate delivery
Rationale: In this scenario, the abrupt drop in fetal heart rate to 60 bpm and its persistence for 5 minutes indicate prolonged severe bradycardia. Immediate delivery is necessary to evaluate and manage the potential cause of this fetal distress. Delay in intervention can lead to irreversible harm to the fetus.

Question 340:
Correct Answer: D) Uterine hyperstimulation.
Rationale: While prolonged decelerations may be associated with various factors such as umbilical cord compression, fetal head compression, and maternal hypotension, they are not typically associated with uterine hyperstimulation. Uterine hyperstimulation, characterized by excessive uterine contractions, may contribute to other fetal heart rate deceleration patterns but is not commonly associated with prolonged decelerations. It is important for healthcare providers to consider and address all potential causes of decelerations to ensure appropriate management and fetal well-being.

Question 341:
Correct Answer: D) Cervical polyp

Rationale: Mrs. Adams' painless vaginal bleeding, non-tender uterus, fundus above the umbilicus, and reassuring fetal heart rate pattern are consistent with a cervical polyp. Cervical polyps are benign growths that arise from the cervical epithelium and can cause painless vaginal bleeding during pregnancy. The bleeding is usually intermittent and not associated with uterine tenderness or fetal compromise. Cervical polyps can be visualized during speculum examination and are managed conservatively unless symptomatic.

Question 342:
Correct Answer: A) Administer tocolytic therapy with terbutaline
Rationale: In this case, tocolytic therapy with terbutaline can be employed to suppress the contractions and delay preterm labor. The closed cervix indicates that delivery is not imminent at this time. Antibiotics are not indicated unless there is a specific concern for infection. Immediate cesarean section is not warranted in this scenario. Magnesium sulfate for fetal neuroprotection is typically indicated in cases of imminent preterm birth.

Question 343:
Correct Answer: A) Ethical considerations in disclosing confidential EFM information
Rationale: Ethical considerations are an important professional issue in EFM. Healthcare providers must handle confidential EFM information appropriately and only disclose it to authorized individuals involved in patient care. This includes protecting patient privacy, ensuring proper consent, and maintaining confidentiality when sharing EFM data and interpretations. Proper positioning of the fetal monitor transducer, technique for sterile vaginal examinations, and guidelines for cesarean sections are important aspects of EFM practice, but they do not specifically address the professional issue of ethical considerations.

Question 344:
Correct Answer: C) It exchanges oxygen and nutrients between the maternal and fetal bloodstreams
Rationale: The placenta acts as a crucial interface between the maternal and fetal blood systems, allowing the transfer of oxygen and nutrients from the mother to the fetus while eliminating waste products. It does not produce fetal red blood cells or maintain the fetal heart rate, although it indirectly affects fetal oxygenation by ensuring an adequate supply of oxygen-rich blood to the fetal circulation.

Question 345:
Correct Answer: D) All of the above
Rationale: Maternal position change, amnioinfusion (the infusion of sterile fluid into the amniotic cavity), and administration of oxygen to the mother can all help promote fetal heart rate variability. Changing the maternal position can improve blood flow to the placenta and subsequently increase variability. Amnioinfusion can improve amniotic fluid volume and reduce umbilical cord compression, leading to better variability. Oxygen administration can increase oxygen supply to the fetus and enhance variability. These interventions are often used in cases of decreased or absent variability.

Question 346:
Correct Answer: D) Base deficit
Rationale: Base deficit is the component in cord blood gases that indicates the presence of fetal hypoxemia. It represents the excess of acid or deficit of base in the fetal blood. A higher base deficit value suggests a greater degree of fetal hypoxemia. Monitoring base deficit helps in

assessing the fetal oxygenation status and guiding interventions to improve oxygen delivery to the fetus.

Question 347:
Correct Answer: A) Assisting with amnioinfusion
Rationale: Amnioinfusion involves infusing isotonic fluid into the uterus to alleviate cord compression and dilute meconium-stained amniotic fluid. This intervention can help improve fetal oxygenation and relieve late decelerations caused by cord compression. Encouraging the mother to bear down during contractions may further compromise fetal oxygenation. Monitoring maternal vital signs every 2 hours is important but does not directly address the management of late decelerations. Administering an epidural analgesia is not specifically indicated for managing late decelerations.

Question 348:
Correct Answer: B) Administering magnesium sulfate
Rationale: Magnesium sulfate is the drug of choice for preventing and treating eclamptic seizures. It is administered to women with severe preeclampsia or those at high risk of developing eclampsia. Magnesium sulfate acts as a central nervous system depressant and helps to prevent seizures by reducing neuronal excitability. Other interventions for managing severe preeclampsia-eclampsia may include bed rest, close monitoring of blood pressure and fetal well-being, and timely delivery of the baby.

Question 349:
Correct Answer: A) Rapid onset and return to baseline.
Rationale: Early fetal heart rate decelerations are characterized by a rapid onset and return to baseline. These decelerations usually occur due to transient head compression during contractions, resulting in a brief reduction in fetal oxygenation. The rapid onset and return to baseline distinguish early decelerations from other types of decelerations, such as late or variable decelerations. It is important for healthcare providers to recognize this pattern to differentiate it from potentially concerning deceleration patterns and provide appropriate interventions.

Question 350:
Correct Answer: D) True labor contractions
Rationale: The regularity, duration, and cervical changes indicate that Mrs. Johnson is experiencing true labor contractions. True labor contractions are regular, increase in frequency, duration, and intensity, and lead to cervical dilation and effacement. Braxton Hicks contractions are irregular, infrequent, and do not cause cervical changes. False labor contractions may be regular but do not lead to cervical changes. Preterm labor contractions occur before 37 weeks gestation, but the consistency of cervical dilation indicates it is not preterm labor in this case.

Question 351:
Correct Answer: A) 15-20 seconds
Rationale: During the latent phase of labor, contractions are usually of shorter duration, lasting around 15-20 seconds. As labor progresses into the active phase, the duration of contractions typically increases.

Question 352:
Correct Answer: A) Acting in the patient's best interest while ensuring no harm is done
Rationale: The principle of beneficence in medical ethics emphasizes the healthcare provider's responsibility to act in the best interest of the patient, promoting their well-being, and ensuring no harm is done. This principle guides medical professionals to prioritize the patient's health and strive for

their overall welfare while providing medical care, treatment, or intervention.

Question 353:
Correct Answer: **C) 40-100 Montvield Units (MU)**
Rationale: During active labor, the normal range of uterine contraction intensity is typically between 40-100 Montvield Units (MU). This range indicates an adequate strength of contractions for efficient cervical dilation and fetal descent. Contractions within this intensity range contribute to optimal progress in labor. Monitoring the intensity of contractions helps healthcare providers assess the strength of contractions, determine the need for interventions, and ensure the well-being of both the mother and the fetus. Overall

Question 354:
Correct Answer: **D) All of the above**
Rationale: Signal ambiguity in electronic fetal monitoring can have significant implications for patient safety and perinatal outcomes. A delay in appropriate interventions due to unclear or misinterpreted fetal heart rate patterns can lead to adverse outcomes for both the mother and the baby. Incorrect interpretation of the fetal heart rate pattern may result in unnecessary interventions or failure to recognize and address fetal distress. These factors can increase the risk of adverse perinatal outcomes, such as hypoxic-ischemic encephalopathy or neonatal acidemia. Therefore, it is crucial for healthcare providers to troubleshoot and resolve signal ambiguity promptly to ensure optimal care and reduce the potential risks associated with inaccurate fetal monitoring.

Question 355:
Correct Answer: **B) Fetal heart rate accelerations are a compensatory response to reduced fetal movements.**
Rationale: The absence of fetal movements is a concerning finding, and further assessment is necessary. However, the presence of fetal heart rate accelerations indicates a compensatory response to reduced fetal movements. Fetal heart rate accelerations are observed when the fetus is stimulated or experiences fetal movement. They indicate a responsive and well-oxygenated fetus. In this scenario, the presence of accelerations suggests that the fetus is compensating for the reduced fetal movements. It is important to investigate the cause of reduced fetal movements further but the presence of accelerations is generally a positive finding.

Question 356:
Correct Answer: **B) Late decelerations**
Rationale: Late decelerations in electronic fetal monitoring occur due to uteroplacental insufficiency and are characterized by a gradual decrease in the fetal heart rate after the peak of a contraction. Early decelerations, on the other hand, are mirror-like decreases in the fetal heart rate that coincide with contractions and are considered benign and normal.

Question 357:
Correct Answer: **D) All of the above**
Rationale: All the mentioned maternal factors, including smoking, advanced maternal age, and substance abuse, are associated with an increased risk of placental abruption. Smoking can lead to vasoconstriction and reduced blood flow to the placenta, increasing the risk of abruption. Advanced maternal age is a known risk factor for placental abruption, possibly due to age-related changes in the placenta. Substance abuse, including illicit drug use, can cause vasoconstriction and placental damage, leading to

abruption. Prompt recognition and management of placental abruption are crucial to prevent maternal and fetal complications.

Question 358:
Correct Answer: **A) Immediate cesarean section**
Rationale: A prolonged deceleration in the FHR tracing lasting more than 3 minutes is considered abnormal and can indicate fetal compromise. Immediate delivery, usually by cesarean section, is the most appropriate intervention to avoid potential fetal injury or death. Administration of oxygen, tocolytic therapy, or performing a vaginal examination are not the primary interventions indicated in this scenario.

Question 359:
Correct Answer: **A) Placenta**
Rationale: The placenta is the main organ responsible for facilitating gas exchange between the fetal and maternal circulations. It acts as a barrier between the maternal and fetal blood supplies, allowing the exchange of oxygen, nutrients, and waste products. The umbilical cord connects the fetus to the placenta and contains blood vessels that transport these substances. Amniotic fluid surrounds the fetus and provides protection, but it does not directly facilitate gas exchange. The decidua refers to the uterine lining during pregnancy and does not play a role in gas exchange between the fetal and maternal circulations.

Question 360:
Correct Answer: **C) Electronic fetal monitoring (EFM)**
Rationale: Electronic fetal monitoring (EFM) is a method used to assess the fetal heart rate and uterine contractions. It can be done non-invasively and is commonly used during labor and delivery in healthcare settings. However, in Jamie's case, if she has concerns about her baby's well-being, she can use a handheld or portable electronic fetal monitor to periodically monitor the fetal heart rate at home. This can provide her with reassurance and peace of mind. Blood tests and amniocentesis are invasive procedures used for different purposes, and ultrasound is primarily used for visualizing the fetus and assessing its growth and development.

Question 361:
Correct Answer: **A) Placenta previa**
Rationale: Mrs. Thompson's painless vaginal bleeding, absence of abdominal pain, closed cervical os, and non-tender uterus along with a non-reassuring fetal heart rate pattern most likely indicate placenta previa. Placenta previa is the abnormal location of the placenta in the lower uterine segment, either partially or completely covering the internal cervical os. This condition can cause painless vaginal bleeding, especially during the third trimester, and carries the risk of fetal compromise due to bleeding. Fetal heart rate abnormalities can occur if the placenta separates further during contractions, leading to decreased oxygen supply to the fetus.

Question 362:
Correct Answer: **C) Applying warm compresses**
Rationale: Applying warm compresses is a non-pharmacological intervention for hypertonus during labor. Warmth can promote relaxation of the uterine muscles and alleviate hypertonus. Administering magnesium sulfate and terbutaline are pharmacological interventions used as tocolytics. Increasing intravenous fluids may help with dehydration but does not directly address hypertonus.

Question 363:
Correct Answer: **A) Decreased platelet count**

Rationale: Severe preeclampsia is associated with multi-system involvement, including hematological changes. Thrombocytopenia, indicated by a decreased platelet count, is commonly observed in severe preeclampsia. The other options mentioned are not characteristic laboratory findings associated with severe preeclampsia.

Question 364:
Correct Answer: A) Sinusoidal pattern
Rationale: Sinusoidal pattern is a distinct fetal heart rate pattern associated with severe fetal hypoxemia. It appears as a smooth, regular wave-like pattern with a frequency of 3-5 cycles per minute. The presence of a sinusoidal pattern indicates an urgent need for intervention as it is highly indicative of severe fetal compromise. The pattern is caused by the release of endogenous opioids due to hypoxemia, which leads to decreased variability and a characteristic wave-like pattern on the fetal heart rate tracing.

Question 365:
Correct Answer: D) Umbilical artery resistance increases in response to maternal hypertension.
Rationale: The umbilical artery carries deoxygenated blood from the fetus to the placenta. During fetal hypoxia, the umbilical artery blood flow increases as a compensatory mechanism to improve oxygen delivery. Umbilical artery resistance increases in response to maternal hypertension, leading to reduced blood flow to the placenta and potentially compromising fetal oxygenation.

Question 366:
Correct Answer: B) Methamphetamine
Rationale: Methamphetamine use during pregnancy has been associated with numerous adverse effects on the developing fetus. These include low birth weight, premature birth, developmental delays, and behavioral problems. Pregnant women who use methamphetamine should seek medical help to reduce the risks to themselves and their unborn baby.

Question 367:
Correct Answer: C) Strong
Rationale: Intensity of uterine contractions is measured in mmHg using an external tocodynamometer. A peak intensity of 70mmHg indicates strong contractions. Weak contractions have a peak intensity of less than 25mmHg, while moderate contractions have a peak intensity between 25-50mmHg. Hyperstimulation refers to excessive uterine contractions, usually induced by administration of oxytocin or prostaglandins.

Question 368:
Correct Answer: C) Hemolysis, elevated liver enzymes, and low platelet count (HELLP) syndrome
Rationale: The clinical features of upper abdominal pain, hypertension, epigastric tenderness, elevated liver enzymes, and low platelet count are consistent with the diagnosis of HELLP syndrome. HELLP syndrome is a severe form of preeclampsia with the additional feature of hematological abnormalities. Severe preeclampsia may present with hypertension and proteinuria, but the presence of elevated liver enzymes and low platelet count indicates HELLP syndrome. Gestational hypertension is characterized by hypertension without the presence of proteinuria or end-organ damage. Eclampsia refers to the occurrence of seizures in a patient with preeclampsia.

Question 369:
Correct Answer: C) Ultrasonography for fetal biophysical profile (BPP)
Rationale: In a situation where the pregnant woman reports decreased fetal movement, it is essential to assess the fetal well-being. Ultrasonography for fetal biophysical profile (BPP) is a comprehensive test that evaluates several parameters including fetal breathing, fetal movements, fetal tone, amniotic fluid volume, and reactive non-stress test (NST). Since minimal fetal movement has been noted on examination, performing a BPP will provide a more detailed assessment of the fetal status and guide further management. Immediate induction of labor may not be warranted in the absence of other abnormal findings. Observation for 48 hours is not recommended due to concerns regarding potential adverse outcomes. Initiation of NST alone may not provide a complete evaluation of the fetal well-being.

Question 370:
Correct Answer: D) All of the above
Rationale: Gestational age, maternal position, and fetal sleep cycles are all factors that can influence fetal heart rate variability. Fetal heart rate variability tends to increase with gestational age, as the fetal nervous system develops. Maternal position can affect blood flow to the placenta and, in turn, affect fetal heart rate variability. Fetal sleep cycles can also impact variability, as the fetal heart rate typically decreases during sleep.

Question 371:
Correct Answer: A) Administering intravenous adenosine
Rationale: The most appropriate initial intervention for a fetus with supraventricular tachycardia (SVT) is administering intravenous adenosine. Adenosine is a medication that can help restore the normal electrical activity of the heart by interrupting the abnormal electrical pathways seen in SVT. It is typically given as a rapid intravenous bolus and can effectively convert SVT back to a normal sinus rhythm. Other interventions, such as administering oxygen to the mother or performing fetal echocardiography, may be considered depending on the specific clinical situation, but administering intravenous adenosine is the first-line treatment for SVT in a fetus.

Question 372:
Correct Answer: D) Biophysical profile
Rationale: The biophysical profile is an appropriate method for assessing fetal movement. It evaluates five parameters: fetal tone, fetal breathing movements, fetal movement, amniotic fluid volume, and reactive fetal heart rate. Each parameter is assigned a score, and a total score of 8-10 is considered reassuring. This assessment is typically performed using ultrasound technology and helps determine the well-being of the fetus. External cephalic version is a procedure to turn a fetus from a breech position to a head-down position. Doppler ultrasound measures blood flow, and a contraction stress test evaluates fetal heart rate response to contractions.

Question 373:
Correct Answer: D) Late decelerations
Rationale: Cord blood acid base testing is indicated when there are signs of fetal compromise, such as late decelerations on the fetal heart rate tracing. Late decelerations suggest inadequate oxygen supply to the fetus and may be associated with fetal acidemia. Cord blood analysis helps determine the extent of acid-base disturbances and guide appropriate interventions for the well-being of the baby.

Question 374:

Correct Answer: D) Internal monitoring devices are recommended for accurate fetal assessment in women with gestational diabetes.

Rationale: Women with gestational diabetes require close monitoring of the fetal heart rate. Internal monitoring devices are recommended in this scenario as they provide more accurate fetal assessment. Gestational diabetes can potentially affect the accuracy of external monitoring devices in determining the fetal heart rate and uterine contractions. Internal monitoring allows for direct measurement of the fetal heart rate using an electrode attached to the baby's scalp, ensuring precise assessment and timely interventions if required.

Question 375:
Correct Answer: D) Perform immediate cesarean section

Rationale: When cord compression is suspected during labor, the immediate intervention should be to perform a cesarean section. This is because cord compression can lead to fetal hypoxia and potential life-threatening complications. Administering terbutaline could help in managing uterine contractions but does not directly address cord compression. Applying a fetal scalp electrode and administering oxygen may provide information about fetal well-being but do not alleviate the immediate risk of cord compression.

Question 376:
Correct Answer: C) Irregular rhythm

Rationale: Normal fetal heart rate variability is characterized by an irregular rhythm. This means that there are fluctuations in the fetal heart rate, with no set pattern or intervals between beats. This irregularity is a sign of a healthy and well-oxygenated fetus. The absence of variability or the presence of minimal fluctuations can indicate fetal distress or other underlying issues. Accelerations in the fetal heart rate are an additional positive sign of fetal well-being and should not be absent. A smooth baseline, without any fluctuations, is also abnormal and may indicate fetal distress.

Question 377:
Correct Answer: B) Maternal fever

Rationale: A sustained baseline FHR greater than 160 bpm is indicative of maternal fever. Fetal tachycardia would present with a baseline FHR consistently above 160 bpm, not sustained elevations. Fetal arrhythmias would show irregularities in the FHR pattern. Maternal anxiety may cause transient increases in the FHR, but not sustained elevations.

Question 378:
Correct Answer: A) Sinusoidal pattern

Rationale: A sinusoidal pattern is commonly seen during supraventricular tachycardia (SVT) in a fetus. A sinusoidal pattern on the fetal heart rate tracing appears as a smooth, regular, and symmetric waveform resembling a sine wave. It is characterized by a consistent amplitude and frequency and is typically seen during sustained, rapid heart rates. This pattern is a non-reassuring sign and may indicate fetal distress. Accelerations, variable decelerations, and early decelerations are not specific to SVT and can be seen in various other fetal heart rate patterns.

Question 379:
Correct Answer: B) Nonreactive

Rationale: A nonreactive nonstress test is characterized by an absence of accelerations despite fetal movement. In this scenario, Mrs. Smith's test shows a fetal heart rate baseline of 110 bpm with minimal variability, indicating a lack of oxygenation or fetal well-being. As no accelerations or decelerations are observed, the test result is nonreactive.

Question 380:
Correct Answer: B) Contractions occurring more than five minutes apart

Rationale: During early labor, the uterine contractions are typically irregular and occur at an interval of more than five minutes apart. These contractions are of low intensity and shorter duration, usually lasting around 30-45 seconds. The palpation of contractions can be felt on both sides of the abdomen, signifying a coordinated effort of the uterine muscle. Contractions during this stage are usually manageable and not associated with severe pain or discomfort.

Question 381:
Correct Answer: B) Moderate to marked variability.

Rationale: During early decelerations, there is often a presence of moderate to marked variability in the fetal heart rate. This variability refers to the fluctuations in the baseline fetal heart rate that indicate a healthy autonomic nervous system and adequate fetal oxygenation. The presence of variability during early decelerations is a reassuring sign and suggests that the fetus is tolerating the transient head compression well. Absent or minimal variability, non-reassuring variability, or unpredictable variability are not characteristic of early decelerations.

Question 382:
Correct Answer: C) Performing a cesarean section.

Rationale: In cases of prolonged decelerations on the fetal heart rate tracing, if other intervention measures fail to resolve the deceleration or if there are signs of fetal compromise, the healthcare provider may consider performing a cesarean section. This surgical intervention provides a prompt delivery method to minimize potential harm to the fetus. The decision for a cesarean section should be based on a thorough assessment of the maternal and fetal condition along with careful consideration of individual circumstances.

Question 383:
Correct Answer: C) Fetal dysrhythmias are benign and do not require any intervention.

Rationale: Fetal dysrhythmias refer to abnormal variations in the fetal heart rate. While they may cause concern for healthcare providers, it is important to note that most fetal dysrhythmias are benign and do not require any intervention. They often resolve on their own without causing harm to the fetus. However, it is still important to monitor the fetal heart rate and promptly investigate any concerning findings. The other options are incorrect as fetal dysrhythmias are not always cause for concern, do not occur as a result of increased heart rate variability, and are not characterized by a regular rhythm in the fetal heart rate.

Question 384:
Correct Answer: B) Arterioarterial anastomosis

Rationale: In monochorionic-diamniotic twin pregnancies, where the twins share one placenta and two amniotic sacs, the most common type of placental vascular anastomosis is arterioarterial (AA) anastomosis. AA anastomosis refers to direct connections between the arterial circulation of the two twins. These anastomoses can lead to imbalances in blood flow between the twins and contribute to complications such as twin-to-twin transfusion syndrome (TTTS) or selective intrauterine growth restriction (sIUGR). Arteriovenous anastomosis, venovenous anastomosis, and venous-arterial anastomosis are less commonly observed in monochorionic-diamniotic twin pregnancies. Understanding the type of placental vascular anastomosis is crucial for managing the pregnancy and monitoring for potential complications.

Question 385:
Correct Answer: D) Autoimmune destruction of thyroid tissue
Rationale: The symptoms and laboratory findings described in the scenario are consistent with hyperthyroidism caused by autoimmune destruction of thyroid tissue, also known as Graves' disease. In this condition, autoantibodies stimulate the thyroid gland to produce excess thyroid hormones, leading to weight loss, palpitations, and increased sweating. The elevated TSH levels represent a feedback mechanism attempting to stimulate thyroid hormone production, but it is ineffective due to the destruction of thyroid tissue.

Question 386:
Correct Answer: A) Induction of labor
Rationale: The management approach for postdates pregnancy involves the induction of labor. Induction is recommended to reduce the risk of stillbirth and other complications associated with prolonged pregnancy. Methods of induction may include mechanical methods like balloon catheters or pharmacological methods using medications such as prostaglandins or oxytocin. The choice of method depends on various factors, including the Bishop score, maternal and fetal well-being, and the presence of cervical ripening. Induction of labor should be carefully planned and monitored, taking into consideration the individual circumstances of the mother and the baby.

Question 387:
Correct Answer: B) To assess the fetal well-being
Rationale: The purpose of the fetal heart rate (FHR) baseline in electronic monitoring is to assess the fetal well-being. It provides a reference point for evaluating changes in the fetal heart rate pattern and serves as a basis for identifying abnormalities. The fetal heart rate variability is assessed by measuring the fluctuations in the baseline, and decelerations and accelerations are deviations from the baseline that help in detecting fetal distress or other complications. However, the primary purpose of the FHR baseline is to evaluate the overall fetal well-being.

Question 388:
Correct Answer: C) Umbilical artery pH
Rationale: Cord blood gas analysis evaluates the metabolic and acid-base status of the newborn. It measures parameters such as umbilical artery pH, partial pressure of carbon dioxide (pCO2), and bicarbonate (HCO3-) levels. These parameters reflect the fetal oxygenation, ventilation, and acid-base balance.

Question 389:
Correct Answer: A) Pre-eclampsia
Rationale: The patient is presenting with symptoms of hypertensive disorders of pregnancy, including right upper quadrant pain, headache, visual disturbances, and elevated blood pressure. Additionally, laboratory results indicate elevated liver enzymes and low platelet count, which are consistent with the diagnosis of HELLP syndrome, a severe form of pre-eclampsia characterized by Hemolysis, Elevated Liver enzymes, and Low Platelet count.

Question 390:
Correct Answer: D) Variable decelerations
Rationale: Calcium channel blockers are commonly used in the management of hypertension during pregnancy. These medications may cause a decrease in placental perfusion by reducing vascular resistance. Fetal heart rate tracings can show variable decelerations, indicating intermittent umbilical cord compression. It is essential to monitor the fetal heart rate closely when calcium channel blockers are administered to pregnant women to detect and manage any potential adverse effects on fetal oxygenation.

Question 391:
Correct Answer: A) Check the connection between the transducer and the monitor
Rationale: When there is a loss of signal from the FHR monitor, the first step in troubleshooting is to check the connection between the transducer and the monitor. A loose or disconnected connection can cause a loss of signal. Changing the mother's position, increasing the volume, and restarting the EFM system are important steps but should be done after checking the connection.

Question 392:
Correct Answer: D) All of the above
Rationale: Umbilical blood flow can be influenced by various factors. Maternal hypotension reduces blood flow to the placenta, compromising oxygen and nutrient delivery to the fetus through the umbilical vein. Fetal hypoxia can lead to vasoconstriction of the umbilical vessels, reducing blood flow. Umbilical cord compression, such as during contractions, can also impede blood flow through the umbilical vessels. Therefore, all the options mentioned can influence umbilical blood flow.

Question 393:
Correct Answer: A) Toxoplasmosis
Rationale: Toxoplasmosis, caused by the parasite Toxoplasma gondii, can be transmitted to the fetus if a pregnant woman contracts the infection. Infection during pregnancy can lead to fetal hydrocephalus, which is the abnormal accumulation of fluid in the brain. This condition can result in intellectual disabilities, vision problems, and seizures in the affected child. Pregnant women are advised to avoid handling cat feces and to ensure proper food safety to prevent toxoplasmosis infection.

Question 394:
Correct Answer: A) Administer intravenous tocolytic therapy
Rationale: Hypertonic contractions can lead to decreased uteroplacental perfusion, resulting in decreased fetal oxygenation. Administering intravenous tocolytic therapy helps to reduce uterine activity, improve placental blood flow, and enhance fetal well-being. This intervention is necessary to prevent further fetal compromise and promote a favorable fetal heart rate pattern.

Question 395:
Correct Answer: B) Prepare for an immediate emergency cesarean section
Rationale: The described pattern is consistent with a sinusoidal pattern. Sinusoidal patterns are concerning and often associated with severe fetal anemia, hypoxia, or other fetal distress. An immediate emergency cesarean section should be prepared to ensure the safety and well-being of the fetus. Other actions, such as fetal scalp stimulation, monitoring the mother's vital signs, or measuring contractions, may not address the underlying cause of the sinusoidal pattern.

Question 396:
Correct Answer: B) Gestational hypertension
Rationale: Pregnant women with diabetes have a higher risk of developing gestational hypertension. This condition is

characterized by high blood pressure during pregnancy and can lead to complications such as preeclampsia. Preterm labor, placenta previa, and ectopic pregnancy are not specifically associated with diabetes.

Question 397:
Correct Answer: D) Midazolam
Rationale: Midazolam is a commonly used benzodiazepine for intravenous sedation during local anesthesia in pregnant patients. It provides anxiolysis, amnesia, and sedation without compromising the maternal or fetal well-being. Propofol, ketamine, and nitrous oxide are not routinely used for intravenous sedation during local anesthesia in pregnancy.

Question 398:
Correct Answer: C) External tocodynamometer
Rationale: The external tocodynamometer is a commonly used method to monitor uterine contractions electronically during labor. It is a non-invasive device that is placed on the maternal abdomen to measure the frequency, duration, and intensity of contractions. Leopold maneuvers are used to determine the fetal position and engagement. Auscultation with a Pinard stethoscope is a method of listening to the fetal heart rate. Vaginal examination is used to assess cervical dilation and effacement.

Question 399:
Correct Answer: A) Administer a bolus of intravenous fluids
Rationale: In this scenario, the patient presents with type 1 diabetes and an abnormal FHR tracing characterized by absent variability, no accelerations, and no decelerations. The initial intervention should include administering a bolus of intravenous fluids to address potential hypovolemia, which can be a causative factor for the abnormal fetal heart rate pattern. Adequate hydration can improve uteroplacental perfusion and subsequent fetal well-being.

Question 400:
Correct Answer: D) Notify the healthcare provider in charge and assist in updating Emily's medical record immediately.
Rationale: Patient safety and quality care are paramount in healthcare settings. Missing important information, such as blood type and medical history, can significantly impact patient care and jeopardize their well-being. In this scenario, it is essential to notify the healthcare provider in charge and assist in updating Emily's medical record immediately. This proactive approach ensures that accurate and complete information is available for clinical decision-making, ensuring the delivery of high-quality care to the patient. Ignoring or delaying the resolution of missing information can hinder effective treatment and compromise patient safety.

Question 401:
Correct Answer: D) Prolactin
Rationale: Prolactin is the hormone responsible for the development and growth of the milk-producing glands in the breasts. It is primarily secreted by the anterior pituitary gland and plays a vital role in lactation. Once the baby is born, suckling stimulates the release of prolactin, leading to milk production. Prolactin levels increase during pregnancy and reach their peak after childbirth to promote milk production and support breastfeeding.

Question 402:
Correct Answer: B) Encouraging the mother to lie on her left side

Rationale: Maternal hypotension can adversely affect fetal oxygenation by reducing placental blood flow. Lying on the left side improves blood flow to the placenta by relieving pressure on major blood vessels and enhancing uterine perfusion. Administering oxygen may be beneficial in some cases, but it does not directly address the underlying cause of maternal hypotension. Increasing fluid intake may be helpful in certain situations, but lying on the left side is the most appropriate immediate intervention. Administering beta-blockers may further lower maternal blood pressure and is not recommended in this scenario.

Question 403:
Correct Answer: D) All of the above.
Rationale: Signal ambiguity in electronic fetal monitoring can be resolved by employing various strategies. Repositioning the mother can help eliminate external interference, such as moving away from electrical equipment or turning off nearby mobile devices. Adjusting the placement of the ultrasound transducer on the mother's abdomen can improve signal quality by ensuring proper contact and minimizing artifacts. Reducing maternal movement during monitoring can also contribute to a clearer fetal heart rate signal. By employing all of these strategies, healthcare providers can optimize signal clarity and ensure accurate interpretation of the fetal heart rate pattern.

Question 404:
Correct Answer: C) Proteinuria
Rationale: Preeclampsia is a disorder characterized by hypertension and the presence of proteinuria after 20 weeks of gestation. Proteinuria is an important diagnostic criterion for preeclampsia. Hypotension, edema of the lower extremities, and bradycardia are not typically associated with preeclampsia.

Question 405:
Correct Answer: B) Normal pH
Rationale: A cord blood pH of 7.39 is within the normal range, indicating a normal pH. The prolonged deceleration followed by a slow return to baseline with reduced variability may suggest fetal distress, but the pH value itself indicates a normal acid-base balance.

Question 406:
Correct Answer: D) Umbilical vein
Rationale: The umbilical vein is the primary vessel responsible for carrying oxygenated blood from the placenta to the fetus. It carries oxygen and nutrient-rich blood, allowing for fetal oxygenation and nutrition. The blood flows directly into the fetus's liver through the ductus venosus, bypassing the liver sinusoids. From there, it joins the systemic venous circulation.

Question 407:
Correct Answer: A) Placental abruption
Rationale: HELLP syndrome is associated with various complications, and placental abruption is one of them. Placental abruption occurs when the placenta separates from the uterus before delivery, leading to significant bleeding and compromising fetal oxygenation. Other potential complications of HELLP syndrome include liver hematoma, disseminated intravascular coagulation (DIC), acute renal failure, and perinatal mortality. Polyhydramnios, gestational diabetes, and preeclampsia are not direct complications of HELLP syndrome.

Question 408:
Correct Answer: C) False labor contractions

Rationale: Contractions that stop with a change in position or activity are indicative of false labor contractions. False labor contractions typically do not increase in intensity or frequency and can be alleviated by changes in activity or position. Preterm labor contractions would not stop with a change in position or activity. True labor contractions would persist regardless of position or activity. Intestinal gas contractions do not occur in the context of uterine contractions during pregnancy.

Question 409:
Correct Answer: B) Insulin therapy began at the onset of labor
Rationale: During labor and delivery, it is typically recommended to discontinue oral hypoglycemic agents and initiate insulin therapy due to concerns of prolonged fasting and the potential for maternal hypoglycemia. Insulin therapy allows for better glycemic control and flexibility in managing blood glucose levels during labor. Blood glucose levels should be monitored closely, ideally every 1-2 hours, to maintain tight glycemic control and prevent adverse outcomes.

Question 410:
Correct Answer: B) Uteroplacental insufficiency
Rationale: Uteroplacental insufficiency refers to a reduction in the blood flow to the placenta, compromising the fetal oxygen and nutrient supply. This can lead to fetal hypoxia, resulting in the observed changes in FHR tracing including decreased variability and late decelerations. Fetal structural abnormalities or medication side effects are less likely to cause these specific findings.

Question 411:
Correct Answer: C) Umbilical cord compression
Rationale: Prolonged decelerations with a slow return to baseline are typically indicative of umbilical cord compression. Uteroplacental insufficiency would present with repetitive variable decelerations. Fetal sleep states can cause periodic breathing patterns or nonreactive tracings, but not prolonged decelerations. Maternal hypotension would present with late decelerations, not prolonged decelerations.

Question 412:
Correct Answer: D) Placenta accreta
Rationale: Placenta accreta is a condition in which the placenta attaches too deeply into the uterine wall, leading to impaired placental function and subsequent fetal growth restriction. It is the most commonly associated uteroplacental complication in cases of fetal growth restriction. Placental abruption, uterine rupture, and placenta previa may cause other pregnancy complications but are less frequently associated with fetal growth restriction.

Question 413:
Correct Answer: A) Cord prolapse
Rationale: Persistent variable decelerations with rapid return to baseline are typically indicative of cord prolapse. Maternal hypertension would present with late decelerations, not variable decelerations. Fetal bradycardia would show a consistently low baseline FHR. Premature rupture of membranes may have variable decelerations, but not necessarily rapid returns to baseline.

Question 414:
Correct Answer: A) It allows for continuous monitoring of the fetal heart rate.
Rationale: Internal fetal heart rate monitoring involves the placement of an electrode on the baby's scalp, which provides a more accurate and continuous measurement of the fetal heart rate compared to external monitoring methods. This allows healthcare providers to closely monitor any changes in the baby's heart rate and make timely interventions if necessary. Internal monitoring is more invasive than external monitoring, but the benefits of continuous monitoring outweigh the risks in certain situations, such as when accurate assessment of the fetal heart rate is crucial.

Question 415:
Correct Answer: D) Decreased fetal respiratory movements
Rationale: Opioid pain medications can cross the placenta and affect the fetus. One of the effects associated with opioid use during pregnancy is the suppression of fetal respiratory movements. These medications can depress the central nervous system, including the respiratory centers in the brain, leading to decreased respiratory efforts in the fetus. This can potentially result in inadequate oxygenation and compromised fetal well-being. Monitoring fetal movements and overall fetal well-being is crucial in pregnant women receiving opioid pain medications.

Question 416:
Correct Answer: D) Initiate immediate delivery by emergency cesarean section
Rationale: The EFM findings of absent fetal heart rate variability and recurrent late decelerations indicate fetal compromise and the need for immediate intervention. Emergency cesarean section delivery should be initiated to expedite the birth and prevent further fetal compromise.

Question 417:
Correct Answer: C) Administering a tocolytic medication.
Rationale: Tachysystole is often managed by administering a tocolytic medication, such as terbutaline or nifedipine, to decrease uterine activity. Increasing oxytocin infusion rate would further exacerbate tachysystole. Encouraging maternal position changes can offer temporary relief, but it may not be sufficient for managing tachysystole. Administering a medication to stimulate contractions would be contraindicated in this situation.

Question 418:
Correct Answer: B) GDM
Rationale: Gestational diabetes mellitus (GDM) is associated with fetal macrosomia (large size) due to increased transfer of glucose from the mother. Macrosomia can lead to impaired umbilical blood flow due to the increased demand for oxygen and nutrients by the larger fetus. This condition increases the risk of placental insufficiency and compromised umbilical blood flow, leading to variable decelerations on fetal heart rate monitoring.

Question 419:
Correct Answer: B) Hypotonic contractions
Rationale: Hypotonic contractions refer to contractions that occur less frequently than normal during labor. These contractions are often weak and ineffective, leading to slower cervical dilation and prolonged labor. Tachysystole, on the other hand, is the term used to describe excessive uterine activity with more than 5 contractions in 10 minutes. Montevideo units are a measurement used to assess the strength of contractions, and uterine atony refers to the lack of uterine tone after childbirth.

Question 420:
Correct Answer: C) Maintenance of adequate blood volume

Rationale: Adequate maternal fluid intake is crucial for maintaining adequate blood volume, which in turn optimizes placental perfusion and fetal oxygenation. Insufficient blood volume can lead to reduced blood flow to the placenta and compromise fetal oxygen supply. Maternal hydration does not directly affect fetal lung development, prevent preterm labor, or enhance fetal hemoglobin production. It primarily ensures optimal circulation and blood flow to support the needs of both the mother and the fetus.

Question 421:
Correct Answer: B) Vaginal bleeding
Rationale: Vaginal bleeding is a common symptom of preterm labor and should be promptly assessed by a healthcare provider. It can indicate various conditions such as cervical changes, placenta previa, or placental abruption, all of which can lead to preterm labor. Other signs and symptoms of preterm labor may include regular contractions occurring every 10 minutes or less, pelvic pressure, low backache, abdominal cramping, and an increase in vaginal discharge. Any concerns or symptoms related to preterm labor should be reported to a healthcare provider for further evaluation and management.

Question 422:
Correct Answer: B) 25-35 mmHg
Rationale: During electronic fetal monitoring, the resting tone represents the baseline uterine pressure between contractions. A normal resting tone typically ranges between 25-35 mmHg. This value indicates the pressure exerted by the uterus when it is at rest. A resting tone below 25 mmHg may suggest uterine hypotonia, which could lead to ineffective contractions. On the other hand, a resting tone above 35 mmHg may indicate uterine hypertonia, which could impede fetal oxygenation. Therefore, maintaining a normal resting tone within the range of 25-35 mmHg is crucial for optimal uterine activity and fetal well-being.

Question 423:
Correct Answer: C) Fetal bradycardia
Rationale: Congenital heart block is characterized by fetal bradycardia, which is defined as a persistent fetal heart rate less than 110 beats per minute. This is considered a serious condition and requires close monitoring and intervention. Decreased fetal heart rate variability, intermittent acceleration of the fetal heart rate, and U-shaped decelerations are not specific features of congenital heart block.

Question 424:
Correct Answer: C) Recommending left lateral positioning during sleep
Rationale: Maternal obesity can cause increased pressure on the diaphragm and decreased lung compliance, leading to dyspnea. To alleviate symptoms, recommending left lateral positioning during sleep is important as it reduces the pressure on the diaphragm and improves breathing mechanics. Sleeping in a supine position can further exacerbate dyspnea due to the weight of the uterus compressing the diaphragm, causing reduced lung capacity. Referring the patient for a sleep study may be indicated if there are signs of sleep apnea. Prescribing bronchodilator medication is not the primary intervention for dyspnea related to maternal obesity.

Question 425:
Correct Answer: A) Administer oxygen to the pregnant woman
Rationale: Prolonged fetal heart rate decelerations lasting more than 2 minutes indicate fetal compromise.

Administering oxygen to the pregnant woman increases oxygen delivery to the fetus and may help improve fetal well-being.

Question 426:
Correct Answer: D) Notify the healthcare provider
Rationale: The presence of normal baseline variability, accelerations, and no decelerations on the EFM tracing indicate that fetal well-being is reassuring. However, the patient's symptoms of a swollen and tender leg should raise concern for possible DVT. The nurse should notify the healthcare provider promptly to ensure appropriate evaluation and management of this maternal complication.

Question 427:
Correct Answer: C) Elevate the presenting fetal part
Rationale: In the case of a visible cord prolapse, immediate action is crucial to prevent fetal compromise. The most appropriate initial intervention is to manually elevate the presenting fetal part off the cord to relieve compression, thereby improving fetal oxygenation. This can be done by pushing the fetus upwards during a sterile vaginal exam or repositioning the woman into the knee-chest or Trendelenburg position. These actions buy time to prepare for an immediate cesarean delivery, if necessary.

Question 428:
Correct Answer: B) It evaluates the adequacy of placental perfusion
Rationale: Cord blood acid-base testing serves as an indirect measure of placental perfusion and fetal oxygenation during labor and delivery. It provides valuable information about the newborn's acid-base balance, reflecting the adequacy of oxygen delivery and exchange. Deviations from normal acid-base values can suggest compromised placental perfusion and potential fetal hypoxia or acidosis.

Question 429:
Correct Answer: A) Fetal hemoglobin has a higher affinity for oxygen compared to adult hemoglobin
Rationale: Fetal hemoglobin has a higher affinity for oxygen compared to adult hemoglobin, allowing it to extract oxygen more efficiently from the maternal blood supply. Fetal oxygen saturation is typically higher than maternal oxygen saturation due to this increased affinity. Fetal oxygenation primarily occurs through active transport rather than diffusion across the placenta. Furthermore, fetal oxygen supply is independent of maternal carbon dioxide levels as the fetus has its own mechanisms for regulating oxygen and carbon dioxide exchange.

Question 430:
Correct Answer: A) Fetal distress
Rationale: A fetal baseline heart rate below 120 bpm for a prolonged period may indicate fetal distress. It is important to closely monitor the fetus and consider appropriate interventions to ensure the well-being of the baby.

Question 431:
Correct Answer: C) Legal implications arise from the interpretation and actions taken based on the fetal monitoring findings.
Rationale: In the context of electronic fetal monitoring, legal implications primarily arise from the interpretation of the fetal monitoring findings and the subsequent actions taken by the healthcare provider. The healthcare provider has the legal responsibility to accurately interpret the fetal heart rate patterns and make appropriate decisions based on them. The expectant father also has the right to be informed and

involved in the process, forming part of the shared decision-making.

Question 432:
Correct Answer: B) Maternal infections
Rationale: Various factors can affect the fetal heart rate variability, and one such factor is maternal infections. Infections can lead to fetal inflammation, compromising the autonomic nervous system's function, and subsequently decreasing the variability. Fetal sleep cycles, fetal movement, and placental abruption can all contribute to changes in fetal heart rate, but they are not specifically associated with decreased variability. It is important to consider these factors and incorporate them into the overall assessment to ensure accurate interpretation and appropriate interventions.

Question 433:
Correct Answer: B) Perform an emergency cesarean section
Rationale: Sudden loss of FHR tracing and fetal movements, along with advanced cervical dilation, may indicate fetal distress and the need for immediate delivery to avoid potential injury or death. Performing an emergency cesarean section is the most appropriate action in this scenario. Performing a fetal scalp stimulation test, administering oxytocin augmentation, or changing the mother's position are not the primary interventions indicated in this situation.

Question 434:
Correct Answer: B) Non-reactive NST with persistent absence of accelerations
Rationale: A non-reactive NST with the persistent absence of accelerations would suggest uteroplacental insufficiency. This pattern indicates that the fetus is not receiving adequate oxygenation and nutrient supply, leading to a non-reactive NST. Absence of fetal movements during the NST, presence of early decelerations, and reactive NST with the presence of late decelerations are not specific findings associated with uteroplacental insufficiency.

Question 435:
Correct Answer: C) Assessing the accuracy and reliability of new EFM devices
Rationale: Technological advancements in EFM introduce new devices and equipment. A professional issue in this context is assessing the accuracy and reliability of these new devices. Healthcare providers need to evaluate the performance of the equipment and ensure that it provides accurate and reliable fetal monitoring data for effective clinical decision-making. Understanding fetal heart rate patterns, interpreting uterine activity, and collaborating with the obstetrician are all important aspects of EFM practice but do not specifically focus on the professional issue of assessing new EFM devices.

Question 436:
Correct Answer: C) By visual inspection during a vaginal examination
Rationale: After the insertion of an Intrauterine Pressure Catheter (IUPC), the position is typically verified by visual inspection during a vaginal examination. Healthcare providers check the position of the catheter's tip and ensure that it is appropriately placed within the uterine cavity. Options A, B, and D are incorrect as they do not accurately describe the method of verifying the position of an IUPC after insertion.

Question 437:

Correct Answer: D) Glucose gel or solution
Rationale: Neonatal hypoglycemia is a common concern in infants born to mothers with diabetes. In such cases, it is recommended to administer glucose gel or solution to maintain euglycemia in the newborn. Fentanyl is an analgesic, oxytocin is used for labor induction, and betamethasone is given to enhance fetal lung maturation. None of these medications specifically address neonatal hypoglycemia.

Question 438:
Correct Answer: C) Hypoglycemia
Rationale: Maternal hypoglycemia can significantly impact fetal oxygenation. When a pregnant mother experiences low blood glucose levels, it can lead to inadequate oxygen supply to the fetus. This occurs because glucose is the primary source of energy for fetal growth and development. Hypoglycemia can result in alterations in placental blood flow and compromise fetal oxygenation. Therefore, it is essential to closely monitor blood glucose levels in pregnant patients with diabetes to prevent fetal hypoxia and related complications.

Question 439:
Correct Answer: D) Variable decelerations
Rationale: Placental abruption, the premature separation of the placenta, can cause variable decelerations in the fetal heart rate due to compromised blood flow. Tachycardia is an increased heart rate, bradycardia is a decreased heart rate, and late decelerations are associated with uteroplacental insufficiency.

Question 440:
Correct Answer: D) Facilitating immediate delivery
Rationale: In cases of suspected decreased blood flow to the fetus, facilitating immediate delivery is the most appropriate intervention to prevent further compromise. Administering tocolytic agents may be considered to delay delivery in specific situations, but it is not an intervention for decreased blood flow. Increasing maternal oxygenation and encouraging maternal hydration may have some benefits but are not the primary interventions in cases of decreased blood flow.

Question 441:
Correct Answer: A) Preeclampsia
Rationale: Preeclampsia, a pregnancy-related hypertensive disorder, is associated with an increased risk of preterm birth. Gestational diabetes, placenta previa, and urinary tract infection may have other complications but are not directly linked to preterm birth.

Question 442:
Correct Answer: C) It is non-invasive and does not require cervical dilation.
Rationale: An external tocodynamometer is a non-invasive device used to assess uterine activity during labor. It is placed on the maternal abdomen and measures changes in uterine activity without requiring cervical dilation. While it provides an indirect measurement of intrauterine pressure, it is not as accurate as an internal uterine pressure catheter (IUPC) in measuring the exact pressure exerted by contractions. Continuous monitoring of fetal heart rate is typically achieved using electronic fetal monitoring (EFM), which involves separate devices. Real-time visualization of uterine contractions is not a feature of an external tocodynamometer.

Question 443:

Correct Answer: C) Monitor closely and repeat blood pressure measurements
Rationale: In this scenario, Mrs. Anderson has a history of gestational hypertension, and her blood pressure is consistently elevated on this occasion. As she is asymptomatic, the initial step in management would be to monitor her closely and repeat blood pressure measurements. Asymptomatic gestational hypertension without severe features does not usually require immediate induction of labor or antihypertensive medication. Proteinuria measurement is essential for diagnosing preeclampsia but is not indicated solely for managing gestational hypertension.

Question 444:
Correct Answer: C) 140-160 beats per minute
Rationale: The normal baseline fetal heart rate during labor is considered to be between 140-160 beats per minute. This range indicates that the fetus is well-oxygenated and is tolerating labor well. Deviations from this range may indicate fetal distress or other complications.

Question 445:
Correct Answer: D) Previous cesarean delivery
Rationale: A previous cesarean delivery is associated with a higher risk of uterine rupture during labor. This is due to the potential weakening of the uterine scar from the previous surgical incision. Uterine rupture can result in severe maternal and fetal complications, including hemorrhage, hypoxia, and fetal demise. Therefore, careful monitoring and prompt intervention are necessary in women with a history of cesarean delivery to detect signs of uterine rupture and ensure a safe delivery.

Question 446:
Correct Answer: C) Fetal biophysical profile (BPP)
Rationale: In a patient with a reassuring non-stress test (NST) but requiring further assessment of fetal well-being, a fetal biophysical profile (BPP) should be performed. BPP evaluates multiple parameters including fetal breathing, fetal movements, fetal tone, amniotic fluid volume, and NST. It provides a comprehensive evaluation of fetal well-being and can guide further management decisions. Fetal kick count may be recommended for cases with decreased fetal movements but is not indicated in this scenario. Amniotic fluid index (AFI) measurement and Doppler velocimetry of umbilical artery are useful in specific situations such as suspected oligohydramnios or intrauterine growth restriction, respectively, but are not the next appropriate step in this case.

Question 447:
Correct Answer: C) Uterine contractions with relaxation in-between
Rationale: A CTG tracing records both the fetal heart rate and uterine activity. The most common pattern seen for uterine activity is regular contractions with relaxation in-between, as represented by rhythmic peaks and troughs on the tracing. Uterine tachysystole refers to an excessive number of contractions within a specified time period, which can lead to fetal heart rate changes and reduced placental perfusion. Uterine hypertonus is a term used to describe excessive uterine contractility during labor. Uterine retraction is not specifically related to uterine activity but refers to the occurrence of intermittent contractions or retraction of the uterus during the postpartum period.

Question 448:
Correct Answer: C) Variable decelerations
Rationale: Variable decelerations are a common fetal heart rate pattern associated with cord compression. These decelerations are characterized by an abrupt decrease in fetal heart rate below the baseline, often with an erratic shape. They can occur during or after contractions and are caused by the compression of the umbilical cord, leading to transient interruption of blood flow to the fetus. Early decelerations are related to head compression, accelerations are an indication of fetal well-being, and late decelerations are associated with uteroplacental insufficiency.

Question 449:
Correct Answer: C) Administer steroids for fetal lung maturation
Rationale: Persistent late decelerations on EFM usually indicate uteroplacental insufficiency and potential fetal hypoxemia. In the context of preterm labor, the initial intervention should be to administer steroids for fetal lung maturation, given the risk of preterm birth. Tocolytic medication may be considered in combination with other interventions to address preterm labor, but it does not directly address the hypoxemia. Vaginal examination and placement of a scalp electrode may be necessary but should be secondary to addressing the risk of preterm birth and fetal well-being.

Question 450:
Correct Answer: C) Preeclampsia
Rationale: Preeclampsia, a hypertensive disorder, can lead to decreased placental perfusion resulting in fetal compromise. It is characterized by hypertension, proteinuria, and end-organ damage. Gestational diabetes, although associated with increased fetal weight, does not have a direct impact on fetal well-being during labor. Placenta previa can cause bleeding but does not directly affect fetal well-being. Urinary tract infection may lead to maternal discomfort but does not usually pose a significant risk to the fetus.

Question 451:
Correct Answer: D) Evaluation for abruptio placentae
Rationale: The combination of decreased fetal movements, vaginal bleeding, and contractions raises concerns regarding the possibility of abruptio placentae, a potentially life-threatening condition. Immediate evaluation for abruptio placentae should be performed, which may include laboratory tests, ultrasound examination, and close maternal and fetal monitoring. Immediate cesarean section may be necessary if there are signs of fetal compromise or maternal instability. Fetal kick count alone is insufficient in this scenario and does not address the underlying etiology. Ultrasonography for fetal biophysical profile (BPP) is not the most appropriate initial step given the clinical presentation and suspicion of abruptio placentae.

Question 452:
Correct Answer: C) Left lateral tilt position
Rationale: The left lateral tilt position is preferred during anesthesia as it improves uteroplacental blood flow and prevents compression of the inferior vena cava, ensuring optimal fetal oxygenation. Supine position can lead to compression of the vena cava, compromising blood flow and oxygenation. The Trendelenburg position may increase maternal blood pressure, impacting fetal oxygenation. Prone position is not suitable during anesthesia as it can compromise ventilation and airway management.

Question 453:
Correct Answer: B) Epidural analgesia
Rationale: Epidural analgesia is a safe and effective technique for labor anesthesia, providing pain relief while maintaining optimal fetal oxygenation. Intrathecal opioids can occasionally lead to fetal respiratory depression. Systemic

opioids may cause neonatal respiratory depression and sedation. Intravenous ketamine should be used cautiously, as it can result in uterine hypertonicity and compromise fetal oxygenation. Epidural analgesia remains the preferred choice for labor pain management.

Question 454:
Correct Answer: C) Expectant management with close fetal monitoring
Rationale: In the scenario described, the presence of variable decelerations suggests umbilical cord compression. However, immediate delivery by cesarean section may not be warranted unless there are other signs of fetal distress or non-reassuring fetal heart rate patterns persist. Administration of IV fluids may improve uteroplacental perfusion but is not the most appropriate initial intervention. Initiation of magnesium sulfate for fetal neuroprotection is indicated in certain situations, such as preterm labor, but is not the first-line intervention in this scenario. Therefore, expectant management with close fetal monitoring is the most appropriate course of action to assess and ensure the well-being of the fetus.

Question 455:
Correct Answer: A) Body Mass Index (BMI) ? 30 kg/m◆
Rationale: Maternal obesity is commonly defined by a Body Mass Index (BMI) ? 30 kg/m◆. BMI is calculated by dividing an individual's weight in kilograms by their height in meters squared. A BMI of 30 or above indicates obesity. It is important to identify and classify maternal obesity accurately as it is a significant risk factor for adverse pregnancy outcomes. Healthcare providers can use this criterion to screen and monitor pregnant women for obesity, assess their associated risks, and provide appropriate interventions and care to improve outcomes for both the mother and fetus.

Question 456:
Correct Answer: C) Minimal Variability
Rationale: Minimal variability is characterized by an amplitude of less than 5 beats per minute and suggests fetal compromise. It indicates poor oxygenation and is associated with an abnormal fetal acid-base balance. Absent variability is a concerning finding and indicates fetal hypoxia or acidemia. Marked variability is characterized by a sinusoidal pattern with a frequency of 2-5 cycles per minute, indicating a well-oxygenated and healthy fetus. Moderate variability is considered to be a reassuring pattern and is associated with a normal fetal acid-base balance.

Question 457:
Correct Answer: A) Administer oxygen via facemask
Rationale: Repetitive late decelerations on fetal heart rate monitoring suggest hypoxemia. The initial intervention should be to increase oxygen supply to the fetus. Administering oxygen via facemask will help improve the oxygenation status of the fetus. It is important to rule out other causes, such as maternal hypotension or hypovolemia, before considering interventions like amnioinfusion or fetal scalp electrode placement. Assessing cervical dilation or discontinuing oxytocin infusion, although important, will not directly address the hypoxemia in this scenario.

Question 458:
Correct Answer: A) Smoking during pregnancy
Rationale: Smoking during pregnancy is a significant risk factor for preterm labor. It has been shown to increase the likelihood of preterm birth by constricting blood vessels, decreasing blood flow to the placenta, and reducing the transfer of nutrients and oxygen to the fetus. Additionally, smoking can lead to cervical insufficiency, premature rupture

of membranes, and intrauterine growth restriction, all of which can contribute to preterm labor. It is crucial for healthcare providers to educate and support pregnant individuals in quitting smoking to reduce the risk of preterm labor and improve maternal and fetal outcomes.

Question 459:
Correct Answer: B) Frequent blood glucose monitoring
Rationale: Glycemic control in pregnant women with diabetes is achieved through frequent blood glucose monitoring. This allows for adjusting insulin doses as needed to maintain optimal blood sugar levels. Monitoring fetal heart rate is important for assessing fetal well-being but does not directly address glycemic control. Administration of corticosteroids may be necessary in certain obstetric situations but does not target blood sugar management. Increasing carbohydrate intake can lead to uncontrolled blood sugar levels.

Question 460:
Correct Answer: A) External monitoring
Rationale: External monitoring is considered a noninvasive method of electronic fetal monitoring. It involves the use of sensors placed on the mother's abdomen to measure the fetal heart rate and uterine contractions. Internal monitoring, on the other hand, involves the insertion of instruments (such as an internal fetal scalp electrode or an intrauterine pressure catheter) into the mother's cervix or uterus. Wireless monitoring and Doppler monitoring are different technologies used in electronic monitoring but do not determine invasiveness.

Question 461:
Correct Answer: B) Document the finding and inform the primary care provider
Rationale: In the case of a prolonged deceleration, which lasts longer than 3 minutes but less than 10 minutes, the nurse should document the finding and immediately inform the primary care provider. Prolonged decelerations are not within the normal range and can be indicative of fetal distress. Prompt communication with the healthcare provider is essential to determine further actions, such as potential interventions or emergency cesarean delivery, to ensure the well-being of both the mother and the baby.

Question 462:
Correct Answer: C) Endometritis
Rationale: Maternal obesity is a risk factor for endometritis, an infection of the uterine lining. The increased adipose tissue in obese women can impair wound healing and increase the risk of surgical site infections. Endometritis can manifest as fever, abdominal pain, uterine tenderness, and foul-smelling vaginal discharge following delivery. Prompt recognition and treatment with appropriate antibiotics are essential to reduce morbidity. Postpartum hemorrhage, deep vein thrombosis, and preterm labor are not directly associated with an increased risk of surgical site infection in maternal obesity.

Question 463:
Correct Answer: C) Continue to monitor the patient and observe the fetal heart rate pattern.
Rationale: Fetal heart rate accelerations occurring during contractions are called "accelerations with contractions" and are typically a reassuring sign. In this scenario, it is important to continue monitoring the patient and observe the fetal heart rate pattern. Fetal heart rate accelerations during contractions indicate a responsive and well-oxygenated fetus. There is no immediate need for intervention or preparation for emergency cesarean section based solely on

the presence of accelerations during contractions. Continuous monitoring and further assessment of the fetal heart rate pattern will provide valuable information regarding fetal well-being.

Question 464:
Correct Answer: A) Fetal bradycardia.
Rationale: Tachysystole can lead to decreased fetal heart rate variability and potential fetal bradycardia. Decreased uterine activity, maternal hypotension, and prolonged intercontraction intervals are not typically associated with tachysystole.

Question 465:
Correct Answer: D) Sinusoidal pattern
Rationale: An abnormal variability pattern in fetal heart rate is characterized by a sinusoidal pattern. This pattern appears as a smooth, undulating waveform with a consistent amplitude and frequency, resembling a sine wave. It is associated with severe fetal anemia, fetal hemorrhage, or other fetal conditions affecting oxygenation. Accelerations, decelerations, and transient tachycardia are all normal components of fetal heart rate and do not represent abnormal variability patterns. The presence of abnormal patterns requires immediate medical intervention to prevent further harm to the fetus.

Question 466:
Correct Answer: D) To measure uterine contractions
Rationale: The primary purpose of using an IUPC is to directly measure the strength and frequency of uterine contractions. This information is crucial in monitoring the progress of labor, ensuring optimal uterine activity, and assessing the need for intervention. The IUPC provides more accurate and objective measurements compared to external monitoring methods such as tocodynamometry. It does not measure cervical dilation, monitor fetal heart rate, or assess fetal movement.

Question 467:
Correct Answer: D) Irregular rhythm
Rationale: Ectopic beats refer to abnormal beats that occur outside the normal sinus rhythm. In fetal monitoring, ectopic beats are characterized by an irregular rhythm, which means there is a deviation from the expected pattern of regular beats. This can be identified by observing the variability in the timing and strength of the fetal heartbeats. It is essential to recognize ectopic beats as they may indicate underlying fetal dysrhythmias or other cardiac abnormalities that require appropriate intervention and further evaluation. Regular rhythm, increase, or decrease in fetal heart rate are not the characteristic features of ectopic beats.

Question 468:
Correct Answer: D) Administer an antihypertensive medication
Rationale: The signs and symptoms presented by Mrs. Smith are indicative of severe preeclampsia, a serious maternal complication. Prioritizing the control of her elevated blood pressure is crucial to minimize the risk of maternal and fetal complications. Administering an antihypertensive medication under the guidance of the healthcare provider is the first step in the management of severe preeclampsia.

Question 469:
Correct Answer: C) Administer oxygen via a non-rebreather mask
Rationale: Late decelerations indicate uteroplacental insufficiency and fetal hypoxemia. Administering oxygen via non-rebreather mask will help improve fetal oxygenation by increasing maternal oxygen levels. This is the most appropriate immediate action to take in order to improve fetal well-being. Administering oxytocin could worsen the situation by further compromising the fetal oxygen supply. Placing the patient in the Trendelenburg position is not recommended as it may decrease placental blood flow. Proceeding with a vaginal examination is not indicated as it does not address the underlying cause of the late decelerations.

Question 470:
Correct Answer: A) Variable decelerations
Rationale: Variable decelerations in electronic fetal monitoring are caused by umbilical cord compression, resulting in a sudden and transient decrease in the fetal heart rate. They are characterized by rapid onset and recovery, with variable shapes and depths. Early decelerations are normal and caused by fetal head compression, while late decelerations indicate uteroplacental insufficiency.

Question 471:
Correct Answer: D) All of the above
Rationale: Signal ambiguity in electronic fetal monitoring can be caused by various factors, including maternal obesity, placental position, and external electrical interference. Maternal obesity can make it challenging to obtain a clear and accurate fetal heart rate signal due to increased layers of subcutaneous tissue. The position of the placenta, especially if it is anterior, can also interfere with signal clarity. Additionally, external electrical interference from sources such as electrocautery devices or mobile phones can disrupt the accuracy of the fetal heart rate signal. It is important for healthcare providers to be aware of these factors and take appropriate measures to minimize signal ambiguity during electronic fetal monitoring.

Question 472:
Correct Answer: B) 20 minutes
Rationale: Nonstress testing (NST) is typically performed for a duration of 20 minutes. During this time, fetal heart rate changes and accelerations are assessed to determine fetal well-being. In some cases, NST may need to be extended to 40 or 60 minutes depending on the clinical scenario.

Question 473:
Correct Answer: D) Induce labor
Rationale: The patient is presenting with symptoms of pre-eclampsia, including right upper quadrant pain, headache, peripheral edema, and elevated blood pressure. However, the absence of elevated liver enzymes and normal platelet count suggests that this patient does not meet the criteria for the diagnosis of HELLP syndrome. The most appropriate management for this patient is to induce labor as it is consistent with the current gestational age and the presence of hypertension.

Question 474:
Correct Answer: B) Intracranial hemorrhage
Rationale: A decrease in fetal heart rate variability is commonly associated with intracranial hemorrhage. This injury occurs when there is bleeding within the skull, leading to increased pressure on the brain and potential damage to brain tissue. The decrease in heart rate variability indicates fetal distress and the need for immediate medical intervention to prevent further complications.

Question 475:
Correct Answer: D) Placental abruption
Rationale: Late decelerations in the fetal heart rate can be caused by placental abruption, a condition where the

placenta separates from the uterus before delivery. The separation of the placenta can compromise blood flow to the fetus, leading to late decelerations.

Question 476:
Correct Answer: A) Accelerations
Rationale: Gestational hypertension usually does not have a direct effect on the fetal heart rate (FHR) patterns. In fact, in uncomplicated cases, the FHR patterns are often normal. Accelerations on the FHR tracing reflect a healthy and responsive fetal autonomic nervous system. Therefore, when monitoring Mrs. Johnson's FHR patterns, it is expected to see accelerations.

Question 477:
Correct Answer: B) The ductus arteriosus connects the aorta and the pulmonary artery in the fetal heart.
Rationale: The ductus arteriosus is a blood vessel that connects the pulmonary artery and the aorta in the fetal heart. It allows most of the blood to bypass the fetal lungs, as they are not yet functional. Option A is incorrect as the umbilical artery carries deoxygenated blood from the fetus to the placenta. Option C is incorrect as oxygenated blood from the placenta enters the fetus through the umbilical vein, not the right atrium. Option D is incorrect as the foramen ovale connects the right and left atria, not the left ventricle to the aorta.

Question 478:
Correct Answer: D) Continuous fetal monitoring
Rationale: When ectopic beats are detected in fetal monitoring, continuous fetal monitoring should be carried out to assess the fetal heart rate and rhythm comprehensively. This allows healthcare professionals to closely monitor the fetal well-being and detect any further abnormalities. Immediate delivery, administration of tocolytic agents, and maternal repositioning are not specific interventions for ectopic beats. The appropriate course of action will depend on the underlying cause, severity, and overall clinical condition of the fetus. Continuous fetal monitoring ensures ongoing surveillance and enables prompt intervention if necessary.

Question 479:
Correct Answer: A) Administer tocolytic therapy with nifedipine
Rationale: In this scenario, tocolytic therapy with nifedipine would be appropriate in order to delay preterm labor and promote fetal lung maturity through corticosteroid administration. The presence of occasional early decelerations in the fetal heart tracing indicates a favorable status of the fetus. Intrauterine pressure catheter placement is not necessary at this time. Immediate cesarean section would only be indicated if there were signs of fetal distress or other complications. Magnesium sulfate for neuroprotection is typically indicated in cases of imminent preterm birth.

Question 480:
Correct Answer: C) Late decelerations
Rationale: Late decelerations are a common finding in pregnant women with obesity. Maternal obesity is associated with chronic inflammation and impaired placental perfusion, leading to uteroplacental insufficiency. Late decelerations occur due to inadequate oxygen supply to the fetus during contractions, resulting in a delayed recovery of the fetal heart rate. It is important to closely monitor maternal blood pressure and fetal heart rate in pregnant women with obesity to detect any signs of fetal distress.

Question 481:

Correct Answer: B) 30 seconds
Rationale: During the active phase of labor, a normal uterine contraction typically lasts for around 30 seconds. Longer durations may indicate hyperstimulation of the uterus, while shorter durations may suggest insufficient uterine activity.

Question 482:
Correct Answer: A) Decreased fetal hemoglobin production
Rationale: Maternal smoking during pregnancy can lead to decreased fetal hemoglobin production due to lower oxygen availability. Carbon monoxide from cigarette smoke binds to fetal hemoglobin more readily than oxygen, reducing oxygen-carrying capacity. This can lead to fetal hypoxia and negatively impact fetal development. Maternal smoking is not associated with increased fetal cardiac output or respiratory rate. Fetal oxygen saturation may be decreased rather than increased due to reduced oxygen availability.

Question 483:
Correct Answer: D) To assess the well-being of the fetus
Rationale: External fetal heart rate monitoring is primarily done during labor to assess the well-being of the fetus. By monitoring the fetal heart rate, healthcare providers can detect any changes or abnormalities that may indicate fetal distress or compromise. This allows for timely intervention and appropriate management to ensure the safety and well-being of the baby. Other parameters, such as the mother's blood pressure, uterine contractions, and cervical dilation, may be monitored separately but are not the primary focus of external fetal heart rate monitoring.

Question 484:
Correct Answer: B) Uterine contractions
Rationale: Decreased fetal heart rate variability is often associated with uterine contractions. As the uterus contracts, it can compress the placenta and reduce fetal oxygenation, leading to changes in fetal heart rate patterns. Maternal hyperglycemia can also affect fetal oxygenation, but it is not directly related to decreased variability. Fetal anemia and maternal hypertension may have other effects on fetal heart rate patterns, but they are not the primary factor contributing to decreased variability in this scenario.

Question 485:
Correct Answer: B) Tocodynamometer
Rationale: The tocodynamometer is a non-invasive device used for external uterine monitoring. It measures the frequency, duration, and intensity of contractions by detecting changes in uterine pressure. The intrauterine pressure catheter (IUPC) is an invasive method that directly measures the pressure within the uterus. The fetal scalp electrode (FSE) is used for fetal heart rate monitoring, and phonocardiography (PCG) is a technique to record heart sounds.

Question 486:
Correct Answer: D) All of the above
Rationale: Several factors can affect uteroplacental blood flow. Hypertension can lead to vasoconstriction and decreased blood flow to the placenta, compromising fetal oxygen and nutrient supply. Maternal position can also influence uteroplacental blood flow, with the left lateral position generally being recommended for optimal blood flow. Maternal smoking is associated with vasoconstriction, decreased placental blood flow, and lower birth weight. Therefore, all the options mentioned in A, B, and C can

affect uteroplacental blood flow, making D) All of the above the correct answer.

Question 487:
Correct Answer: **D) Calcium channel blockers**
Rationale: Calcium channel blockers are often used to manage hypertension in pregnancy. These medications work by relaxing blood vessels, improving blood flow to the placenta, and increasing fetal oxygenation. They are considered safe and effective for the treatment of hypertension during pregnancy.

Question 488:
Correct Answer: **B) Documenting all interventions and observations accurately**
Rationale: Accurate documentation is essential for patient safety in electronic fetal monitoring. It helps to ensure that all interventions and observations are properly recorded and can be reviewed by healthcare providers. This documentation allows for better continuity of care, reduces the risk of errors, and enables effective communication among the healthcare team. Regularly monitoring the patient's vital signs is important but not directly related to electronic fetal monitoring. Checking for proper placement of the fetal monitor is also important to ensure accurate monitoring. Administering medication without proper documentation can compromise patient safety.

Question 489:
Correct Answer: **D) All of the above.**
Rationale: Auscultation during fetal assessment involves the use of a stethoscope to listen to fetal heart sounds. It is a non-invasive technique used to evaluate fetal well-being and can help detect abnormal heart rates or rhythm abnormalities in the fetus. By listening to the fetal heart sounds, healthcare providers can gather important information about the baby's cardiac function and assess the overall health of the fetus. Auscultation is a simple and widely accessible method that can provide valuable insights during pregnancy monitoring.

Question 490:
Correct Answer: **C) In all pregnancies regardless of risk**
Rationale: Cord blood acid base testing should ideally be performed in all pregnancies regardless of risk. It provides valuable information about fetal acid-base status and helps identify any potential signs of fetal compromise. While certain situations may increase the likelihood of fetal distress, it is essential to assess fetal well-being in all pregnancies to ensure timely interventions if necessary and prevent adverse outcomes.

Question 491:
Correct Answer: **B) pH greater than 7.4**
Rationale: In cord blood acid base testing, a pH greater than 7.4 indicates metabolic alkalosis. Metabolic alkalosis is characterized by an elevated pH and can be caused by a loss of acid or excessive bicarbonate. This finding may indicate a disruption in the acid-base balance and warrants further evaluation to identify the underlying cause and its potential effects on the fetuses' well-being.

Question 492:
Correct Answer: **A) To increase fetal oxygenation**
Rationale: Administration of oxygen via a face mask to the mother increases oxygen levels in the mother's blood, which, in turn, leads to increased oxygen transfer to the fetus. This intervention helps counteract the effects of variable decelerations, which are often caused by reduced oxygen supply to the fetus.

Question 493:
Correct Answer: **A) Hypertonic uterus**
Rationale: A resting uterine tone of 25 mmHg indicates a hypertonic uterus, suggesting excessive uterine activity. Normal resting tone ranges between 5-20 mmHg. In this scenario, the high resting tone signifies increased uterine contractions, which may be a concern for preterm labor.

Question 494:
Correct Answer: **D) Monitor the fetal heart rate closely**
Rationale: Occasional late decelerations that resolve after the end of contractions are likely associated with benign causes such as maternal hypertension or uterine activity. Monitoring the fetal heart rate closely is the most appropriate action in this situation as it allows for the identification of any changes or worsening patterns. Placing the patient in the Trendelenburg position is not indicated as it may decrease placental blood flow. Administering terbutaline as a tocolytic is not necessary as there is no need to stop or slow down labor. Encouraging the patient to push during contractions may increase intrauterine pressure and potentially exacerbate the late decelerations.

Question 495:
Correct Answer: **D) Encourage Emma to count fetal movements at the same time each day.**
Rationale: Consistency in fetal movement monitoring is key for accurate assessment. By encouraging Emma to count fetal movements at the same time each day, the healthcare provider ensures that she can establish a baseline for what is normal for her baby. Any significant decrease or change in fetal movements from the established baseline can then be promptly addressed and evaluated.

Question 496:
Correct Answer: **B) Decreases contraction strength**
Rationale: A decreased resting tone during electronic fetal monitoring is often associated with uterine hypotonia. Uterine hypotonia refers to inadequate uterine muscle tone during rest or between contractions. This condition can lead to decreased contraction strength, making the contractions less effective in promoting cervical dilation and fetal descent during labor. It does not affect the frequency or duration of contractions. Monitoring and addressing uterine hypotonia is important in order to improve the strength of uterine contractions and facilitate progress in labor. Measures such as ambulation, hydration, and oxytocin administration may be employed to enhance uterine activity.

Question 497:
Correct Answer: **C) Fetal hypoxia**
Rationale: Tachycardia, defined as a fetal heart rate above 160 bpm, can indicate fetal hypoxia. This occurs when the fetus is not receiving enough oxygen, possibly due to uteroplacental insufficiency or cord compression. Maternal fever and anxiety can cause a mild increase in fetal heart rate, but are less likely to result in a sustained baseline tachycardia. Fetal anomalies may cause bradycardia or a variable deceleration pattern, but are not typically associated with tachycardia.

Question 498:
Correct Answer: **A) FHR accelerations are normal and reassuring**
Rationale: In this scenario, the nurse observes accelerations in the FHR tracing, even though they last less than 10 seconds. Accelerations are considered normal and reassuring signs of fetal well-being, regardless of their duration. They indicate fetal responsiveness and intact neurologic pathways. Continuous monitoring for 30 minutes

or suggesting uteroplacental insufficiency is not necessary in this case.

Question 499:
Correct Answer: C) Check the attachment of the transducer to the mother's abdomen
Rationale: Excessive baseline fetal movement artifacts on the EFM tracing can occur if the transducer is not securely attached to the mother's abdomen. Checking the attachment of the transducer is the first step in troubleshooting this issue. Repositioning the mother, assessing her perception of fetal movement, and adjusting the sensitivity setting on the EFM should be done after checking the transducer attachment.

Question 500:
Correct Answer: A) Ventricular septal defect
Rationale: Maternal diabetes, particularly when uncontrolled, is associated with an increased risk of congenital abnormalities. One of the most common abnormalities seen in infants of diabetic mothers is a ventricular septal defect (VSD), which is a hole in the wall separating the two lower chambers of the heart. Other congenital abnormalities associated with maternal diabetes include caudal regression syndrome, sacral agenesis, renal abnormalities, and musculoskeletal anomalies. Down syndrome is caused by chromosomal abnormalities and is not directly related to maternal diabetes. Neural tube defects, such as spina bifida, are associated with folic acid deficiency rather than diabetes. Cleft lip and palate can be multifactorial in etiology and not solely attributed to maternal diabetes.

Question 501:
Correct Answer: B) Maternal hemorrhage
Rationale: Preeclampsia-eclampsia can lead to an increased risk of maternal hemorrhage. This can occur during pregnancy, childbirth, or in the postpartum period. The underlying pathophysiology of preeclampsia, including abnormal placental development and compromised vascular function, can contribute to bleeding complications. Other potential complications of preeclampsia-eclampsia include organ damage (such as liver or kidney), premature birth, fetal growth restriction, and placental abruption. Early recognition and appropriate management are essential to minimize the risks associated with preeclampsia-eclampsia.

Question 502:
Correct Answer: D) Administering antihypertensive medication as ordered
Rationale: In the case of a pregnant woman with chronic hypertension, antihypertensive medication may be required during labor to maintain blood pressure within a normal range and minimize the risk of complications. The other options mentioned may not directly address the management of hypertension during labor.

Question 503:
Correct Answer: A) Maternal diabetes
Rationale: Maternal diabetes is associated with an increased risk of fetal dysrhythmias. Poor glycemic control in diabetic mothers can lead to abnormal fetal heart rate patterns and dysrhythmias. It is important for healthcare providers to closely monitor and manage blood glucose levels in diabetic pregnant women to minimize the risk of fetal dysrhythmias. The other options are not directly associated with an increased risk of fetal dysrhythmias.

Question 504:
Correct Answer: C) Uterine hypertonia

Rationale: An elevated resting tone during electronic fetal monitoring suggests uterine hypertonia. Uterine hypertonia refers to excessive uterine muscle tone during rest or between contractions. This condition can lead to impaired uterine blood flow, resulting in decreased fetal oxygenation and potential fetal distress. Monitoring and identifying an elevated resting tone is crucial for timely intervention to prevent adverse fetal outcomes. Techniques such as relaxation exercises or the use of tocolytic medications may be employed to reduce uterine hypertonia and improve uterine activity.

Question 505:
Correct Answer: D) Fetal sleep cycles.
Rationale: Fetal heart rate accelerations are commonly associated with fetal sleep cycles. They are considered a normal physiological response and are often an indication of a well-oxygenated fetus. Umbilical cord compression, fetal hypoxemia, and maternal fever are not typically associated with accelerations, but rather with decelerations or other abnormal patterns.

Question 506:
Correct Answer: B) To assess fetal heart rate response to sound stimulus
Rationale: Fetal acoustic stimulation is performed during an amniotic fluid assessment to assess the fetal heart rate response to a sound stimulus. The sound stimulus, such as a buzzer or a maternal voice recording, is used to stimulate the fetus and evaluate its cardiac response. This helps in assessing the fetal well-being and responsiveness. The estimation of amniotic fluid volume is performed separately using methods like the amniotic fluid index (AFI) or the single deepest pocket (SDP) measurement. Fetal movements and the presence of meconium in the amniotic fluid are also evaluated during an amniotic fluid assessment but are not directly related to fetal acoustic stimulation.

Question 507:
Correct Answer: C) Metabolic acidosis
Rationale: Metabolic acidosis is characterized by low pH and low bicarbonate (HCO3-) levels in cord blood gases. It results from an excess of acid or a loss of base in the body. Metabolic acidosis in the fetus can be caused by conditions such as hypoxia, placental insufficiency, or fetal distress. Monitoring cord blood gases can help diagnose and manage metabolic acidosis in the fetal circulation.

Question 508:
Correct Answer: C) Moderate variability
Rationale: A moderate variability in fetal heart rate is considered normal and indicates a healthy fetal state. It is characterized by fluctuations in the baseline heart rate that range between 6 and 25 beats per minute. This variability reflects the autonomous functioning of the fetal autonomic nervous system and indicates an absence of metabolic acidemia or acute hypoxia. Absent or minimal variability is abnormal and may suggest fetal compromise, whereas marked variability is excessive and may indicate fetal distress. It is crucial to recognize and interpret the variability patterns to make appropriate clinical decisions during monitoring and intervention.

Question 509:
Correct Answer: A) Fetal acoustic stimulation involves the use of sound to stimulate fetal activity.
Rationale: Fetal acoustic stimulation is a method used to evaluate fetal well-being during a non-stress test (NST). It involves the use of sound, such as a buzzer or a maternal voice recording, to stimulate fetal activity. This stimulation

helps assess the fetus's heart rate and reactivity. Fetal acoustic stimulation is a non-invasive procedure that is safe for both the mother and the fetus. It is not contraindicated after 32 weeks of gestation and can be performed throughout pregnancy as needed.

Question 510:
Correct Answer: A) Metabolic acidosis
Rationale: A base excess value of -5 indicates metabolic acidosis. Base excess reflects the metabolic component of acid-base balance. A negative base excess indicates the presence of excess acid or a metabolic acidosis. In this scenario, the late decelerations, reduced FHR variability, and tachycardia suggest fetal hypoxia, leading to metabolic acidosis.

Question 511:
Correct Answer: B) Ultrasound transducer
Rationale: The ultrasound transducer is a component in electronic monitoring equipment that is used to measure the fetal heart rate. It emits high-frequency sound waves and detects the echoes that bounce back from the fetal heart, allowing for the measurement of the fetal heart rate. The toco transducer measures uterine contractions, the pressure transducer measures intrauterine pressure, and the intrauterine pressure catheter is used to measure the strength of the contractions.

Question 512:
Correct Answer: B) Encourage the mother to change positions
Rationale: Late decelerations on the fetal heart rate tracing suggest uteroplacental insufficiency, which may compromise fetal oxygenation. The most appropriate action to improve the fetal heart rate pattern is to encourage the mother to change positions, as this promotes optimal blood flow to the placenta. Administering oxygen, increasing intravenous fluid rate, and administering terbutaline are not indicated for the management of late decelerations.

Question 513:
Correct Answer: A) Toco transducer
Rationale: The toco transducer is used to measure uterine contractions in electronic monitoring equipment. It is a noninvasive sensor placed on the mother's abdomen that measures the changes in pressure on the surface of the uterus during contractions. The ultrasound transducer is used to measure the fetal heart rate, the pressure transducer measures intrauterine pressure, and the intrauterine pressure catheter is used to measure the strength of the contractions.

Question 514:
Correct Answer: B) Uterine contractions are primarily responsible for cervical dilation.
Rationale: Uterine contractions play a significant role in cervical dilation during labor. The contractions exert pressure on the cervix, leading to its progressive opening. The strength of contractions may vary, with the fundus being the area where contractions are generally the weakest. Uterine contractions are not directly responsible for initiating fetal descent but rather assist in pushing the fetus downward after cervical dilation. Although uterine contractions do aid in the expulsion of the placenta following delivery, they do not increase blood flow to the placenta during labor.

Question 515:
Correct Answer: B) 30-45 seconds
Rationale: The average duration of a uterine contraction during the active phase of labor is typically between 30-45 seconds. This duration allows sufficient time for effective uterine muscle contractions to facilitate cervical dilation and promote progress in labor. Contractions lasting less than 30 seconds may not provide adequate force for cervical dilation, while contractions lasting longer than 45 seconds may compromise fetal oxygenation and increase the risk of uterine hyperstimulation.

Question 516:
Correct Answer: A) Regular monitoring and evaluation
Rationale: Sustaining a quality improvement initiative requires regular monitoring and evaluation of the implemented changes. This allows healthcare professionals to assess the effectiveness of the improvement initiatives, identify areas for further improvement, and make necessary adjustments. Resistance to change can hinder sustainability, so it is important to address any concerns and involve stakeholders in the process. Ignoring feedback from stakeholders can undermine the success and sustainability of the initiative. Patient safety should never be compromised in any improvement initiative. Therefore, regular monitoring and evaluation are essential strategies to sustain a quality improvement initiative.

Question 517:
Correct Answer: D) All of the above.
Rationale: Improper use of electronic fetal monitoring (EFM) tracings can lead to various legal issues. Failure to detect fetal distress due to misinterpretation of tracings may result in delayed intervention and potential harm to the fetus or mother. False-positive interpretations can lead to unnecessary interventions, exposing the patient to risks and potential legal consequences. Failure to implement timely interventions based on accurate EFM interpretations can also result in legal issues if harm or adverse outcomes occur. Thus, all the options mentioned in the Question can arise due to improper use of EFM tracings.

Question 518:
Correct Answer: C) Tocodynamometer probe displacement
Rationale: Tocodynamometer probe displacement can cause signal ambiguity, resulting in erroneous readings of the fetal heart rate. In this scenario, the malfunction in the tocodynamometer is the likely cause of the poor contraction tracing and the sudden decrease in the baseline fetal heart rate. It is important for the nurse to reposition the tocodynamometer probe properly to accurately monitor the contractions and the fetal heart rate.

Question 519:
Correct Answer: B) Decreased variability
Rationale: Maternal hypotension can lead to decreased blood flow to the fetus, resulting in decreased variability in the fetal heart rate. Decreased variability refers to a reduced fluctuation of the heart rate and is indicative of fetal distress. Increased variability, accelerations, and early decelerations are not commonly associated with maternal hypotension.

Question 520:
Correct Answer: A) Admit for immediate induction of labor
Rationale: Mrs. Thompson's elevated blood pressure, urinary protein, laboratory findings of thrombocytopenia and elevated liver enzymes, along with decreased platelet count, suggest the development of severe preeclampsia. In this scenario, the most appropriate next step would be to admit Mrs. Thompson for immediate induction of labor, as prompt delivery is considered the definitive treatment for severe preeclampsia. Monitoring the fetal heart rate and scheduling

a follow-up visit would delay necessary management. Administration of antihypertensive medication alone may not address the potential risks associated with severe preeclampsia.

Question 521:
Correct Answer: D) Hydralazine
Rationale: Hydralazine is the first-line antihypertensive medication recommended for the treatment of severe hypertension in pregnancy. It is a direct vasodilator that helps lower blood pressure and improve maternal and fetal outcomes. Methyldopa, nifedipine, and labetalol are also commonly used antihypertensive medications in pregnancy, but hydralazine is specifically recommended as the initial treatment option for severe hypertension. The choice of medication should be based on the individual patient's condition and preferences, as well as the expertise of the healthcare provider.

Question 522:
Correct Answer: C) Using ultrasound imaging
Rationale: Ectopic beats in fetal monitoring can be detected using ultrasound imaging. Ultrasound allows visualization of the fetal heart and provides real-time information about the fetal heart rate and rhythm. By observing the ultrasound image, healthcare professionals can identify irregularities in the heartbeats, such as ectopic beats. Absence of fetal movement, decreased variability in fetal heart rate, and palpation of the maternal abdomen are not reliable methods for detecting ectopic beats. Ultrasound imaging provides a more accurate and visual representation of the fetal heart's electrical activity.

Question 523:
Correct Answer: C) Variable decelerations
Rationale: Variable decelerations are characterized by abrupt, visually apparent decreases in FHR below the baseline rate. They are commonly associated with cord compression and can occur during contractions or spontaneously. When examining the tracing, variable decelerations exhibit an erratic pattern, without any particular relationship to the uterine contractions. In this scenario, the FHR of 150 bpm with occasional accelerations and decelerations suggests variable decelerations, indicating the need for further evaluation for cord compression and prompt intervention if necessary.

Question 524:
Correct Answer: D) Increased risk of congenital anomalies
Rationale: Maternal obesity can have a detrimental impact on fetal well-being, but it is not directly associated with an increased risk of congenital anomalies. However, there is evidence suggesting that maternal obesity may indirectly contribute to certain congenital anomalies, such as neural tube defects, through its association with inadequate folic acid intake or metabolism. Maternal obesity is associated with an increased risk of other adverse outcomes, including an increased risk of stillbirth, macrosomia (excessive fetal growth), and an increased incidence of complications during labor and delivery. Healthcare providers should be aware of these risks to provide appropriate antenatal, intrapartum, and postpartum care for obese pregnant women.

Question 525:
Correct Answer: C) Umbilical cord compression
Rationale: Umbilical cord compression can lead to a significant decrease in fetal oxygen supply. Compression of the umbilical cord can occur due to factors such as cord prolapse, nuchal cord, or tightening of the cord around fetal body parts. The compression can restrict blood flow and oxygen delivery to the fetus, potentially resulting in fetal distress. Maternal hypotension, decreased fetal heart rate, and maternal hyperglycemia can all have an impact on fetal oxygenation, but umbilical cord compression is more likely to greatly affect fetal oxygenation in this scenario.

Question 526:
Correct Answer: C) Avoiding harm and minimizing risks to the patient
Rationale: Non-maleficence in medical ethics refers to the obligation of healthcare providers to avoid causing harm to the patient and minimize any potential risks associated with their care. This principle highlights the importance of preventing harm, whether physical or psychological, and prioritizing patient safety throughout the medical decision-making and treatment processes.

Question 527:
Correct Answer: B) Uterine rupture
Rationale: The clinical presentation of severe abdominal pain, vaginal bleeding, nonreassuring fetal heart rate pattern, tense and tender uterus, and variable decelerations with minimal spontaneous recovery is highly suggestive of uterine rupture. This is a life-threatening emergency and prompt surgical intervention is required to prevent maternal and fetal morbidity and mortality.

Question 528:
Correct Answer: C) Notify the healthcare provider immediately
Rationale: In this scenario, the nurse detects late decelerations in the FHR tracing, which suggests uteroplacental insufficiency. The nurse should prioritize notifying the healthcare provider immediately, as this finding requires prompt intervention. Administering oxygen via face mask, initiating a continuous pitocin infusion, or performing a pelvic examination do not address the underlying cause of late decelerations and are not the initial priority.

Question 529:
Correct Answer: C) Prepare for immediate delivery
Rationale: In this scenario, the presence of decreased fetal movement and a fetal heart rate of 90 bpm indicates bradycardia. Variable decelerations are signs of cord compression, which can lead to fetal compromise. Immediate delivery is necessary to alleviate the cord compression and prevent further fetal distress.

Question 530:
Correct Answer: D) All of the above
Rationale: Uteroplacental circulation can be impaired by various factors, including maternal hypertension, fetal growth restriction, and placental abnormalities. Maternal conditions such as chronic hypertension or preeclampsia can lead to inadequate perfusion of the placenta, compromising fetal oxygen and nutrient supply. Fetal growth restriction can result in reduced blood flow to the placenta, leading to poor fetal growth. Placental abnormalities, such as placental insufficiency or abruption, can also disrupt uteroplacental circulation and compromise fetal well-being. It is important to identify and manage these factors to optimize uteroplacental circulation and promote a healthy pregnancy outcome.

Question 531:
Correct Answer: D) Order a nonstress test
Rationale: The EFM tracing shows a flat baseline with absent variability. This is concerning for fetal hypoxemia. The most appropriate initial intervention is to order a nonstress test to assess fetal well-being. A biophysical

profile may be considered, but it requires further time for evaluation and may not be readily available in all settings. Tocolytic medication is used to control preterm contractions and is not indicated in this scenario. Continuous fetal scalp stimulation may be used to evaluate for accelerations, but it does not provide immediate information regarding fetal well-being.

Question 532:
Correct Answer: D) Document the finding and continue monitoring
Rationale: In the scenario described, the fetal heart rate is above 160 bpm, but there are no signs of distress such as decelerations or a loss of variability. The presence of accelerations, which are reactive increases in heart rate, suggests a healthy fetus and is reassuring. In this case, there is no immediate need for intervention or emergency cesarean section. The nurse should document the finding and continue monitoring the fetal heart rate. Oxygen administration or position changes are not indicated.

Question 533:
Correct Answer: D) Umbilical artery
Rationale: The umbilical artery is responsible for carrying deoxygenated blood away from the fetus towards the placenta. It carries waste products and deoxygenated blood to be exchanged at the placental interface. Options A, B, and C are incorrect as they carry oxygenated blood. The umbilical vein carries oxygenated blood from the placenta to the fetus, the ductus arteriosus connects the pulmonary artery and the aorta, and the pulmonary artery carries deoxygenated blood from the right ventricle of the heart to the lungs.

Question 534:
Correct Answer: D) Prepare for an immediate delivery
Rationale: Decreased fetal movements and late decelerations on EFM, along with frequent and strong uterine contractions, are suggestive of uteroplacental insufficiency and potential fetal compromise. As an immediate intervention, preparing for an immediate delivery is the most appropriate management to avoid fetal injury or distress. Intravenous magnesium sulfate, a non-stress test, or tocolytic therapy are not the primary interventions indicated in this situation.

Question 535:
Correct Answer: D) All of the above
Rationale: Gestational hypertension carries the risk of various complications, including preterm labor, placental abruption (separation of the placenta from the uterine wall), and fetal growth restriction. These complications can have adverse effects on the well-being of both the mother and the baby. It is crucial for healthcare providers to closely monitor and manage individuals with gestational hypertension to minimize the risks associated with these complications.

Question 536:
Correct Answer: D) Inconsistent intensity with frequent uterine relaxation
Rationale: Hyperstimulation refers to excessive uterine contractions, characterized by inconsistent intensity with frequent uterine relaxation. This pattern is often associated with the administration of oxytocin or prostaglandins. Peak intensity above 50mmHg indicates strong contractions, and intensity between 25-50mmHg suggests moderate contractions. Fluctuating intensity between 70-90mmHg is not specific to hyperstimulation.

Question 537:

Correct Answer: A) Meconium-stained amniotic fluid
Rationale: Severe bradycardia in the fetus is commonly associated with meconium-stained amniotic fluid. Meconium-stained amniotic fluid can occur due to fetal distress, and bradycardia is a sign of compromised fetal well-being. Accelerations of the fetal heart rate are indicative of fetal well-being and are not typically observed in severe bradycardia. Uterine hyperstimulation and fetal tachycardia are not commonly associated with severe bradycardia.

Question 538:
Correct Answer: A) Gradual onset and offset
Rationale: Early decelerations in fetal heart rate are characterized by a gradual onset and offset, mirroring the shape of the uterine contraction. They are caused by head compression during contractions. It is important to differentiate early decelerations from late or variable decelerations, which have different shapes and implications. Early decelerations are not associated with sudden drops in heart rate or variable durations.

Question 539:
Correct Answer: A) pH
Rationale: In cord blood acid base testing, the pH of the umbilical cord blood is primarily used to assess fetal well-being. The pH value reflects the acidity or alkalinity of the blood and provides crucial information about the baby's oxygenation status during labor and delivery. Abnormal values may indicate fetal distress and can help guide interventions to improve the baby's condition.

Question 540:
Correct Answer: B) Perform an immediate emergency cesarean section
Rationale: A sinusoidal fetal heart rate pattern is a concerning finding and indicates severe fetal compromise. It is associated with decreased fetal blood flow and is often seen in cases of fetal hemorrhage, severe fetal anemia, or fetal hypoxia. An immediate emergency cesarean section is the most appropriate intervention to expedite delivery and prevent further harm to the fetus.

Question 541:
Correct Answer: C) Inform the appropriate personnel and document the issue
Rationale: If electronic fetal monitoring equipment malfunctions during a clinical situation, it is crucial to inform the appropriate personnel and document the issue. This ensures that the malfunction is reported and addressed promptly by the responsible parties. Continuing to use the equipment despite the malfunction may compromise patient safety and lead to inaccurate monitoring. Attempting to fix the equipment oneself is not recommended as it could potentially cause further damage. Proper reporting and documentation allow for timely troubleshooting or replacement of the equipment to ensure uninterrupted and reliable fetal monitoring.

Question 542:
Correct Answer: D) Late decelerations.
Rationale: Late decelerations are a concerning fetal heart rate pattern, especially in the presence of tachysystole. Late decelerations indicate uteroplacental insufficiency and can be a sign of fetal compromise. Early decelerations, variable decelerations, and accelerations are generally considered normal or benign patterns in fetal heart rate monitoring.

Question 543:
Correct Answer: D) Prepare for an emergency cesarean section

Rationale: The presence of absent variability and recurrent late decelerations indicates an abnormal fetal heart rate pattern and is highly suggestive of fetal distress. In this situation, immediate delivery is warranted to prevent further compromise to the fetus. The most appropriate management is to prepare for an emergency cesarean section to expedite the delivery and ensure the well-being of the fetus.

Question 544:
Correct Answer: B) "A traditional stethoscope is not capable of detecting the high-frequency sounds of the fetal heart."
Rationale: A traditional stethoscope is not designed to capture the high-frequency sounds of the fetal heart. The Doppler device uses ultrasound technology to amplify and detect these specific sounds, making it a more effective and accurate tool for auscultating the fetal heart rate (FHR).

Question 545:
Correct Answer: B) Administration of tocolytic medications to decrease contractions.
Rationale: If contractions are too frequent and intense during labor, administration of tocolytic medications may be necessary to decrease contractions. Tocolytics help relax the uterus and reduce contractility. Oxytocin infusion is typically used to strengthen contractions if they are not occurring frequently or intensely enough. Epidural anesthesia primarily provides pain relief and does not directly affect contraction frequency or intensity. Continuous fetal monitoring is important to assess fetal well-being but does not directly address the issue of contractions being too frequent and intense.

Question 546:
Correct Answer: D) Assist the client to change positions
Rationale: In this scenario, the nurse observes decreased FHR variability with a normal baseline and occasional decelerations. The appropriate intervention is to assist the client in changing positions. Changes in maternal position can often improve fetal oxygenation and restore normal FHR before further interventions are required. Administering oxygen via face mask, applying an internal fetal scalp electrode, and increasing intravenous fluid rate are not the primary interventions for decreased FHR variability.

Question 547:
Correct Answer: C) 1 contraction every 90 seconds
Rationale: The frequency of contractions is determined by the time interval between the start of one contraction and the start of the next contraction. In this scenario, since each contraction lasts for 90 seconds, there is a 90-second interval between contractions, resulting in a frequency of 1 contraction every 90 seconds.

Question 548:
Correct Answer: C) Sinusoidal pattern
Rationale: A sinusoidal pattern in electronic fetal monitoring is a smooth and regular waveform resembling a sine wave, with a frequency of 3-5 cycles per minute and an amplitude of 5-10 bpm. It is typically associated with severe fetal anemia and requires immediate intervention, such as immediate delivery by cesarean section. Abrupt baseline changes, minimal variability, and prolonged decelerations may indicate fetal compromise but do not require immediate intervention.

Question 549:
Correct Answer: A) Respect the patient's decision and document the refusal

Rationale: Patient autonomy is a fundamental principle in healthcare. In this situation, the nurse should respect the patient's decision and document the refusal. It is the patient's right to make decisions about her own body and healthcare. The nurse should provide the patient with information about the procedure, including its benefits and potential risks, but ultimately, the decision lies with the patient. Respecting the patient's autonomy promotes a patient-centered approach and maintains the integrity of the nurse-patient relationship.

Question 550:
Correct Answer: D) All of the above
Rationale: The intensity of uterine contractions during labor can be influenced by multiple factors including maternal age, fetal position, and the presence of uterine fibroids. Maternal age can affect uterine contractility due to variations in hormone levels and uterine muscle tone. Fetal position plays a role in the effectiveness of contractions by promoting optimal engagement and descent. Uterine fibroids can interfere with uterine contractility, potentially leading to abnormal labor patterns. Considering all these factors is crucial in assessing and managing labor progress effectively.

Question 551:
Correct Answer: C) Elevated AST and ALT levels
Rationale: Severe HELLP syndrome is characterized by elevated liver enzymes, specifically aspartate transaminase (AST) and alanine transaminase (ALT) levels. Platelet count is typically low in HELLP syndrome (less than 100,000/mm◆). Serum lactate dehydrogenase (LDH) level is often elevated in HELLP syndrome due to increased hemolysis. Bilirubin levels may be elevated in severe cases, indicating liver dysfunction. Therefore, options A, B, and D are incorrect.

Question 552:
Correct Answer: A) Sinusoidal pattern
Rationale: The biophysical profile includes the assessment of the fetal heart rate, represented by the reactive fetal heart rate parameter. While accelerations and early decelerations are considered normal findings, variable decelerations are associated with umbilical cord compression and can be a cause for concern. However, a sinusoidal pattern is the most significant abnormal finding in the fetal heart rate and is often indicative of severe fetal anemia or other conditions causing hypoxia. It appears as a smooth, undulating pattern akin to a continuously rocking entity on the fetal heart rate monitoring strip. Identifying a sinusoidal pattern warrants immediate attention and intervention.

Question 553:
Correct Answer: A) Placenta Previa
Rationale: Placenta previa refers to the abnormal implantation of the placenta in the lower uterine segment, partially or completely covering the internal cervical os. It can lead to painless vaginal bleeding in the third trimester and is associated with risk factors such as advanced maternal age, multiparity, and previous cesarean delivery. An ultrasound is used for diagnosis, and management depends on the degree of placental coverage and the presence of bleeding and fetal distress. In severe cases, a cesarean delivery may be necessary.

Question 554:
Correct Answer: A) The fetal baseline heart rate is within the normal range.
Rationale: The normal range for fetal baseline heart rate is 110-160 bpm. A baseline heart rate of 160 bpm falls within this range and indicates a normal finding for the fetus.

Question 555:
Correct Answer: A) Uterine contractions
Rationale: In active labor, uterine contractions play a crucial role in promoting umbilical blood flow. During contractions, the uterine arteries and veins are compressed, reducing blood flow to the uterus. However, the placental intervillous space remains perfused due to the elasticity of the umbilical arteries and veins. This intermittent compression and relaxation of the umbilical vessels facilitate the exchange of oxygen and nutrients between the maternal and fetal circulations. As a result, uterine contractions are essential for maintaining umbilical blood flow and fetal oxygenation during labor.

Question 556:
Correct Answer: A) Normal fetal heart rate pattern
Rationale: Early decelerations are a normal fetal heart rate response to contractions and are considered reassuring. They are characterized by a gradual decrease in the fetal heart rate coinciding with the onset, nadir, and recovery of contractions. The baseline fetal heart rate and minimal variability in this scenario are within the normal range, further supporting a normal fetal heart rate pattern.

Question 557:
Correct Answer: B) Type 2 diabetes
Rationale: Type 2 diabetes is a metabolic disorder characterized by insulin resistance and impaired insulin production. Insulin resistance occurs when the body's cells become less responsive to the effects of insulin, leading to elevated blood sugar levels. Type 2 diabetes is often associated with lifestyle factors such as obesity, sedentary behavior, and poor diet. It is the most common form of diabetes, accounting for approximately 90-95% of all cases. Treatment may include lifestyle modifications, oral medications, and insulin therapy.

Question 558:
Correct Answer: B) Applying a cold compress to the abdomen
Rationale: When faced with a non-reactive fetal heart rate tracing, it is important to stimulate fetal activity to assess fetal well-being. Applying a cold compress to the mother's abdomen can often elicit fetal movement. This can be achieved by using a chilled gel pack or a cold cloth. The cold temperature stimulates the fetus, increasing the chances of demonstrating a reactive tracing. Other methods, such as administering intravenous fluids, changing the maternal position, or decreasing oxygen supplementation, may not be effective in stimulating fetal activity during a non-reactive tracing.

Question 559:
Correct Answer: B) 7.2-7.6
Rationale: The normal range for pH in cord blood gases is between 7.2 and 7.6. This indicates a normal acid-base balance in the fetal blood. Values below 7.2 indicate acidemia, while values above 7.6 indicate alkalemia. Monitoring the pH level in cord blood gases is important to assess the fetal oxygenation and determine any potential acid-base imbalances.

Question 560:
Correct Answer: C) Fetal Acoustic Stimulation involves using sound waves to elicit a response from the fetus.
Rationale: Fetal Acoustic Stimulation is a non-invasive technique that involves using sound waves to stimulate the fetus and evaluate its response. It is commonly used to assess the well-being of the fetus and its ability to mount a healthy physiological response. By exposing the fetus to sound waves, the fetal heart rate can be monitored and analyzed for any abnormalities or variations. This allows healthcare professionals to gather important information about the fetal condition and make appropriate management decisions if necessary.

Question 561:
Correct Answer: C) American College of Obstetricians and Gynecologists (ACOG)
Rationale: The American College of Obstetricians and Gynecologists (ACOG) is a professional organization that sets standards for EFM education and certification. They provide guidelines and recommendations for the use of EFM in obstetric care. ACOG's guidelines are widely adopted and followed by healthcare professionals involved in managing fetal monitoring during labor and delivery. EFM education and certification programs are aligned with ACOG's recommendations and help healthcare providers develop the necessary skills and knowledge for accurate interpretation of fetal heart rate tracings.

Question 562:
Correct Answer: D) Trendelenburg position
Rationale: The Trendelenburg position involves elevating the mother's pelvis higher than her head. This position helps relieve cord compression by utilizing the pull of gravity to guide the fetus away from the compressed cord. It can be an effective intervention to relieve variable decelerations caused by umbilical cord compression.

Question 563:
Correct Answer: D) Referral to a fetal cardiologist for further evaluation and management.
Rationale: In the case of a fetus with a complete heart block, referral to a fetal cardiologist for further evaluation and management is essential. Atropine administration is not effective in improving fetal heart rate in cases of a complete heart block. Immediate delivery is not warranted unless there are other indications for an emergency cesarean section. Monitoring fetal heart rate during labor is important, but further evaluation by a specialist is necessary to develop a comprehensive management plan.

Question 564:
Correct Answer: A) Inform the pregnant woman that it is normal not to hear the fetal heart sounds at this gestational age.
Rationale: It is normal not to hear the fetal heart sounds using a Doppler device at 16 weeks gestation. The fetus is still relatively small, and the location of the heart may make it difficult to detect using external auscultation techniques. It is important to provide reassurance to the pregnant woman and explain the limitations of the examination at this stage of pregnancy.

Question 565:
Correct Answer: B) Supraventricular tachycardia
Rationale: The fetal heart rate pattern described in this scenario is consistent with supraventricular tachycardia (SVT). SVT is characterized by a rapid and irregular fetal heart rate between 200-240 beats per minute. The maternal heart rate is usually normal. Immediate evaluation and management should be initiated to assess the severity and potential risks associated with SVT in the fetus.

Question 566:
Correct Answer: A) Sinusoidal pattern
Rationale: A sinusoidal pattern on fetal heart rate monitoring is commonly associated with decreased blood flow to the fetus. It appears as a smooth, regular, sine-like

wave with no variability and may indicate severe fetal compromise. Accelerations, early decelerations, and variable decelerations are not specific patterns associated with decreased blood flow but rather have different clinical interpretations.

Question 567:
Correct Answer: A) Reactive
Rationale: A reactive nonstress test is characterized by two or more accelerations with fetal heart rate variability. In this scenario, Mrs. Johnson's test shows moderate variability in the fetal heart rate, occasional accelerations, and no decelerations or contractions. These findings indicate a healthy, well-oxygenated fetus, making the test result reactive.

Question 568:
Correct Answer: D) Prepare for immediate cesarean delivery
Rationale: In this scenario, the patient presents with severe vaginal bleeding and a non-reassuring FHR tracing characterized by minimal variability and late decelerations with contractions. These findings are suggestive of placental abruption, a life-threatening condition for both the mother and fetus. The most appropriate immediate action in this case is to prepare for an immediate cesarean delivery, as delivery is the definitive treatment for placental abruption to ensure the timely delivery of the baby and control of maternal bleeding.

Question 569:
Correct Answer: A) Document the finding and continue monitoring the fetal heart rate.
Rationale: Ectopic beats in the fetus can occur and are usually benign. They are a temporary rhythm disturbance and usually resolve. The nurse should document the finding, continue to monitor the fetal heart rate, and assess for any signs of fetal distress. Most often, no intervention is required for ectopic beats.

Question 570:
Correct Answer: D) It is an abnormal finding requiring further evaluation.
Rationale: A baseline variability of more than 25 bpm is considered excessive or increased. It can be associated with fetal hypoxemia, fetal anemia, or a central nervous system abnormality. This finding requires further evaluation to assess the cause and determine appropriate management for the fetus.

Question 571:
Correct Answer: D) Fibroid degeneration
Rationale: The symptoms of abdominal pain, vaginal bleeding, tender and palpable mass in the lower uterine segment, and late decelerations on fetal heart rate tracing are consistent with fibroid degeneration. Uterine rupture is unlikely in this case as the clinical findings suggest a localized uterine process rather than global rupture. Immediate management involves close monitoring of the mother and fetus and timely delivery if indicated.

Question 572:
Correct Answer: D) Fetal arrhythmia
Rationale: An irregular fetal heart rate (FHR) with frequent pauses is suggestive of fetal arrhythmia. Fetal arrhythmias can be caused by various factors, such as structural heart defects, maternal autoimmune disorders, or congenital heart block. Further evaluation and monitoring are required to determine the specific type of arrhythmia and its impact on fetal well-being. Umbilical cord compression, maternal fever,

and fetal tachycardia are less likely to cause the described FHR pattern.

Question 573:
Correct Answer: A) Encourage Olivia to lie on her left side and monitor fetal movements.
Rationale: Maternal positioning can affect fetal movements. Lying on the left side can improve blood flow to the uterus, providing an optimal environment for fetal movement. By encouraging Olivia to lie on her left side and monitor fetal movements, the healthcare provider promotes fetal well-being and encourages a favorable position for optimal blood supply to the fetus.

Question 574:
Correct Answer: A) Decreased sympathetic outflow
Rationale: Spinal anesthesia blocks sympathetic autonomic outflow, resulting in peripheral vasodilation and decreased systemic vascular resistance. This vasodilation leads to a sudden decrease in blood pressure. Cardiac output may initially increase compensatorily, but the main cause of the hypotensive episode during spinal anesthesia is the decreased sympathetic outflow.

Question 575:
Correct Answer: B) Maternal anemia
Rationale: Maternal anemia decreases the oxygen-carrying capacity of the blood, resulting in reduced oxygen availability for transfer to the fetus. Anemic mothers may have a lower level of hemoglobin, leading to decreased oxygen saturation and delivery to the placenta. Maternal hypertension, hyperthyroidism, and obesity can also have an impact on fetal oxygenation but do not directly reduce the availability of oxygen for transfer.

Question 576:
Correct Answer: C) Perform a complete maternal-fetal assessment and consider prompt delivery.
Rationale: Sinusoidal pattern in electronic fetal monitoring is an abnormal finding that requires immediate evaluation and intervention. The recommended intervention is to perform a complete maternal-fetal assessment, including a comprehensive evaluation of fetal well-being and oxygenation. This may involve additional tests, such as fetal blood sampling, ultrasound evaluation, and consideration of prompt delivery if necessary to ensure the best possible outcome for the fetus. No intervention is benign for sinusoidal pattern and it should not be ignored.

Question 577:
Correct Answer: D) Biophysical profile
Rationale: The biophysical profile is an appropriate method for assessing fetal movement. It evaluates five parameters: fetal tone, fetal breathing movements, fetal movement, amniotic fluid volume, and reactive fetal heart rate. Each parameter is assigned a score, and a total score of 8-10 is considered reassuring. This assessment is typically performed using ultrasound technology and helps determine the well-being of the fetus. External cephalic version is a procedure to turn a fetus from a breech position to a head-down position. Doppler ultrasound measures blood flow, and a contraction stress test evaluates fetal heart rate response to contractions.

Question 578:
Correct Answer: D) Maternal hypotension
Rationale: Maternal hypotension is not typically considered a potential cause of fetal demise. However, maternal hypertension, maternal hyperthyroidism, and maternal diabetes are known risk factors that can contribute to fetal

demise. These conditions can lead to placental insufficiency or other complications that may compromise fetal well-being.

Question 579:
Correct Answer: A) Fetal distress
Rationale: A sudden drop in the fetal heart rate (FHR) following a uterine contraction is known as a deceleration and is often indicative of fetal distress. It may be caused by factors such as umbilical cord compression or inadequate blood flow to the fetus. Immediate medical attention should be sought to assess the well-being of the fetus and take appropriate interventions, if necessary.

Question 580:
Correct Answer: A) Inform the patient of your concerns and recommend further evaluation and monitoring.
Rationale: As a healthcare professional, it is your ethical obligation to inform the patient of your concerns and recommend further evaluation and monitoring in cases where there is a potential risk to the patient or her unborn baby. Gestational hypertension can lead to complications such as preeclampsia, which can be life-threatening if not properly managed. Open and honest communication with the patient is essential to ensure her well-being and the best possible outcome for both the patient and her baby.

Question 581:
Correct Answer: C) Radiofrequency interference
Rationale: Radiofrequency interference can cause sharp and uniform spikes on the fetal heart rate tracing. It usually occurs as a result of electronic devices in the vicinity of the monitoring equipment, such as cell phones or walkie-talkies. This interference can cause false accelerations or decelerations in the fetal heart rate, leading to an inaccurate interpretation of the tracing. It is essential to troubleshoot and identify the source of interference to ensure the accuracy of fetal monitoring.

Question 582:
Correct Answer: C) It is primarily regulated by maternal factors
Rationale: Uteroplacental circulation is primarily regulated by maternal factors, such as blood pressure, vascular tone, and oxygen tension. Maternal blood is responsible for delivering oxygen and nutrients to the developing fetus through the placenta. The placenta acts as a site for exchange between maternal and fetal blood, allowing for the transfer of gases, nutrients, and waste products. The fetal cardiovascular system adapts to the maternal environment to ensure efficient placental perfusion and fetal well-being.

Question 583:
Correct Answer: C) Proper communication enhances patient safety, reduces errors, and improves overall healthcare outcomes.
Rationale: Communication is a critical component of quality improvement in healthcare settings. Effective communication plays a vital role in ensuring patient safety, reducing errors, and improving overall healthcare outcomes. It involves clear and concise exchange of information between healthcare providers, patients, and other members of the healthcare team. Proper communication enhances collaboration, reduces misunderstandings, and enables timely interventions. By promoting transparency, effective communication facilitates the identification and resolution of quality issues. It also allows for the dissemination of best practices and the implementation of evidence-based guidelines, ultimately leading to improved patient care and outcomes.

Question 584:
Correct Answer: C) Fetal blood sampling
Rationale: Fetal blood sampling, also known as cordocentesis, is a diagnostic procedure performed during pregnancy to evaluate the fetal condition. It involves the sampling of fetal blood from the umbilical cord for analysis. While fetal blood sampling is useful for assessing fetal well-being and identifying specific conditions, it is not a management option for hypoxemia. Management options for hypoxemia may include maternal repositioning, administration of fluids to optimize maternal blood volume, and if necessary, immediate delivery to improve fetal oxygenation.

Question 585:
Correct Answer: C) Multiple episodes of strong contractions with a frequency of six minutes
Rationale: During external tocodynamometry, a normal pattern of uterine activity would be the presence of multiple episodes of strong contractions occurring approximately every 5-7 minutes. The duration of contractions can vary but generally lasts longer than 30 seconds. Regular contractions lasting 90 seconds or occurring every two minutes would be indicative of an abnormal pattern. Contractions lasting for 30 seconds or less may suggest inadequate uterine activity.

Question 586:
Correct Answer: C) Ultrasound transducer
Rationale: An ultrasound transducer is commonly used for external uterine monitoring. It is placed on the maternal abdomen to detect uterine contractions by bouncing sound waves off the uterine wall. A colposcope and laparoscope are instruments used for visual examination of the cervix and internal pelvic organs, respectively. A fetal blood sampling catheter is used for obtaining a sample of fetal blood during certain procedures.

Question 587:
Correct Answer: B) Progesterone
Rationale: During pregnancy, high levels of progesterone are secreted by the corpus luteum and later by the placenta. Progesterone plays a crucial role in preparing and maintaining the uterine lining for implantation and supports the growth of the fetus throughout pregnancy. It helps to prevent contractions of the uterus and ensures that the uterine lining remains intact to provide a suitable environment for fetal development.

Question 588:
Correct Answer: D) Perform a scalp electrode insertion to assess fetal well-being
Rationale: The described pattern is consistent with a sinusoidal pattern, which is a concerning sign. It is important to assess the fetal well-being more accurately. The insertion of a scalp electrode can provide a direct and continuous measurement of the fetal heart rate, allowing for better assessment and monitoring. Administering oxytocin, preparing for an emergency cesarean section, or administering oxygen may not directly address the underlying cause of the sinusoidal pattern.

Question 589:
Correct Answer: D) All of the above
Rationale: Various external factors can cause interference with electronic fetal monitoring equipment. Mobile phones, fluorescent lights, Wi-Fi routers, and other electronic devices emit electromagnetic waves that can disrupt the signals transmitted by the fetal monitor. This interference can lead to inaccurate readings and affect the reliability of the monitoring data. To minimize interference, it is important to ensure a

safe distance between the equipment and potential sources of electromagnetic waves.

Question 590:
Correct Answer: C) Twin gestation
Rationale: Twin gestation is a contraindication for nonstress testing (NST) as it may limit the ability to accurately assess fetal heart rate abnormalities and fetal well-being. Maternal hypertension, gestational diabetes, and previous cesarean delivery are not contraindications for NST and can still be performed in these cases.

Question 591:
Correct Answer: A) Painful vaginal bleeding
Rationale: The most common clinical manifestation of placental abruption is painful vaginal bleeding. The bleeding is typically dark and may be accompanied by uterine tenderness or contractions. Other symptoms include abdominal pain or cramping, back pain, and signs of fetal distress. Prompt evaluation and management are necessary to ensure the well-being of both the mother and fetus.

Question 592:
Correct Answer: C) Fetal growth restriction
Rationale: Fetal growth restriction can lead to impaired fetal oxygenation due to decreased oxygen exchange in the placenta. In cases of fetal growth restriction, the blood flow to the placenta may be reduced, resulting in reduced oxygen supply to the fetus. Fetal tachycardia, macrosomia, and bradycardia can also affect fetal oxygenation, but they do not directly impair oxygen exchange in the placenta.

Question 593:
Correct Answer: C) Change the mother's position.
Rationale: When a prolonged deceleration pattern is observed on the fetal heart rate tracing, the immediate action of the healthcare provider should be to change the mother's position. This simple intervention can sometimes relieve pressure on the umbilical cord or improve blood flow to the fetus, potentially resolving the deceleration. Other interventions may be necessary depending on the clinical context, but changing the mother's position is a recommended initial step.

Question 594:
Correct Answer: B) Maternal administration of corticosteroids
Rationale: Maternal administration of corticosteroids, such as dexamethasone, is a recommended intervention for a fetus diagnosed with congenital heart block. This intervention aims to suppress maternal antibodies and reduce inflammation, potentially improving fetal heart rate. Fetal heart rate monitoring every 12 hours, intrauterine blood transfusion, and immediate delivery via cesarean section are not standard interventions for congenital heart block.

Question 595:
Correct Answer: A) Administer oxygen via nasal cannula
Rationale: The clinical presentation of sudden onset dyspnea, chest pain, low oxygen saturation, and variable decelerations on EFM is highly suspicious for pulmonary embolism, a life-threatening maternal complication. Administering oxygen via nasal cannula is the initial priority to optimize oxygenation and support the maternal cardiovascular system. The other interventions may be considered as indicated but should not delay the immediate provision of oxygen.

Question 596:

Correct Answer: C) Internal monitoring devices are preferred for accurate fetal assessment in women receiving epidural anesthesia.
Rationale: Women receiving epidural anesthesia for pain management during labor may require accurate fetal assessment. Internal monitoring devices are preferred in this scenario as they provide more accurate measurement of the fetal heart rate. Epidural anesthesia can affect the accuracy of external monitoring devices in assessing the fetal heart rate and uterine contractions. Internal monitoring allows for direct measurement of the fetal heart rate using an electrode attached to the baby's scalp, ensuring accurate assessment and timely interventions if required.

Question 597:
Correct Answer: A) Pregnancy that extends beyond 42 weeks
Rationale: Postdates pregnancy, also known as prolonged pregnancy, is defined as a pregnancy that extends beyond the standard 40 weeks of gestation and continues into or beyond 42 weeks. It is important to monitor postdates pregnancies closely as they are associated with an increased risk of adverse maternal and fetal outcomes, such as macrosomia, meconium aspiration syndrome, and stillbirth. Timely intervention and monitoring are crucial to ensure the well-being of both the mother and the baby.

Question 598:
Correct Answer: C) Fetal heart rate accelerations are an indicator of fetal well-being.
Rationale: Fetal heart rate accelerations are reassuring signs that indicate fetal well-being. They are usually observed in response to fetal movement or stimulation. Fetal heart rate accelerations are characterized by an increase in the baseline heart rate of at least 15 beats per minute, lasting for at least 15 seconds. These accelerations are a positive sign and suggest that the fetus is receiving an adequate oxygen supply. Fetal heart rate accelerations are not related to contractions or the phase of labor and should be considered a reassuring finding in antenatal monitoring.

Question 599:
Correct Answer: D) All of the above actions should be undertaken by Dr. Thompson.
Rationale: In the context of legal considerations, Dr. Thompson, as the obstetrician responsible for interpreting fetal heart rate tracings, should undertake all of the listed actions. Clear documentation of the interpretation and any concerns is crucial for legal compliance and continuity of care. Promptly informing the nursing staff helps facilitate communication and timely interventions. Additionally, involving the expectant mother in the decision-making process ensures patient autonomy and shared responsibility. Thus, all of these actions are essential for legal compliance and optimal care.

Question 600:
Correct Answer: A) Preterm birth
Rationale: Chronic hypertension in pregnancy is associated with an increased risk of complications, including preterm birth. Preterm birth refers to the delivery of a baby before 37 weeks of gestation. Oligohydramnios, hyperglycemia, and fetal macrosomia are not directly associated with chronic hypertension. However, it is important to monitor and manage these conditions to prevent further complications and ensure the well-being of both the mother and the baby.

Question 601:
Correct Answer: C) Blood pressure

Rationale: Preeclampsia is characterized by high blood pressure during pregnancy. Elevated blood pressure in the mother can cause placental insufficiency, reducing blood flow to the fetus and compromising fetal oxygenation. Preeclampsia can result in poor placental perfusion, impaired nutrient and oxygen exchange, and decreased fetal growth. Close monitoring of blood pressure and effective management of preeclampsia are essential to maintain adequate fetal oxygenation and prevent further complications.

Question 602:
Correct Answer: C) Elevated serum creatinine levels
Rationale: In preeclampsia-eclampsia, there is often impaired kidney function, leading to elevated serum creatinine levels. The kidneys are affected by the underlying pathophysiology, resulting in reduced glomerular filtration rate and impaired renal function. Other laboratory findings that may be seen in preeclampsia-eclampsia include proteinuria, thrombocytopenia, and elevated liver function tests.

Question 603:
Correct Answer: D) When the cervix is fully dilated and delivery is imminent.
Rationale: Internal fetal heart rate monitoring is typically discontinued when the cervix is fully dilated and delivery is imminent. Once the baby's head is engaged in the birth canal, the electrode may become dislodged or interfere with the delivery process. At this stage, the healthcare provider may switch to external monitoring methods or rely on intermittent auscultation to continue monitoring the fetal heart rate until delivery. Continuous monitoring is not necessary during the pushing stage of labor, as the progress of labor and well-being of the baby can be assessed through other means.

Question 604:
Correct Answer: D) Close monitoring of fetal well-being
Rationale: In the management of chronic essential hypertension during pregnancy, close monitoring of fetal well-being is essential. Sarah's blood pressure is moderately elevated, and initiation of antihypertensive medication is not indicated unless her blood pressure exceeds 160/110 mmHg. Dietary modification and increased physical activity are important aspects of lifestyle management but do not address the immediate need for fetal monitoring. While monitoring serum creatinine and uric acid levels can provide information on renal function and markers of preeclampsia, these tests are not specific to managing hypertension. Therefore, the most appropriate intervention for Sarah is close monitoring of fetal well-being to ensure optimal outcomes for both mother and baby.

Question 605:
Correct Answer: D) Doppler velocimetry of umbilical artery
Rationale: In the scenario mentioned, the combination of reduced fetal movements and a fundal height measurement indicating decreased growth raises concerns regarding fetal well-being. Doppler velocimetry of the umbilical artery is a useful tool to assess fetal blood flow and placental function. It can provide insights into the presence of placental insufficiency and associated risks. Immediate induction of labor may not be warranted based solely on these findings. Fetal kick count for 2 hours may be considered if there are no other concerning features, but given the reduced growth and decreased fetal movements, further evaluation is necessary. Ultrasonography for fetal biophysical profile

(BPP) evaluates multiple parameters and may be performed if Doppler velocimetry yields abnormal results.

Question 606:
Correct Answer: A) Placental abruption
Rationale: Placental abruption is a condition in which the placenta prematurely separates from the uterine wall, leading to abdominal pain, vaginal bleeding, uterine tenderness, and hemodynamic instability. It is typically associated with a sudden onset of symptoms and may be life-threatening. Uterine rupture, placenta previa, and placenta accreta may cause bleeding, but they are less likely to present with severe abdominal pain and hemodynamic instability.

Question 607:
Correct Answer: D) Prepare for immediate instrumental delivery
Rationale: The presence of late decelerations in fetal heart rate associated with reduced baseline variability and a fully dilated cervix indicates an urgent need for delivery. In this scenario, preparing for immediate instrumental delivery, such as vacuum or forceps, would be the most appropriate next step to expedite delivery and reduce the risk of prolonged fetal hypoxia. Performing a biophysical profile, administering intravenous fluids, or administering terbutaline would not address the urgency of the situation.

Question 608:
Correct Answer: D) Preparing for immediate cesarean delivery
Rationale: Repetitive and severe variable decelerations indicate persistent umbilical cord compression. This can be a sign of fetal distress, and immediate cesarean delivery may be necessary to prevent further compromise to the fetus.

Question 609:
Correct Answer: A) Fetal bradyarrhythmia
Rationale: The fetal heart rate pattern described in this scenario is consistent with fetal bradyarrhythmia. Fetal bradyarrhythmia is characterized by a fetal heart rate consistently below 100 beats per minute. It is important to evaluate the underlying cause of bradyarrhythmia and consider appropriate management to ensure the well-being of the fetus.

Question 610:
Correct Answer: D) Both A and B
Rationale: In this scenario, Nurse Roberts should document the deceleration and nursing actions in Mrs. Brown's medical record, ensuring that there is a clear record of the event. Additionally, since Nurse Roberts was interrupted and could not pass on the information about the prolonged deceleration, it is crucial for her to immediately inform the obstetrician again. These actions demonstrate legal compliance, documentation, and effective communication for the safety and well-being of the patient.

Made in the USA
Middletown, DE
05 January 2024